This book examines renal disease from an immunological perspective; it has been designed to be suitable both as an introductory overview of the area, as well as a guide to further reading. Following an introductory chapter, which discusses general immunological principles of particular relevance to autoimmunity and immunological mechanisms of renal injury, each of the major forms of renal disease with a significant immunopathogenesis is considered. The immunogenetics of each condition are reviewed, followed by a discussion of the immunopathology in animal models and in human disease. A section on therapeutic aspects of immunological relevance is followed by a concluding section which contains more speculative material. A final chapter summarises the various therapeutic strategies available, with particular emphasis on current experimental and possible future approaches.

The volume is suitable for consultants and clinicians in training, particularly in the areas of nephrology and immunology, and for basic scientists working on relevant animal models.

Immunological aspects of renal disease

CAMBRIDGE REVIEWS IN CLINICAL IMMUNOLOGY

Series editors:

D.B.G. OLIVEIRA
Lister Institute Research Fellow, University of Cambridge, Addenbrooke's Hospital, Cambridge.

D.K. PETERS
Regius Professor of Physic, University of Cambridge, Addenbrooke's Hospital, Cambridge.

A.P. WEETMAN
Professor of Medicine, University of Sheffield Clinical Sciences Centre.

Recent advances in immunology, particularly at the molecular level, have led to a much clearer understanding of the causes and consequences of autoimmunity. The aim of this series is to make these developments accessible to clinicians who feel daunted by such advances and require a clear exposition of the scientific and clinical issues. The various clinical specialities will be covered in separate volumes, which will follow a fixed format: a brief introduction to basic immunology followed by a comprehensive review of recent findings in the autoimmune conditions which, in particular, will compare animal models with their human counterparts. Sufficient clinical detail, especially regarding treatment, will also be included to provide basic scientists with a better understanding of these aspects of autoimmunity. Thus each volume will be self-contained and comprehensible to a wide audience. Taken as a whole the series will provide an overview of all the important autoimmune disorders.

ALSO IN THIS SERIES:

A. P. WEETMAN **Autoimmune endocrine disease**

Immunological aspects of renal disease

DAVID B. G. OLIVEIRA
Lister Institute Research Fellow and Honorary Consultant
Nephrologist
Addenbrooke's Hospital, Cambridge, UK

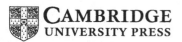

CAMBRIDGE
UNIVERSITY PRESS

Published by the Press Syndicate of the University of Cambridge
The Pitt Building, Trumpington Street, Cambridge CB2 1RP
40 West 20th Street, New York, NY 10011–4211, USA
10 Stamford Road, Oakleigh, Victoria 3166, Australia

First published 1992

Printed in Great Britain at the University Press, Cambridge

A catalogue record for this book is available from the British Library

Library of Congress cataloguing in publication data
Oliveira, D. B. G.
  Immunological aspects of renal disease / David B. G. Oliveira.
    p.   cm. – (Cambridge reviews in clinical immunology)
  Includes index.
  ISBN 0-521-40174-7 (hardback)
  1. Kidneys – Diseases – Immunological aspects.   I. Title.
II. Series.
  [DNLM: 1. Kidney Diseases – immunology.   WJ 300 0483i]
RC903.045   1992
616.6'1079 – dc20   91-29634   CIP

ISBN 0 521 40174 7 hardback

Contents

Preface

Immunology is a large and rapidly expanding field, and as such often appears intimidating to outsiders. However, its clinical importance lies in the fact that many of the more fundamental advances are of increasing relevance to disease. Although this process has a long way to go, there is no doubt that some familiarity with present immunological concepts is useful clinically, and particularly in an area such as nephrology in which a substantial proportion of disease has a significant immunopathogenesis.

I have attempted in this book to examine renal disease from an immunological perspective. Constraints of length and intelligibility have meant that this is not a comprehensive account; I have made free use of references to review articles and textbook chapters as a guide to those who do require more background. When citing primary references, I have tried to use those that provide good references to the preceding literature, or important earlier papers that will allow later relevant work to be retrieved using citation indices. I hope in this way to have provided an introductory overview of the area which will also serve as a starting point for a more detailed study.

Certain topics were felt to be beyond the scope of this book, notably the effects of renal failure on the immune system, and transplantation. Coverage of other areas, where possible, follows a common layout, with a general introductory section followed by sections on immunogenetics, immunopathogenesis (animal models as well as human disease), therapeutic aspects and concluding remarks. Subject to the constraints mentioned above, the sections on immunogenetics do attempt to be more comprehensive, as this is an area that is often not well covered elsewhere. The concluding sections allow me to indulge in a more speculative treatment of the chapter topic; any ideas expressed here should be treated with caution.

Finally, I would like to thank my colleagues who have helped with constructive criticism, and above all my wife and family for allowing me the time.

D. B. G. Oliveira, October 1991

–1–
Autoimmunity and immunopathogenesis in renal disease

This introductory chapter will attempt to cover some of the basic immunology which underlies our present understanding of autoimmunity and immunopathogenesis. In broad terms, there are two main areas to be considered. First, much immunologically mediated renal disease is probably autoimmune in nature, and this implies a breakdown in the normal mechanisms of tolerance. The discussion of tolerance and the aetiology of autoimmunity will be fairly general, and will not attempt to treat the subject in depth; the first volume in this series (*Autoimmune Endocrine Disease*, A. P. Weetman) has covered this area, and in particular the immunogenetics of autoimmunity. This section will also consider the extent to which immunoregulatory abnormalities may contribute to a breakdown in self-tolerance. Secondly, the immunopathogenic mechanisms that are particularly relevant to renal disease will be considered. Not all renal disease that has a significant immunopathological component is necessarily autoimmune (e.g. poststreptococcal glomerulonephritis), and this section is therefore more general in scope.

These two areas can be viewed as the afferent and efferent limbs, respectively, of the immune response in the context of renal disease. To date, much work has been done on the efferent side and relatively little attention has been paid to the afferent side, with the exception of certain animal models. It is to be hoped that the recent advances in the understanding of tolerance will allow progress to be made in this area with respect to human disease.

Tolerance and the aetiology of autoimmunity

It is only necessary to acquire tolerance to self-antigens that are visible to the immune system, and it seems likely that, for many such antigens, effective

1

sequestration from the immune system is all that is required. For self-antigens that are so exposed, then, in general terms, two types of tolerance (which are not mutually exclusive) can be envisaged. First, tolerance may be due to actual elimination, or functional silencing without elimination, of autoreactive components of the immune system; such mechanisms are essentially passive in nature. Secondly, autoreactive cells may be present, but tissue damage is prevented by active immunoregulatory mechanisms.

Sequestration of autoantigens

Autoimmunity can certainly result when a normally sequestered antigen is exposed by tissue damage. The classic example is lens-induced uveitis (Wright, 1982) but this is clearly a general mechanism that could exacerbate autoimmune damage due to any cause. In the context of renal disease, it is possible that the occasional reports of anti-glomerular basement membrane antibody disease following various forms of renal damage (Hume et al., 1970; Guerin et al., 1990; Weber, Pullig & Boesken, 1990) are examples of this mechanism.

There are a number of more recent variants on the theme of sequestration of self-antigens from the immune system. B cells, via their antigen receptors (antibody molecules), can recognise free antigens. T cells, on the other hand, cannot see antigens unless they are presented in the context of a product of the major histocompatibility complex (MHC). In general, cytotoxic (usually CD8$^+$) T cells see antigen in the context of class I MHC molecules, whereas helper/inducer (usually CD4$^+$) T cells use class II molecules. Class I MHC molecules have a wide tissue distribution, occurring essentially on all nucleated cells. Class II molecule expression is normally confined to antigen-presenting cells, such as B cells, macrophages, Langerhans cells, etc. As a consequence, the key regulatory cell, the helper/inducer T cell, is effectively blind to other tissues. The observation that thyroid cells undergoing an autoimmune attack aberrantly express class II MHC molecules led to the hypothesis (Bottazzo et al., 1983) that an initial stimulus, such as a viral infection causing gamma interferon production, could cause up-regulation of MHC class II expression. This would unblind helper/inducer T cells to thyroid autoantigens presented in the context of the aberrantly expressed class II MHC molecules. As these autoantigens are normally effectively sequestered, tolerance to them does not exist, and an autoimmune response could thus be initiated. This initial observation of aberrant class II MHC molecule expression has since been made in other autoimmune diseases (e.g. Bottazzo et al., 1989), suggesting that this could be a general mechanism. Further support is provided by the demonstration that MHC class II positive thyroid epithelial cells can indeed act as antigen-presenting cells in vitro (Londei, Bottazzo & Feldmann, 1985). However, in many cases it is possible that the aberrant expression is secondary to the autoimmune process, which is likely to be accompanied by the production of cytokines with the ability to up-regulate class II MHC expression. There is evidence for this sequence of events in an animal model of autoimmune thyroid disease in which T cell infiltration precedes class II MHC expression (Cohen, Dijkstra & Weetman, 1988). Further, the ability of mouse class II molecule-positive thyroid cells to present antigen has been questioned (Minami *et al.*, 1987), and such cells may, in fact, suppress thyroid autoantibody production, suggesting that they may have a protective effect *in vivo* (Iwatani *et al.*, 1988). The possibility remains that small numbers of contaminating classical antigen presenting cells may explain the positive results obtained with human thyroid cells *in vitro*. In fact, as suggested above, it is entirely possible that class II MHC expression may play a role in down-regulating the autoimmune response. The transgenic mouse lines mentioned below in the context of peripheral T cell tolerance were in many cases produced to test the hypothesis that aberrant MHC molecule expression could initiate autoimmunity. Although many of these strains, with aberrant expression on beta cells in pancreatic islets, do indeed develop diabetes, this is not due to autoimmune attack, but probably reflects interference with insulin secretion (Parham, 1988). Indeed, the animals are usually tolerant of the aberrant MHC molecules and presumably therefore of any pancreatic autoantigens that are being presented by them. It is therefore unclear how important aberrant class II MHC molecule expression is in the initiation of autoimmunity.

The final variation on sequestration involves the role of the complement system in the normal disposal of immune complexes. Such complexes may contain self-antigens produced by normal cell turnover, and their efficient disposal prevents further stimulation of the immune system, which might result in an amplified and potentially damaging autoimmune response. As predicted by this concept, defects of the complement system do indeed result in autoimmunity, and this mechanism is considered further in Chapter 4 on lupus nephritis.

Passive maintenance of tolerance

This form of tolerance is passive in the sense that autoreactive cells are absent, due to elimination or anergy, and that therefore no active mechanisms are required to prevent tissue damage. It is probable that this form of tolerance is particularly critical for T cells. Although some autoreactive B cells are subject to tolerisation (Goodnow *et al.*, 1988), there are a number of self-proteins to which autoantibodies can readily be induced by a variety of experimental manoeuvres (Mitchison, 1985); furthermore, autoantibodies are present in healthy individuals (Mackay, 1983) and may even be required for the normal development of the antibody repertoire (Vakil & Kearney, 1986). In these cases, tolerance may be largely maintained by the absence (due to tolerance) of an autoreactive T cell, which would be required to provide help for autoantibody production. Furthermore, the process of somatic hypermutation, whereby mutations in the combining site of an antibody lead to the generation and selection of higher affinity antibodies during an immune response, must constantly generate new potentially autoreactive B cell clones. These new clones could, in their turn, be tolerised (Goodnow et al., 1989), but in addition they may be relatively harmless without help from linked autoreactive T cells. These considerations focus attention on the T cell as a key cell for the maintenance of self-tolerance, and it may well be for this reason that an analogous process of somatic mutation does not appear to operate on the T cell antigen receptor (Toyonaga & Mak, 1987).

There is now a wealth of evidence from the mouse that elimination of autoreactive T cell clones occurs during T cell development within the thymus (Kappler, Roehm & Marrack, 1987; Kappler et al., 1988; McDonald et al., 1988). This process of negative selection is dependent upon recognition by the T cell of self-components in the context of products of the MHC (discussed further below), and is probably one of the mechanisms explaining the well-known link between the MHC and autoimmunity (Svejgaard, Platz & Ryder, 1983). It should be noted that any association produced by this mechanism will probably be a protective one, the opposite to the usual situation in which possession of a particular MHC allele predisposes to autoimmunity. In man, the best example of such a protective association is probably insulin diabetes mellitus (Baisch et al., 1990, and see first volume in this series), but there are hints that certain MHC antigens are associated with a more rapid disappearance of autoantibodies in systemic vasculitis (see Chapter 8).

As a brief diversion, it is worth considering at this point other mechanisms by which the MHC may influence the development of autoimmunity. Our present understanding of the function of the products of the class I and II loci of the MHC is that these molecules bind antigens, or fragments of antigens, and present them to T cells. The interaction between MHC molecule and antigen has a degree of specificity, and in some experimental systems only MHC molecules that are linked with the ability to respond to a particular antigen can form the MHC molecule–antigen complex (Babbitt et al., 1985; Buus et al., 1987; Sette et al., 1989). This is one way in which possession of a particular MHC allele may predispose to the development of autoimmunity: the MHC product can bind to, and present, a critical autoantigen. Another, and not mutually exclusive, possibility is that the predisposing MHC molecule *positively* selects the developing T cell repertoire within the thymus so that potentially autoreactive T cells are preferentially allowed out into the periphery. Again, there is accumulating evidence for this process of positive selection in the mouse (Marrack, McCormack & Kappler, 1989; Kisielow et al., 1988; Blackman, Marrack & Kappler, 1989), but at present no examples of its involvement in autoimmunity. These mechanisms are discussed more concretely in the context of anti-glomerular basement membrane disease in Chapter 2.

Returning now to T cell tolerance, although the thymus appears to play a key role in the negative and positive selection of the T cell repertoire, peripheral mechanisms may also be important. The development of transgenic lines of mice (mice that have had extra genes introduced into their germ line) that express 'foreign' MHC molecules in the periphery (typically in the pancreas) but not in the thymus has shown that in some cases (Lo et al., 1988; Morahan, Allison & Miller, 1989), but not all (Böhme et al., 1989), the mice are tolerant of these transgenic MHC molecules. Other evidence shows that T cells can be rendered anergic when presented with antigen and MHC molecules on lipid membranes (Quill & Schwartz, 1987) or 'non-professional' antigen presenting cells (Gaspari, Jenkins & Katz, 1988), which presumably cannot supply critical accessory functions. All this suggests that post-thymic T cells in the periphery may be rather susceptible to tolerisation if they receive incomplete activation signals. The potential importance of this as a fail safe device guarding against autoimmunity is clear.

Active maintenance of tolerance

Despite the mechanisms considered above, autoreactive T cells can be isolated from normal individuals with apparent ease (Glimcher et al., 1981; Pereira et al., 1986); this would seem to imply that some form of regulation is required in order to prevent uncontrolled autoreactivity. Two main mechanisms have been proposed, namely suppression and idiotypic–antiidiotypic regulation.

The extent to which suppression contributes to self-tolerance is controversial, as indeed is the very existence of a discrete lineage of suppressor cells (Möller, 1988). Evidence for the importance of suppression in this context is provided by certain experimental systems in which manipulations that are thought to interfere with the generation of suppression lead to an exaggerated autoimmune response (Gibson et al., 1985). On the other hand, attempts to demonstrate a role for suppression in tolerance to simple peptides have been unsuccessful (Gammon et al., 1986), and it is fair to say, particularly in the light of our increased understanding concerning clonal deletion in the thymus, that it is rather unfashionable to invoke a significant role for suppression in the maintenance of self tolerance.

Despite this current climate, a defect in suppression has been claimed as a factor in the aetiology of a number of autoimmune diseases (Corazza et al.,

1986; Shinomiya, Yata & Sasazuki, 1984; Okita, Row & Volpé, 1981; Topliss *et al.*, 1983; Vento *et al.*, 1987). The assays involved are technically difficult, and the findings have not been universally reproducible (Ludgate *et al.*, 1985). However, the importance of a defect of suppression, at least in the aetiology of autoimmune thyroid disease, has been robustly defended (Volpé, 1988), and there is a considerable body of data in some animal models of renal disease that also supports a role for suppression in the maintenance of self tolerance (see Chapter 9 on interstitial nephritis). The issue remains controversial.

Another regulatory mechanism is idiotype–antiidiotype interaction, which expresses the direct interaction between the antigen receptor (idiotype) on one cell with a complementary receptor (antiidiotype) on another cell. Following the original network hypothesis of Jerne (Jerne, 1974), this is usually thought of in terms of antibodies. However, similar interactions can certainly occur between T cells (Martinez *et al.*, 1988), and, at least in some experimental systems, this seems to be an important mode of action of suppressor cells (Mitchison & Oliveira, 1986). Evidence for a close connection between antibodies and suppressor cells in one experimental system is provided by the marked perturbation of suppressor cell development that follows modulation of B cell development (Hayglass, Benacerraf & Sy, 1986). The potential importance of antiidiotypes is suggested by their presence, apparently with a specificity for a wide range of autoantibodies, in pooled normal human immunoglobulin. This preparation has been used to treat a number of autoimmune diseases (Imbach *et al.*, 1981; Newland *et al.*, 1988; Veys *et al.*, 1988), and although other actions are possible, e.g. non-specific blockade of the reticulo-endothelial system, in at least one case, spontaneous antifactor VIII disease, there is good evidence for the role of antiidiotypes (Sultan *et al.*, 1984). This example is also interesting because the down-regulation of the autoantibody induced by infusion of the pooled immunoglobulin preparation appears long lasting, and certainly longer than is explicable by persistence of the infused material (Sultan, Rossi & Kazatchkine, 1987). However, in other autoimmune diseases, attempts to demonstrate the existence of antiidiotypic antibodies have been unsuccessful, e.g. anti-glomerular basement membrane disease (Savage, 1986) and myasthenia gravis (Vincent, 1988).

The possible therapeutic implications of harnessing these endogenous immunoregulatory mechanisms are considered in the final chapter of this volume.

The aetiology of autoimmunity

The above brief survey of tolerance mechanisms has indicated some of the ways in which tolerance might be circumvented. To conclude this section, some other mechanisms that may cause autoimmunity will be mentioned.

The normal importance of the T cell in regulating the B cell means that any escape of the latter from the control of the former is potentially hazardous. This is typified by autonomous proliferation of a B cell clone. The resulting disease may range from a relatively benign condition such as mixed essential cryoglobulinaemia, in which the abnormal clone produces a monoclonal rheumatoid factor (Gorevic *et al.*, 1980), to a frankly malignant process such as chronic lymphatic leukaemia, which may be associated with the production of a number of autoantibodies (Bröker *et al.*, 1988). The lack of an autoreactive T cell may also be circumvented by direct polyclonal activation. The Epstein Barr virus has this property, and this is the probable explanation for the variety of autoantibodies that may be found in infectious mononucleosis. Alternatively, T cell help may be supplied, but it is directed to foreign T cell epitopes on a molecule that shares B cell epitopes with self components. These T cells, behaving correctly in responding to non-self antigens, can then provide help via the classical hapten-carrier mechanism (Mitchison, 1971) to the linked autoreactive B cell. There are now many examples of mimicry by pathogens of self-antigens (Oldstone, 1987), and one experimental example in which immunisation with a viral peptide leads to autoreactivity (Fujinami & Oldstone, 1985). In man, many of the manifestations of rheumatic fever could be related to the close antigenic mimicry by the streptococcus of a wide range of host tissues (Zabriskie, 1982).

There are undoubtedly many other factors involved in the aetiology of autoimmunity. These include variations in the target organ (Wick, 1987), the influence of sex, and the polygenic contributions to high and low immune responsiveness as demonstrated in Biozzi mice (Biozzi *et al.*, 1979). Although there may be examples of autoimmunity that have a relatively 'pure' aetiology, this is likely in most cases to be multifactorial.

Immunopathogenic mechanisms in renal disease

This section will not deal with non-immunological processes, notably the progressive sclerosis that follows many forms of glomerular injury (Klahr, Schreiner & Ichikawa, 1988), although they are of undoubted importance in pathogenesis. In some cases, just a simple overview will be given, with reference to a more detailed discussion in later chapters.

The immunological mechanisms involved in pathogenesis can be considered at two main levels. First, there are the specific processes involved in immune recognition by antibody on the humoral side and T cells on the cellular side. Secondly, these specific mechanisms employ, or recruit, a variety of non-specific factors that directly mediate tissue damage. Conceptually there is overlap between these levels. Thus deposition of immune complexes, although clearly involving specific antibody–antigen systems, can in some circumstances be non-specific in the sense that the resulting damage does not depend on the particular specificity of the antibody. Similarly, the damage caused by cytotoxic T cells is presumably mediated at the molecular level by non-specific molecules such as perforin, but this is so closely bound up with specific recognition that it is of little help to attempt to separate the two. However, the distinction between specific and non-specific mechanisms does have some force and is useful for discussion purposes.

Specific mechanisms

Historically, antibody-mediated damage has always been considered as the main specific mechanism in immunologically mediated renal disease, and this is still reflected in major textbooks of nephrology (Wilson & Dixon, 1986). No doubt this reflects, to some extent, the importance of such mechanisms, but it is also true that the tools to study T cell involvement are only just becoming available. Because of the arguably more important role of T cells, at least in the initiation of autoimmunity, this will be an area of great interest in the future.

Humoral

Stress has been laid on two major mechanisms of antibody-mediated damage, namely reactions with insoluble or tissue-fixed antigens on the one hand, and reactions with soluble antigens, with resulting immune complex deposition, on the other (Wilson & Dixon, 1986). The tissue-fixed antigens may either be intrinsic components of the kidney (typically of the glomerular or tubular basement membrane) or extrinsic 'planted' antigens. The distinction between these two mechanisms is not always clear cut. Many examples that were originally regarded as due to deposition of circulating immune complexes are in fact due to interaction with fixed antigens, either intrinsic (Heymann nephritis; see Chapter 3) or planted, e.g. cationic bovine serum albumin (Border et al., 1982; Adler et al., 1983) and DNA (Izui, Lambert & Miescher, 1976). Furthermore, antigen–antibody complexes, even if deposited preformed in the kidney, are still exposed to other circulating molecules. This may lead, on the one hand, to further accumulation of material with the initial deposits now acting as planted antigen (Ford & Kosatka, 1981), and on the other, in conditions of suitable antigen excess, to dissolution of the deposits (Wilson & Dixon, 1971; Mannik & Striker, 1980). Clearly, the deposition of antigen and antibody in the kidney is a fluid process, with considerable scope for flexibility in the order with which the components are laid down, and further potential for dynamic modification of deposits once formed. The rest of this section on antibody-mediated damage will consist of a brief discussion of the general principles involved in glomerular deposition, localisation and handling of immune complexes, an area that has been the subject of much work. Models that involve antibody reacting with fixed antigens are of direct relevance to particular human diseases, and further aspects of such models are therefore considered in Chapters 2 and 3.

The classical models of acute (one-shot) and chronic serum sickness, produced by a single or multiple injections of antigen respectively, have produced a considerable body of data on the nephritogenicity of immune complexes (for review see Wilson & Dixon, 1986). As a general point, although acute serum sickness in rabbits produces a proliferative nephritis, chronic serum sickness may cause a variety of histological appearances. These include mesangial proliferation, a membranous nephropathy, a proliferative necrotising crescentic glomerulonephritis, or combinations of these. Therefore the particular histological pattern depends on factors other than the particular antigen–antibody system involved; this is almost certainly true of some human glomerulonephritides as well.

Considering first the events that lead to deposition of immune complexes in the kidney, non-immunological processes are also involved. Interference with urinary drainage or with the blood supply, in both experimental systems (Germuth, Kelemen & Pollack, 1967) and following renal artery stenosis in man (Salyer & Salyer, 1974), provides considerable protection from immune complex deposition. On the other hand, an increase in glomerular permeability exacerbates immune glomerular damage (Kniker & Cochrane, 1968). Considering the immunological factors, it is clear that the quantity and quality of the immune response play a major role. Animals that make a poor response, or that are maintained in a state of relative antigen excess, experience less glomerular injury (Wilson & Dixon, 1971). This may, in part, reflect the size of the resulting complexes, in that, under these conditions, only small complexes are formed, and there is some evidence that large complexes are more nephritogenic (Cochrane & Hawkins, 1968). However, in other cases, smaller complexes appeared to be associated with the more severe lesion (Germuth, Senterfit & Dreesman, 1972), and it has been suggested that large amounts of high affinity antibody are protective, because they result in the formation of large complexes that are more easily eliminated (Noble *et al.*, 1987). The problem in interpreting most studies stems from the difficulty of knowing the extent to which circulating complexes are an accurate reflection of deposited complexes. In general, the antibody–antigen ratio, rather than the absolute concentration of either component, is probably the important variable in determining complex size and resultant handling. The influence of antibody affinity is complex. High affinity antibody is usually said to be associated with a more severe glomerular lesion in serum sickness (Wilson & Dixon, 1986), but, on the other hand, low affinity antibody may allow the persistence of antigen, which may also lead to a more severe lesion (Devey *et al.*, 1982). The charge of the antibody, as well as influencing the site of deposition (see below), may also be instrumental in determining whether an immune complex will be deposited in the glomerulus at all: even a small proportion of cationic species within a complex will enable deposition of the entire complex, including the non-cationic component (Gauthier & Mannik, 1990). In addition to the characteristics of the antigen–antibody complex, other factors that influence deposition include the complement and mononuclear phagocytic systems (Mannik, 1982), and glomerular haemodynamics and permeability. It is now clear that the complement system plays a major role in the solubilization of immune complexes, and then, via the CR1 receptor on erythrocytes, their transport to, and disposal by, the mononuclear phagocytic system (Pusey, Venning & Peters, 1988). Interruption of this mechanism may play an important part in the pathogenesis of human immune complex diseases such as systemic lupus erythematosus (see Chapter 4). Another important clearance mechanism is provided by the glomerulus itself, but the effect of prior deposition of complexes on subsequent accumulation is unclear. In chronic serum sickness, mesangial uptake is enhanced (Ward & Wilson, 1977), but, on the other hand, mesangial deposition in another model appears to inhibit mesangial egress but not uptake (Keane & Raij, 1980), whilst glomerular capillary deposition may inhibit uptake (Schneeberger *et al.*, 1980).

Some of the above factors, involved in determining whether immune complexes will deposit in the kidney or not, are also involved in determining the initial site of deposition of such complexes. If such complexes are being produced with fixed or planted antigens, clearly the site is predetermined. The important variables that determine the localisation of circulating immune complexes seem to be charge, size of complex, and affinity of antibody involved; these latter two are probably closely connected. The anionic charge of the glomerular basement membrane will favour the subepithelial and subendothelial localisation of cationic complexes (Gallo, Caulin-Glaser & Lamm, 1981). This effect is particularly well demonstrated by the shift from a mesangial to a glomerular capillary wall localisation of the same species when its charge is altered (Border *et al.*, 1982). Smaller complexes, as formed with low affinity IgG antibodies, preferentially localise to the subepithelial area, whereas larger insoluble complexes, formed from IgM or high affinity IgG, deposit in subendothelial and mesangial areas (Lew, Staines & Steward, 1984; Iskander & Jennette, 1983; Cameron & Clark, 1982). The load of immune complexes is also important:

the initial site of mesangial deposition in chronic serum sickness is followed by glomerular capillary deposition as the quantity of immune complexes increases (Wilson & Dixon, 1971). This effect is probably not due simply to the overloading of mesangial clearance mechanisms, because of the evidence mentioned above of enhanced mesangial function in this model (Ward & Wilson, 1977).

The modification and clearance of immune complexes, once deposited, will depend on both extrarenal factors and intrinsic renal mechanisms. The existence of a dynamic equilibrium between deposited complexes and circulating antigen, antibody and complexes has already been mentioned, together with the possibilities for augmentation or dissolution of the deposits. In addition to the primary antigen–antibody system, rheumatoid factors (Penner et al., 1979; Miyazaki et al., 1990) and antiidiotypic antibodies (Zanetti & Wilson, 1983) may also participate in these interactions. Both glomerular mesangial cells and bone marrow derived monocytes may be involved in the uptake and processing of immune deposits, and their relative importance varies from system to system; in some cases, bone marrow-derived cells appear to be exclusively involved (Striker, Mannik & Tung, 1979).

Cellular

The initial part of this chapter concentrated particularly on the importance of T cells in the maintenance of tolerance. It is therefore unfortunate that little is known about the role of T cells in human glomerulonephritis. For the reasons outlined above, it is likely that they will be involved in the initiation of the autoimmune process, even for diseases that are principally autoantibody mediated, such as anti-glomerular basement membrane disease. This is discussed further in Chapter 2, but it is worth making the point here that the MHC associations of this disease strongly suggest an important role for T cells, as MHC products are in general concerned with T cell and not with B cell activation. The presence of T cells within inflamed glomeruli is further indirect evidence for their importance in man (Nolasco et al., 1987; Neale et al., 1988), and a number of animal models of autoimmune renal disease provide direct evidence for this (Mann et al., 1987; Bannister, Ulich & Wilson, 1987; Mihara et al., 1988; Bolton et al., 1988; Oite et al., 1989). Further progress in man will probably require the in vitro isolation and growth of the relevant autoantigen-specific T cells. This is technically very difficult and has only been achieved for a small number of autoimmune diseases (De Berardinis et al., 1988; Hohlfeld et al., 1984; Londei, Bottazzo & Feldmann, 1985). The difficulty is compounded by, and closely related to, our practically complete ignorance (myasthenia gravis is a possible exception: Hohlfeld et al., 1987) of the nature of the autoantigens recognised by

T cells. Although there is rapid progress in the identification of autoantigens as recognised by autoantibodies (e.g. Gershwin *et al.*, 1987; Doble *et al.*, 1988, and see chapters on anti-glomerular basement membrane disease and systemic vasculitis) there is no guarantee that the T cell autoantigen will be the same (Lake & Mitchison, 1976), although this does appear to be the case in myasthenia. Despite our ignorance, there is no doubt that therapy aimed empirically at the T cell can be very effective in animal models of glomerulo-nephritis and in some cases of human disease; this aspect is considered further in the final chapter.

Non-specific mechanisms

The specific mechanisms discussed above may be capable of causing tissue damage directly: antibody alone is sufficient to induce proteinuria in guinea pig nephrotoxic nephritis (Simpson *et al.*, 1975, and see Chapter 2), and, although the involvement of T cells is less well defined, such cells are certainly capable of direct cytotoxicity. However, in many cases a variety of mediator systems (complement, the clotting system, arachidonic acid metabolites, reactive oxygen species) and non-specific cells (polymorpho-nuclear leukocytes, macrophages, platelets) are recruited (Wilson & Dixon, 1986).

The complement system, mentioned above in its protective role as a mechanism for the safe disposal of immune complexes, may also cause damage in a number of ways. The terminal components of the complement cascade, triggered via either the classical or alternative pathways, can assemble to form the membrane attack complex (MAC) which is directly cytotoxic (Biesecker, 1983). The importance of MAC is suggested both by its presence in a variety of renal lesions (Biesecker, Katz & Koffler, 1981) and by the fact that full expression of injury in many cases requires a complete complement system (Groggel *et al.*, 1983, 1985; Couser, Baker & Adler, 1985; de Heer *et al.*, 1985). In some situations, however, complement deficiency appears to exacerbate damage, perhaps due to inefficient complement-mediated disposal of immune complexes (Groggel & Terreros, 1990). Other products of the complement cascade include anaphylatoxins, chemotactic factors for polymorphonuclear leukocytes (PMN) and activators of macrophages (Lachmann & Peters, 1982).

Activation of the coagulation system is prominent in acute glomerulo-nephritis, and may, in many cases, reflect macrophage procoagulant activity (Brentjens, 1987); macrophages are also capable of augmenting endogenous glomerular procoagulant activity (Tipping, Lowe & Holdsworth, 1988). Activated neutrophils, via the production of reactive oxygen species (see page 13), may also be capable of initiating glomerular thrombosis (Poelstra *et al.*, 1990). It seems likely that deposition of fibrin is a major factor in the formation of crescents, and interruption of this process with ancrod ameliorates renal damage in models of crescentic nephritis (see Chapter 8). Fibrin deposition may also play an important role in lupus nephritis, and some impressive therapeutic results of ancrod treatment have been reported in man (see Chapter 4).

The products of arachidonic acid metabolism (prostaglandins, thromboxanes, leukotrienes) are important inflammatory and vasoactive mediators (Levenson, Simmons & Brenner, 1982). Direct administration of prostaglandin E1 has a beneficial effect in a number of renal lesions, both experimental (Kelly *et al.*, 1987; Clark *et al.*, 1987) and human (Nagayama *et al.*, 1988; Lin, 1990), and manipulation of the arachidonic acid system by alteration of dietary lipids is also an effective therapeutic approach, at least in some animal models (Kelley *et al.*, 1985). Antagonism of leukotriene D4, a product of activated leukocytes, can preserve the glomerular ultrafiltration coefficient during nephrotoxic nephritis (see Chapter 2), suggesting an important role for this mediator in pathogenesis (Badr *et al.*, 1988).

The production of reactive oxygen species as an important final common pathway of tissue injury has attracted recent interest (Johnson, Klebanoff & Couser, 1988*b*; Shah, 1989). Immune complexes can trigger the production of reactive oxygen species by PMN and macrophages (Ward *et al.*, 1983) and inhibitors of such species can ameliorate renal damage (Jennette, Hyson & Iskander, 1982; Riehan, Wiggins & Johnson, 1984). The production of hydroxyl radicals, catalysed by iron present in tubules as a result of glomerular leakage of transferrin, may be a major cause of the tubulointerstitial damage found in models of primary glomerular injury (Alfrey, Froment & Hammond, 1989). Myeloperoxidase, a product of PMN, can bind to the glomerular basement membrane by virtue of its cationic charge, and once there can catalyse oxidant injury by hydrogen peroxide and halide ions (Johnson *et al.*, 1988*a*).

PMN and macrophages are the most prominent of the non-specific cellular mechanisms. PMN accumulation is strongly influenced by the complement system. This is shown by the prevention of such accumulation in complement-depleted animals during the heterologous phase of nephrotoxic nephritis (Cochrane, Unanue & Dixon, 1965); other factors (e.g. adherence via receptors for the Fc portion of immunoglobulin) are also involved, as complement depletion does not affect PMN accumulation in the autologous phase (Thomson *et al.*, 1976, and see Chapter 2 for more on nephrotoxic nephritis models). Once on site, PMN are capable of releasing a range of destructive enzymes (Janoff, 1972) and, via the action of myeloperoxidase, generating damaging reactive oxygen species (see above). The importance of PMN in at least one model is elegantly demonstrated by the fact that beige mice, which have a congenital abnormality of PMN, are protected from the effects of nephrotoxic antiserum (Schrijver *et al.*, 1989).

Macrophages, attracted by a variety of stimuli such as complement and fibronectin fragments, lymphokines and Fc receptor-mediated mechanisms, typically tend to dominate experimental inflammatory glomerular conditions following the initial influx of PMN (Schreiner *et al.*, 1978). They make a major contribution to glomerular hypercellularity (Becker *et al.*, 1982; Atkins *et al.*, 1982) and are probably the dominant cell involved in extra-capillary proliferation (crescent formation; Atkins & Thomson, 1988), at least when this is associated with breaches in the glomerular basement membrane (Boucher *et al.*, 1987). The ability of macrophages to produce procoagulant activity has already been mentioned and they are also capable of secreting a multitude of potentially damaging enzymes (Werb, Bainton & Jones, 1980), and the generation of reactive oxygen species (Boyce, Tipping & Holdsworth, 1989). They produce a variety of cytokines (IL-1, tumour necrosis factor) which may play an important role in mediating renal injury (Tomosugi *et al.*, 1989). In distinction from PMN, and by virtue of their constitutive expression of MHC class II molecules, macrophages can also act as antigen-presenting cells for CD4$^+$ T cells. They could thus play an important role in activating the autoreactive T cells that are probably the key cells involved in initiating autoimmune renal disease (see discussion earlier in chapter). As with PMN, direct evidence for the importance of macrophages in the mediation of damage is provided by the amelioration of such damage when macrophages are depleted (Lavelle, Durland & Yum, 1981; Holdsworth, Neale & Wilson, 1981).

The role of platelets in glomerular disease has been reviewed (Cameron, 1984). Platelet factors can stimulate the proliferation of glomerular cells (Nakashima, Hirose & Hamashima, 1980) and act as chemotactic agents for PMN and macrophages (Devel *et al.*, 1982). Despite this, the therapeutic effect of anti-platelet drugs, in both experimental models (Ogawa & Naruse, 1982) and human disease (see Chapter 6), has been disappointing.

References

Adler, S. G., Wang, H., Ward, H. J., Cohen, A. H. & Border, W. A. (1983). Electrical charge: its role in the pathogenesis and prevention of experimental membranous nephropathy in the rabbit. *Journal of Clinical Investigation*, **71**, 487–99.

Alfrey, A. C., Froment, D. H. & Hammond, W. S. (1989). Role of iron in the tubulo-interstitial injury in nephrotoxic serum nephritis. *Kidney International*, **36**, 753–9.

Atkins, R. C., Holdsworth, S. R., Hancock, W. W., Thomson, N. M. & Glasgow, E. F. (1982). Cellular immune mechanisms in human glomerulonephritis: the role of mononuclear leucocytes. *Springer Seminars in Immunopathology*, **5**, 269–96.

Atkins, R. C. & Thomson, N. M. (1988). Rapidly progressive glomerulonephritis. In *Diseases of the Kidney*, 4th edn, ed. R. W. Schrier & C. W. Gottschalk, pp. 1903–27. Boston/Toronto: Little, Brown and Company.

Babbitt, B. P., Allen, P. M., Matsueda, G., Haber, E. & Unanue, E. R. (1985). Binding of immunogenic peptides to Ia histocompatibility molecules. *Nature*, **317**, 359–61.

Badr, K. F., Schreiner, G. F., Wasserman, M. & Ichikawa, I. (1988). Preservation of the glomerular capillary ultrafiltration coefficient during rat nephrotoxic serum nephritis by a specific leukotriene D_4 receptor antagonist. *Journal of Clinical Investigation*, **81**, 1702–9.

Baisch, J. M., Weeks, T., Giles, R., Hoover, M., Stastny, P. & Capra, D. J. (1990). Analysis of HLA-DQ genotypes and susceptibility in insulin-dependent diabetes mellitus. *New England Journal of Medicine*, **322**, 1836–41.

Bannister, K. M., Ulich, T. R. & Wilson, C. B. (1987). Induction, characterization, and cell transfer of autoimmune tubulointerstitial nephritis. *Kidney International*, **32**, 642–51.

Becker, G. J., Hancock, W. W., Stow, J. L., Glasgow, E. F., Atkins, R. C. & Thomson, N. M. (1982). Involvement of the macrophage in experimental chronic immune complex glomerulonephritis. *Nephron*, **32**, 227–33.

Biesecker, G. (1983). Membrane attack complex of complement as a pathologic mediator. *Laboratory Investigation*, **49**, 237–49.

Biesecker, G., Katz, S. & Koffler, D. (1981). Renal localization of the membrane attack complex in systemic lupus erythematosus. *Journal of Experimental Medicine*, **154**, 1779–94.

Biozzi, G., Mouton, D., Heumann, A. M., Bouthillier, Y., Stiffel, C. & Mevel, J. C. (1979). Genetic analysis of antibody responsiveness to sheep erythrocytes in crosses between lines of mice selected for high and low antibody synthesis. *Immunology*, **36**, 427–38.

Blackman, M. A., Marrack, P. & Kappler, J. (1989). Influence of the major histocompatibility complex on positive selection of $V\beta17a^+$ T cells. *Science*, **244**, 214–17.

Böhme, J., Haskins, K., Stecha, P. *et al.* (1989). Transgenic mice with I-A on islet cells are normoglycaemic but immunologically intolerant. *Science*, **244**, 1179–83.

Bolton, W. K., Chandra, M., Tyson, T. M., Kirkpatrick, P. R., Sadovnic, M. J. & Sturgill, B. C. (1988). Transfer of experimental glomerulonephritis in chickens by mononuclear cells. *Kidney International*, **34**, 598–610.

Border, W. A., Ward, H. J., Kamis, E. S. & Cohen, A. H. (1982). Induction of membranous nephropathy in rabbits by administration of an exogenous cationic antigen. Demonstration of a pathogenic role for electrical charge. *Journal of Clinical Investigation*, **69**, 451–61.

Bottazzo, G. F., Pujol-Borrell, R., Hanafusa, T. & Feldmann, M. (1983). Role of aberrant HLA-DR expression and antigen presentation in the induction of endocrine autoimmunity. *Lancet*, **ii**, 1115–19.

Bottazzo, G. F., Bosi, E., Bonifacio, E., Mirakian, R., Todd, I. & Pujol-Borrell, R. (1989). Pathogenesis of type I (insulin-dependent) diabetes: possible mechanisms of autoimmune damage. *British Medical Bulletin*, **45**, 37–57.

Boucher, A., Droz, D., Adafer, E. & Noel, L. H. (1987). Relationship between the integrity of Bowman's capsule and the composition of cellular crescents in human crescentic glomerulonephritis. *Laboratory Investigation*, **56**, 526–33.

Boyce, N. W., Tipping, P. G. & Holdsworth, S. R. (1989). Glomerular macrophages produce reactive oxygen species in experimental glomerulonephritis. *Kidney International*, **35**, 778–82.

Brentjens, J. R. (1987). Glomerular procoagulant activity and glomerulonephritis. *Laboratory Investigation*, **57**, 107–11.

Bröker, B. M., Klajman, A., Youinou, P. *et al.* (1988). Chronic lymphocytic leukemic (CLL) cells secrete multispecific autoantibodies. *Journal of Autoimmunity*, **1**, 469–81.

Buus, S., Sette, A., Colon, S. M., Miles, C. & Grey, H. M. (1987). The relation between major histocompatibility complex (MHC) restriction and the capacity of Ia to bind immunogenic peptides. *Science*, **235**, 1353–8.

Cameron, J. S. (1984). Platelets in glomerular disease. *Annual Review of Medicine*, **35**, 175–80.

Cameron, J. S. & Clark, W. F. (1982). A role for insoluble antibody–antigen complexes in glomerulonephritis? *Clinical Nephrology*, **18**, 55–61.

Clark, W. F., Parbtani, A., McDonald, J. W. D., Taylor, N., Reid, B. D. & Kreeft, J. (1987). The effects of a thromboxane synthase inhibitor, a prostacyclin analog and PGE$_1$ on the nephritis of the NZB/W F$_1$ mouse. *Clinical Nephrology*, **28**, 288–94.

Cochrane, C. G. & Hawkins, D. (1968). Studies on circulating immune complexes. III. Factors governing the ability of circulating complexes to localize in blood vessels. *Journal of Experimental Medicine*, **127**, 137–54.

Cochrane, C. G., Unanue, E. R. & Dixon, F. J. (1965). A role of polymorphonuclear leukocytes and complement in nephrotoxic nephritis. *Journal of Experimental Medicine*, **122**, 99–116.

Cohen, S. B., Dijkstra, C. D. & Weetman, A. P. (1988). Sequential analysis of experimental autoimmune thyroiditis induced by neonatal thymectomy in the Buffalo strain rat. *Cellular Immunology*, **114**, 126–36.

Corazza, G. R., Sachielli, P., Londei, M., Frisoni, M. & Gasbarrini, G. (1986). Gluten specific suppressor T cell dysfunction in coeliac disease. *Gut*, **27**, 392–8.

Couser, W. G., Baker, P. J. & Adler, S. (1985). Complement and the direct mediation of immune glomerular injury: a new perspective. *Kidney International*, **28**, 879–90.

De Berardinis, P., Londei, M., James, R. F. L., Lake, S. P., Wise, P. H. & Feldmann, M. (1988). Do CD4-positive cytotoxic T cells damage islet β cells in type I diabetes? *Lancet*, **ii**, 823–4.

de Heer, E., Daha, M. R., Bhakdi, S., Bazin, H. & Van Es, L. A. (1985). Possible involvement of terminal complement complex in active Heymann nephritis. *Kidney International*, **27**, 388–93.

Devel, T. F., Senior, R. M., Huang, J. S. & Griffin, G. L. (1982). Chemotaxis of monocytes and neutrophils to platelet-derived growth factor. *Journal of Clinical Investigation*, **69**, 1046–9.

Devey, M. E., Bleasdale, K., Collins, M. & Steward, M. W. (1982). Experimental antigen–antibody complex disease in mice. The role of antibody levels, antibody affinity and circulating antigen–antibody complexes. *International Archives of Allergy and Applied Immunology*, **68**, 47–53.

Doble, N. D., Banga, J. P., Pope, R., Lalor, E., Kilduff, P. & McGregor, A. M. (1988). Autoantibodies to the thyroid microsomal/thyroid peroxidase antigen are polyclonal and directed to several distinct antigenic sites. *Immunology*, **64**, 23–9.

Ford, P. M. & Kosatka, I. (1981). A mechanism of enhancement of immune complex deposition following *in situ* immune complex formation in the mouse glomerulus. *Immunology*, **43**, 433–9.

Fujinami, R. S. & Oldstone, M. B. A. (1985). Aminoacid homology between the encephalitogenic site of myelin basic protein and virus: mechanism for autoimmunity. *Science*, **230**, 1043–5.

Gallo, G. R., Caulin-Glaser, T. & Lamm, M. E. (1981). Charge of circulating immune complexes as a factor in glomerular basement membrane localization in mice. *Journal of Clinical Investigation*, **67**, 1305–13.

Gammon, G., Dunn, K., Shastri, N., Oki, A., Wilbur, S. & Sercarz, E. E. (1986). Neonatal T-cell tolerance to minimal immunogenic peptides is caused by clonal inactivation. *Nature, London*, **319**, 413–15.

Gaspari, A. A., Jenkins, M. K. & Katz, S. I. (1988). Class II MHC-bearing keratinocytes induce antigen-specific unresponsiveness in hapten-specific TH1 clones. *Journal of Immunology*, **141**, 2216–20.

Gauthier, V. J. & Mannik, M. (1990). A small proportion of cationic antibodies in immune complexes is sufficient to mediate their deposition in glomeruli. *Journal of Immunology*, **145**, 3348–52.

Germuth, F. G., Kelemen, W. A. & Pollack, A. D. (1967). Immune complex disease. II. The role of circulatory dynamics and glomerular filtration in the development of experimental glomerulonephritis. *Johns Hopkins Medical Journal*, **120**, 252–61.

Germuth, F. G., Senterfit, L. B. & Dreesman, G. R. (1972). Immune complex disease. V. The nature of the circulating complexes associated with glomerular alterations in the chronic BSA-rabbit system. *Johns Hopkins Medical Journal*, **130**, 344–57.

Gershwin, M. E., Mackay, I. R., Sturgess, A. & Coppel, R. L. (1987). Identification and specificity of a cDNA encoding the 70 kD mitochondrial antigen recognised in primary biliary cirrhosis. *Journal of Immunology*, **138**, 3525–31.

Gibson, J., Basten, A., Walker, K. Z. & Loblay, R. H. (1985). A role for suppressor T cells in induction of self-tolerance. *Proceedings of the National Academy of Sciences, USA*, **82**, 5150–4.

Glimcher, L. H., Longo, D. L., Green, I. & Schwartz, R. H. (1981). Murine syngeneic mixed lymphocyte response. I. Target antigens are self Ia molecules. *Journal of Experimental Medicine*, **154**, 1652–70.

Goodnow, C. C., Crosbie, J., Adelstein, S. *et al.* (1988). Altered immunoglobulin expression and functional silencing of self-reactive B lymphocytes in transgenic mice. *Nature*, London, **334**, 676–82.

Goodnow, C. C., Crosbie, J., Jorgensen, H., Brink, R. A. & Basten, A. (1989). Induction of self-tolerance in mature peripheral B lymphocytes. *Nature*, London, **342**, 385–91.

Gorevic, P. D., Kassab, H. J., Levo, Y. *et al.* (1980). Mixed cryoglobulinemia: clinical aspects and long-term follow-up of 40 patients. *American Journal of Medicine*, **69**, 287–308.

Groggel, G. C., Adler, S., Rennke, H. G., Couser, W. G. & Salant, D. J. (1983). Role of terminal complement pathway in experimental membranous nephropathy in the rabbit. *Journal of Clinical Investigation*, **72**, 1948–57.

Groggel, G. C., Salant, D. J., Darby, C., Rennke, H. G. & Couser, W. G. (1985). Role of terminal complement pathway in the heterologous phase of antiglomerular basement membrane nephritis. *Kidney International*, **27**, 643–51.

Groggel, G. C. & Terreros, D. A. (1990). Role of the terminal complement pathway in accelerated autologous anti-glomerular basement membrane nephritis. *American Journal of Pathology*, **136**, 533–40.

Guerin, V., Rabian, C., Noel, L. H. *et al.* (1990). Anti-glomerular-basement-membrane disease after lithotripsy. *Lancet*, **335**, 856–7.

Hayglass, K. T., Benacerraf, B. & Sy, M-S. (1986). T cell development in B cell-deficient mice. V. Stopping anti-μ treatment results in Igh-restricted expansion of the T suppressor cell repertoire concomitant with the development of normal immunoglobulin levels. *Journal of Experimental Medicine*, **164**, 36–49.

Hohlfeld, R., Toyka, K. V., Heininger, K., Grosse-Wilde, H. & Kalies, I. (1984). Autoimmune human T lymphocytes specific for acetylcholine receptor. *Nature*, London, **310**, 244–6.

Hohlfeld, R., Toyka, K. V., Tzartos, S. J., Carson, W. & Conti-Tronconi, B. M. (1987). Human T-helper lymphocytes in myasthenia gravis recognize the nicotinic receptor α subunit. *Proceedings of the National Academy of Sciences, USA*, **84**, 5379–83.

Holdsworth, S. R., Neale, T. J. & Wilson, C. B. (1981). Abrogation of macrophage-dependent injury in experimental glomerulonephritis in the rabbit. Use of an antimacrophage serum. *Journal of Clinical Investigation*, **68**, 686–98.

Hume, D. M., Sterling, W. A., Weymouth, R. J., Siebel, H. R., Madge, G. E. & Lee, H. M. (1970). Glomerulonephritis in human renal homotransplants. *Transplantation Proceedings*, 2, 361–412.

Imbach, P., Barandun, S., d'Apuzo, V. *et al.* (1981). High-dose intravenous gammaglobulin for idiopathic thrombocytopenic purpura in childhood. *Lancet*, i, 1228–31.

Iskander, S. S. & Jennette, J. C. (1983). Influence of antibody avidity on glomerular immune complex localization. *American Journal of Pathology*, 112, 155–9.

Iwatani, Y., Iitaka, M., Row, V. V. & Volpé, R. (1988). Effect of HLA-DR positive thyrocytes on *in vitro* thyroid autoantibody production. *Clinical and Investigative Medicine*, 11, 279–85.

Izui, S., Lambert, P-H. & Miescher, P. A. (1976). *In vitro* demonstration of a particular affinity of glomerular basement membrane and collagen for DNA. A possible basis for a local formation of DNA–anti-DNA complexes in systemic lupus erythematosus. *Journal of Experimental Medicine*, 144, 428–43.

Janoff, A. (1972). Neutrophil proteases in inflammation. *Annual Review of Medicine*, 23, 177–90.

Jennette, J. C., Hyson, C. P. & Iskander, S. S. (1982). Palliative effect of superoxide dismutase (SOD) on heterologous protein induced glomerulonephritis. *Federation Proceedings*, 41, 325.(Abstract)

Jerne, N. K. (1974). Towards a network theory of the immune system. *Annales d'Immunologie (Paris)*, 125C, 373–89.

Johnson, R. J., Guggenheim, S. J., Klebanoff, S. J. *et al.* (1988a). Morphologic correlates of glomerular oxidant injury induced by the myeloperoxidase–hydrogen peroxide–halide system of the neutrophil. *Laboratory Investigation*, 58, 294–301.

Johnson, R. J., Klebanoff, S. J. & Couser, W. G. (1988b). Oxidants in glomerular injury. In *Immunopathology of Renal Disease. Contempory Issues in Nephrology. 18*, ed. C. B. Wilson, B. M. Brenner & J. H. Stein, pp. 87–110. New York, Edinburgh, London, Melbourne: Churchill Livingstone.

Kappler, J. W., Roehm, N. & Marrack, P. (1987). T cell tolerance by clonal elimination in the thymus. *Cell*, 49, 273–80.

Kappler, J. W., Staerz, U., White, J. & Marrack, P. C. (1988). Self-tolerance eliminates T cells specific for Mls-modified products of the major histocompatibility complex. *Nature*, London, 332, 35–40.

Keane, W. F. & Raij, L. (1980). Impaired mesangial clearance of macromolecules in rats with chronic mesangial ferritin-antiferritin immune complex deposition. *Laboratory Investigation*, 43, 500–8.

Kelley, V. E., Ferreti, A., Izui, S. & Strom, T. B. (1985). A fish oil diet rich in eicosapentaenoic acid reduces cyclooxygenase metabolites, and suppresses lupus in MRL-lpr mice. *Journal of Immunology*, 134, 1914–19.

Kelly, C. J., Zurier, R. B., Krakaver, K. A., Blanchard, N. & Neilson, E. G. (1987). Prostaglandin E_1 inhibits effector T cell induction and tissue damage in experimental murine interstitial nephritis. *Journal of Clinical Investigation*, 79, 782–89.

Kisielow, P., Teh, H. S., Blüthmann, H. & Von Boehmer, H. (1988). Positive selection of antigen-specific T cells in thymus by restricting MHC molecules. *Nature*, London, 335, 730–3.

Klahr, S., Schreiner, G. & Ichikawa, I. (1988). The progression of renal disease. *New England Journal of Medicine*, 318, 1657–66.

Kniker, W. T. & Cochrane, C. G. (1968). The localization of circulating immune complexes in experimental serum sickness. The role of vasoactive amines and hydrodynamic forces. *Journal of Experimental Medicine*, 127, 119–36.

Lachmann, P. J. & Peters, D. K. (1982). Complement. In *Clinical Aspects of Immunology*, 4th edn, ed. P. J. Lachmann & D. K. Peters, pp. 18–49. Oxford: Blackwell Scientific Publications.

Lake, P. & Mitchison, N. A. (1976). Associative control of the immune response to cell surface antigens. *Immunological Communications*, 5, 795–805.

Lavelle, K. J., Durland, B. D. & Yum, M. N. (1981). The effect of antimacrophage antiserum on immune complex glomerulonephritis. *Journal of Laboratory and Clinical Medicine*, 98, 195–205.

Levenson, D. J., Simmons, C. E. & Brenner, B. M. (1982). Arachidonic acid metabolism, prostaglandins and the kidney. *American Journal of Medicine*, 72, 354–74.

Lew, A. M., Staines, N. A. & Steward, M. W. (1984). Glomerulonephritis induced by preformed immune complexes containing monoclonal antibodies of defined affinity and isotype. *Clinical and Experimental Immunology*, 57, 413–22.

Lin, C. Y. (1990). Improvement in steroid and immunosuppressive drug resistant lupus nephritis by intravenous prostaglandin E1 therapy. *Nephron*, 55, 258–64.

Lo, D., Burkly, L. C., Widera, G. *et al.* (1988). Diabetes and tolerance in transgenic mice expressing class II MHC molecules in pancreatic beta cells. *Cell*, 53, 159–68.

Londei, M., Bottazzo, G. F. & Feldmann, M. (1985). Human T-cell clones from autoimmune thyroid glands: specific recognition of autologous thyroid cells. *Science*, 228, 85–9.

Ludgate, M. E., Ratanachaiyavong, S., Weetman, A. P., Hall, R. & McGregor, A. M. (1985). Failure to demonstrate cell-mediated immune responses to thyroid antigens in Graves' disease using *in vitro* assays of lymphokine-mediated migration inhibition. *Journal of Clinical Endocrinology and Metabolism*, 60, 98–102.

Mackay, I. R. (1983). Natural autoantibodies to the fore – forbidden clones to the rear? *Immunology Today*, 4, 340–2.

Mann, R., Kelly, C. J., Hines, W. H. *et al.* (1987). Effector T cell differentiation in experimental interstitial nephritis. I. The development and modulation of effector lymphocyte maturation by I-J$^+$ regulatory T cells. *Journal of Immunology*, 138, 4200–8.

Mannik, M. (1982). Pathophysiology of circulating immune complexes. *Arthritis and Rheumatism*, 25, 783–7.

Mannik, M. & Striker, G. E. (1980). Removal of glomerular deposits of immune complexes in mice by administration of excess antigen. *Laboratory Investigation*, 42, 483–9.

Marrack, P., McCormack, J. & Kappler, J. (1989). Presentation of antigen, foreign major histocompatibility complex proteins and self by thymus cortical epithelium. *Nature*, London, 338, 503–5.

Martinez, C., Pereira, P., Toribio, M-L. *et al.* (1988). The participation of B cells and antibodies in the selection and maintenance of T cell repertoires. *Immunological Reviews*, 101, 191–215.

McDonald, H. R., Schneider, R., Lees, R. K. *et al.* (1988). T-cell receptor Vβ use predicts reactivity and tolerance to Mls^a-encoded antigens. *Nature*, London, 332, 40–5.

Mihara, M., Ohsugi, Y., Saito, K. *et al.* (1988). Immunologic abnormality in NZB/NZW F$_1$ mice. Thymus-independent occurrence of B cell abnormality and requirement for T cells in the development of autoimmune disease, as evidenced by an analysis of the athymic nude individuals. *Journal of Immunology*, 141, 85–90.

Minami, M., Ebner, S. A., Stadecker, M. K. & Dorf, M. (1987). The effects of phorbol ester on alloantigen presentation. *Journal of Immunology*, 138, 393–400.

Mitchison, N. A. (1971). The carrier effect in the secondary response to hapten-carrier conjugates. I. Measurement of the effect with transferred cells and objections to the local environment hypothesis. *European Journal of Immunology*, 1, 10–17.

Mitchison, N. A. (1985). Four intermediate concentration proteins and their message for self-tolerance, autoimmunity, and suppressor epitopes. *Clinical Immunology Newsletter*, **6**, 12–14.

Mitchison, N. A. & Oliveira, D. B. G. (1986). Epirestriction and a specialised subset of T helper cells are key factors in the regulation of T suppressor cells. In *Progress in Immunology VI. Sixth International Congress of Immunology*, ed. B. Cinader & R. G. Miller, pp. 326–34. London: Academic Press.

Miyazaki, M., Endoh, M., Suga, T. *et al.* (1990). Rheumatoid factors and glomerulonephritis. *Clinical and Experimental Immunology*, **81**, 250–5.

Möller, G. (1988). Do suppressor T cells exist? *Scandinavian Journal of Immunology*, **27**, 247–50.

Morahan, G., Allison, J. & Miller, J. F. A. P. (1989). Tolerance of class I histocompatibility antigens expressed extrathymically. *Nature, London*, **339**, 622–4.

Nagayama, Y., Namura, Y., Tamura, T. & Muso, R. (1988). Beneficial effect of prostaglandin E_1 in three cases of lupus nephritis with nephrotic syndrome. *Annals of Allergy*, **61**, 289–95.

Nakashima, Y., Hirose, S. & Hamashima, Y. (1980). Proliferation of cultured rabbit renal glomerular cells stimulated by platelet factor. *Acta Pathologica Japonica*, **30**, 1–7.

Neale, T. J., Tipping, P. G., Carson, S. D. & Holdsworth, S. R. (1988). Participation of cell-mediated immunity in deposition of fibrin in glomerulonephritis. *Lancet*, **ii**, 421–4.

Newland, A. C., Veys, P. A., Macey, M. G., Gutteridge, C. N., Bussel, S. B. & Cunningham-Rundles, C. (1988). Use of intravenous immunoglobulin in autoimmune haemolytic anaemia. In *Prospective Indications for Intravenous Immunoglobulins*, Medicine Publishing Foundation Symposium Series 24, pp. 3–11. Oxford: The Medicine Group (UK) Ltd.

Noble, B., Steward, M. W., Vladutiu, A. & Brentjens, J. R. (1987). Relationship of the quality and quantity of circulating anti-BSA antibodies to the severity of glomerulonephritis in rats with chronic serum sickness. *Clinical and Experimental Immunology*, **67**, 277–82.

Nolasco, F. E. B., Cameron, J. S., Hartley, B., Coelho, A., Hildreth, G. & Reuben, R. (1987). Intraglomerular T cells and monocytes in nephritis: study with monoclonal antibodies. *Kidney International*, **31**, 1160–6.

Ogawa, S. & Naruse, T. (1982). Effect of various antiplatelet drugs and a defibrinating agent on experimental glomerulonephritis in rats. *Journal of Laboratory and Clinical Medicine*, **99**, 428–41.

Oite, T., Shimizu, F., Kagami, S. & Morioka, T. (1989). Hapten-specific cellular immune response producing glomerular injury. *Clinical and Experimental Immunology*, **76**, 463–8.

Okita, N., Row, V. W. & Volpé, R. (1981). Suppressor T lymphocyte deficiency in Grave's disease and Hashimoto's thyroiditis. *Journal of Clinical Endocrinology and Metabolism*, **52**, 528–33.

Oldstone, M. B. A. (1987). Molecular mimicry and autoimmune disease. *Cell*, **50**, 819–20.

Parham, P. (1988). Intolerable secretion in tolerant transgenic mice. *Nature*, **333**, 500–3.

Penner, E., Albini, B., Andres, G. A. & Milgrom, F. (1979). Dissociation of immune complexes in kidney biopsies by antigen excess. *Federation Proceedings*, **38**, 1412.(Abstract)

Pereira, P., Forni, L., Larsson, E-L., Cooper, M. D., Heusser, C. & Coutinho, A. (1986). Autonomous activation of B and T cells in antigen-free mice. *European Journal of Immunology*, **16**, 685–8.

Poelstra, K., Hardonk, M. J., Koudstaal, J. & Bakker, W. W. (1990). Intraglomerular platelet aggregation and experimental glomerulonephritis. *Kidney International*, **37**, 1500–8.

Pusey, C. D., Venning, M. C. & Peters, D. K. (1988). Immunopathology of glomerular and interstitial disease. In *Diseases of the Kidney*, 4th edn, ed. R. W. Schrier & C. W. Gottschalk, pp. 1827–83. Boston/Toronto: Little, Brown and Company.

Quill, H. & Schwartz, R. H. (1987). Stimulation of normal inducer T cell clones with antigen presented by purified Ia molecules in planar lipid membranes: specific induction of a long-lived state of proliferative nonresponsiveness. *Journal of Immunology*, **138**, 3704–12.

Riehan, A., Wiggins, R. C. & Johnson, K. J. (1984). Hydrogen peroxide induced proteinuria in rats caused by injection of phorbol myristate acetate (PMA) into the renal artery. *Kidney International*, **25**, 217.(Abstract)

Salyer, W. R. & Salyer, D. C. (1974). Unilateral glomerulonephritis. *Journal of Pathology*, **113**, 247–51.

Savage, C. O. S. (1986). Regulation of autoantibody production in man. The role of idiotype–antiidiotype network interactions in anti-glomerular basement membrane antibody mediated disease. University of London: PhD Thesis.

Schneeberger, E. E., Collins, A. B., Stavrakis, G. & McCluskey, R. T. (1980). Diminished mesangial accumulation of intravenously injected soluble immune complexes in rats with autologous immune complex nephritis. *Laboratory Investigation*, **42**, 440–9.

Schreiner, G. F., Cotran, R. S., Pardo, V. & Unanue, E. R. (1978). A mononuclear cell component in experimental immunological glomerulonephritis. *Journal of Experimental Medicine*, **147**, 369–84.

Schrijver, G., Schalkwijk, J., Robben, J. C. M., Assman, K. J. M. & Koene, R. A. P. (1989). Antiglomerular basement membrane nephritis in beige mice. Deficiency of leukocytic neutral proteinases prevents the induction of albuminuria in the heterologous phase. *Journal of Experimental Medicine*, **169**, 1435–48.

Sette, A., Buus, S., Appella, E. *et al.* (1989). Prediction of major histocompatibility complex binding regions of protein antigens by sequence pattern analysis. *Proceedings of the National Academy of Sciences, USA*, **86**, 3296–300.

Shah, S. V. (1989). Role of reactive oxygen metabolites in experimental glomerular disease. *Kidney International*, **35**, 1093–106.

Shinomiya, N., Yata, J. & Sasazuki, T. (1984). T-cell subsets regulating anti-acetylcholine–receptor–antibody formation in myasthenia gravis and characterization of suppressor T-cell factors involved. *Clinical Immunology and Immunopathology*, **33**, 182–90.

Simpson, I. J., Amos, N., Evans, D. J., Thomson, N. M. & Peters, D. K. (1975). Guinea-pig nephrotoxic nephritis. I. The role of complement and polymorphonuclear leucocytes and the effect of antibody subclass and fragments in the heterologous phase. *Clinical and Experimental Immunology*, **19**, 499–511.

Striker, G. E., Mannik, M. & Tung, M. Y. (1979). Role of marrow-derived monocytes and mesangial cells in removal of immune complexes from renal glomeruli. *Journal of Experimental Medicine*, **149**, 127–36.

Sultan, Y., Kazatchkine, M. D., Maisonneuve, P. & Nydegger, U. E. (1984). Anti-idiotypic suppression of autoantibodies to factor VIII (anti-haemophilic factor) by high dose intravenous gammaglobulin. *Lancet*, **ii**, 765–8.

Sultan, Y., Rossi, F. & Kazatchkine, M. D. (1987). Recovery from anti-VII:c (anti-haemophilic factor) autoimmune disease is dependent on generation of anti-idiotypes against anti-VIII:c autoantibodies. *Proceedings of the National Academy of Sciences, USA*, **84**, 828–31.

Svejgaard, A., Platz, P. & Ryder, L. P. (1983). HLA and disease 1982 – a survey. *Immunological Reviews*, **70**, 193–218.

Thomson, N. M., Naish, P. F., Simpson, I. J. & Peters, D. K. (1976). The role of C3 in the autologous phase of nephrotoxic nephritis. *Clinical and Experimental Immunology*, **24**, 464–73.

Tipping, P. G., Lowe, M. G. & Holdsworth, S. R. (1988). Glomerular macrophages express augmented procoagulant activity in experimental fibrin-related glomerulonephritis in rabbits. *Journal of Clinical Investigation*, **82**, 1253–9.

Tomosugi, N. I., Cashman, S. J., Hay, H. *et al.* (1989). Modulation of antibody-mediated glomerular injury *in vivo* by bacterial lipopolysaccharide, tumour necrosis factor, and IL-1. *Journal of Immunology*, **142**, 3083–90.

Topliss, D., How, J., Lewis, M., Row, V. & Volpé, R. (1983). Evidence for cell-mediated immunity and specific suppressor T lymphocytes in Grave's disease and diabetes mellitus. *Journal of Clinical Endocrinology and Metabolism*, **57**, 700–5.

Toyonaga, B. & Mak, T. W. (1987). Genes of the T-cell antigen receptor in normal and malignant T cells. *Annual Review of Immunology*, **5**, 585–620.

Vakil, M. & Kearney, J. F. (1986). Functional characteristics of monoclonal auto-anti-idiotype antibodies isolated from the early B cell repertoire of BALB/c mice. *European Journal of Immunology*, **16**, 1151–8.

Vento, S., O'Brien, C. J., McFarlane, I. G., Williams, R. & Eddleston, A. L. W. F. (1987). T-cell inducers of suppressor lymphocytes control liver-directed autoreactivity. *Lancet*, **i**, 886–8.

Veys, P. A., Macey, M. G., Gutteridge, C. N. & Newland, A. C. (1988). Autoimmune neutropenia and intravenous immunoglobulin. In *Prospective indications for intravenous immunoglobulins*, Medicine Publishing Foundation Symposium Series 24, pp. 13–18. Oxford: The Medicine Group (UK) Ltd.

Vincent, A. C. (1988). Are spontaneous anti-idiotypic antibodies against anti-acetylcholine receptor antibodies present in myasthenia gravis? *Journal of Autoimmunity*, **1**, 131–42.

Volpé, R. (1988). Hypothesis: the immunoregulatory disturbance in autoimmune thyroid disease. *Autoimmunity*, **2**, 55–72.

Ward, D. M. & Wilson, C. B. (1977). Mesangial function during chronic serum sickness (CSS) glomerulonephritis (GN). *Federation Proceedings*, **36**, 1055.(Abstract)

Ward, P. A., Duque, R. E., Sulavik, M. C. & Johnson, K. J. (1983). *In vitro* and *in vivo* stimulation of rat neutrophils and alveolar macrophages by immune complexes. *American Journal of Pathology*, **110**, 297–309.

Weber, M., Pullig, O. & Boesken, W. H. (1990). Anti-glomerular basement membrane disease after renal obstruction (letter). *Lancet*, **336**, 512–13.

Werb, Z., Bainton, D. F. & Jones, P. A. (1980). Degradation of connective tissue matrices by macrophages. III. Morphological and biochemical studies on extracellular, pericellular, and intracellular events in matrix proteolysis by macrophages in culture. *Journal of Experimental Medicine*, **152**, 1537–53.

Wick, G. (1987). Concept of a multigenic basis for the pathogenesis of spontaneous auto-immune thyroiditis. *Acta Endocrinologia*, **115** (suppl. 281), 63–9.

Wilson, C. B. & Dixon, F. J. (1971). Quantitation of acute and chronic serum sickness in the rabbit. *Journal of Experimental Medicine*, **134**, 7s–18s.

Wilson, C. B. & Dixon, F. J. (1986). The renal response to immunological injury. In *The Kidney*, 3rd edn, ed. B. M. Brenner & F. C. Rector, pp. 800–89. Philadelphia: W.B.Saunders Company.

Wright, P. (1982). The eye. In *Clinical Aspects of Immunology*, 4th edn, ed. P. J. Lachmann & D. K. Peters, pp. 1151–8. Oxford: Blackwell Scientific Publications.

Zabriskie, J. B. (1982). Streptococcal diseases and their relationship to antigenic mimicry in the group A streptococcus. In *Clinical Aspects of Immunology*, 4th edn, ed. P. J. Lachmann & D. K. Peters, pp. 1428–44. Oxford: Blackwell Scientific Publications.

Zanetti, M. & Wilson, C. B. (1983). Participation of auto-anti-idiotypes in immune complex glomerulonephritis in rabbits. *Journal of Immunology*, **131**, 2781–3.

–2–
Anti-glomerular basement membrane disease

Anti-glomerular basement membrane (GBM) disease is of considerable interest, as it has perhaps the best understood immunopathology of all human autoimmune renal disease. It is, however, rare, occurring with an incidence of approximately 0.5 per million per annum (Rees & Lockwood, 1988) and accounting for about 2% of renal biopsy series (Beirne *et al.*, 1977) and 2% of end stage renal failure (Disney, 1986). The disease usually presents as a rapidly progressive glomerulonephritis, often in association with pulmonary haemorrhage. This combination is known as Goodpasture's syndrome, and anti-GBM disease is a major cause (but not the only one; see Chapter 8) of this syndrome. Anti-GBM disease is distinguished by the presence of an autoantibody to GBM, both in the circulation and bound in linear fashion along the GBM.

The renal histology may show only a mild focal proliferative nephritis, but more usually there is severe glomerular inflammation with crescent formation and necrosis, often with interstitial inflammation. These appearances are not specific for anti-GBM disease but the findings on indirect immunofluorescence are very characteristic. There is bright linear staining along the GBM, in almost all cases for IgG, and in about two-thirds of cases for C3. These are occasionally accompanied by IgA and IgM, and very rarely these immunoglobulins may be the only ones found (Savage *et al.*, 1986a). There is usually similar staining of the distal tubule basement membrane. This typical pattern may not be so obvious in advanced cases associated with considerable disruption and distortion of the GBM. Occasional confusion may also result from the occurrence of linear fluorescence along the GBM in conditions such as SLE and diabetes (Wilson & Dixon, 1974). Electron microscopy may reveal discontinuities in the GBM. Electron dense deposits are usually absent, but may occasionally be visible within, or adjacent to, the GBM (Rees & Lockwood, 1988).

Immunogenetics

The MHC

The association between anti-GBM disease and the MHC was the first such association described for a renal disease (Rees *et al.*, 1978), and remains one of the strongest. The initial report found that DR2 was present in 88% of patients in whom DR status could be determined, compared with 32% in a control population. Extension of the series confirmed the frequency of DR2 and gave a relative risk of 36 and an aetiological fraction of 0.86 associated with this allele (Rees *et al.*, 1984). A very similar frequency of DR2 was noted in a series from Australia (Perl *et al.*, 1981), whereas American data found a frequency of 50% (Garovoy, 1982). Although this decreased frequency probably partly reflects a more heterogeneous study population, it may well be that the initial estimates were unduly high. Thus the most recent analysis of MHC class II alleles from the United Kingdom showed a frequency of 69% for DR2 in patients versus 30% in controls (relative risk 4.9, aetiological fraction 0.55; A.J.Rees, personal communication, and in abstract: Burns *et al.*, 1990). There was also a significant association with DR4 (60% versus 37%, relative risk 2.55, aetiological fraction 0.36).

The only class I allele that has been found associated with anti-GBM disease is B7 (Rees *et al.*, 1984). Although B7 is in linkage disequilibrium with DR2, linkage analysis demonstrated that the increased frequency of B7 in patients was greater than could be accounted for by an effect purely secondary to the increased frequency of DR2. Furthermore, categorisation of patients into three groups by severity of disease demonstrated that the 'excess' linkage with B7 (over and above that due to linkage disequilibrium with DR2) was most significant for the most severely affected group, and not at all significant for the least affected group. This type of subgroup analysis must be treated with some caution, but the magnitude of the effect in the most severely affected group, and the consistent relationship between significance and severity, provide strong support for the reality of the phenomenon.

Other loci

An association has been shown with Gm allotypes (Rees, Demaine & Welsh, 1984). This was found both in the form of an increased incidence of the haplotype Gm 1,2,21 (54% in patients versus 17% in controls; relative risk 5.75), and as an increased titre of anti-GBM antibodies in patients heterozygous at the Gm complex.

The genetic contribution to the aetiology of anti-GBM disease is emphasised by the number of reports of concordance in close relatives, and in particular in two sets of identical twins (d'Apice *et al.*, 1978; Simonsen *et al.*, 1982). However, there are at least as many reported examples of identical twins discordant for the disease (Almkuist *et al.*, 1981). The rarity of anti-GBM disease precludes any precise calculation of concordance rate, but these reports allow some comparison with insulin dependent diabetes mellitus (IDDM). In this disease, a concordance rate of 50% in identical twins reflects a probable genetic contribution of 5–40% to the aetiology (Diabetes Epidemiology Research International, 1987).

Immunopathology

Animal studies

Animal models relevant to anti-GBM disease can be considered in three groups. In the first group (nephrotoxic nephritis, Masugi nephritis), disease is produced by the injection of heterologous anti-GBM antibodies. This leads to a biphasic disease, in which the initial pathology caused by the heterologous antibodies is followed by an autologous immune response to the foreign immunoglobulin, now acting as a planted antigen on the GBM. The second group, typified by Steblay nephritis, involves the induction of an autoimmune response to the GBM by immunisation with heterologous or homologous GBM. The final group represents the spontaneous occurrence of anti-GBM antibodies, or their induction by relatively non-specific stimuli such as polyclonal activation.

Nephrotoxic nephritis

Studies of models in the first group give no insight into the causation of spontaneous anti-GBM disease, but have been very informative with respect to the pathogenicity of anti-GBM antibodies. A major factor in such pathogenicity is the amount of antibody deposited (Unanue & Dixon, 1965). Below a certain threshold, which is species dependent, antibody binds to the GBM but does not result in injury. Above this threshold there is a steep dose-dependent increase in damage. Other relevant variables include the rate at which antibody is deposited (van Zyl Smit, Rees & Peters, 1983), the class and subclass of the antibody and thus its ability to fix complement (Unanue & Dixon, 1964), and the affinity of the antibodies (Unanue, Dixon & Lees, 1966), with rapid deposition of high affinity, complement-fixing antibodies being the most damaging. The binding of antibody on its own can cause heavy proteinuria, as exemplified by nephrotoxic nephritis in the guinea-pig (Simpson *et al.*, 1975). However, in most models, the major acute injury in the heterologous phase is due to fixation of complement (Tipping, Boyce & Holdsworth, 1989), attraction of polymorphs, and subsequent proteolytic damage (Schrijver *et al.*, 1989). The release of reactive oxygen species by the polymorphs is also probably an important pathogenetic mechanism (Johnson, Klebanoff & Couser, 1988). The importance of polymorphs, at least in mouse nephrotoxic nephritis, is demonstrated by the fact that injury in this model is independent of complement (Schrijver *et al.*, 1990). This dependence on factors other than simple binding of anti-GBM antibodies is illustrated by the exacerbation of injury in rabbits with a constant amount of bound antibody by intercurrent infection (Rees, Amos & Peters, 1981) or the administration of inflammatory cytokines (Tomosugi *et al.*, 1989). Other elements of the cellular immune system are also important. The presence of pre-sensitized lymphocytes exacerbates the effects of antibody (Bhan *et al.*, 1978), and T cells can be observed accumulating in the glomeruli (Tipping, Neale & Holdsworth, 1985). Later in the course of the disease, during the autologous phase, macrophages appear and make a major contribution to crescent formation, probably secondary to the deposition of fibrin in Bowman's space (Thomson *et al.*, 1976); further aspects of crescent formation are considered in Chapter 8. Evidence for the pathogenetic importance of T cells and macrophages is provided by the beneficial effect of therapy directed at these cells (Tipping, Neale & Holdsworth, 1985; Holdsworth, Neale & Wilson, 1981).

The antigens recognised by the anti-GBM antibodies in these models are diverse (Neale & Wilson, 1982), and it is unclear whether there is any relationship with the antigen recognised by human anti-GBM antibodies. One study showed that rabbit anti-human GBM antibodies bound to a separate part of the GBM as compared to human anti-GBM antibodies (Fish, Carmody & Michael, 1979); antibodies eluted from the immunised rabbit's kidneys, however, showed the same binding pattern as the human antibodies.

Although pulmonary haemorrhage has been noted in a number of models of nephrotoxic nephritis, much less is known of the factors involved in the pathogenesis of this aspect. At least in the mouse, the antibodies do not normally have access to the alveolar basement membrane, and accessory factors in the form of cytokines are required to increase permeability, to allow binding and subsequent production of pulmonary haemorrhage (Queluz *et al.*, 1990).

Induced autoimmune anti-GBM disease

The second group of models involves the induction of an autoimmune response to the GBM and is thus potentially more informative with respect to the breakdown in tolerance that must underlie human anti-GBM disease.

The classical model is Steblay nephritis, a proliferative, crescentic glomeru-lonephritis of sheep induced by immunisation with heterologous or homolo-gous but, importantly, not autologous GBM in complete Freund's adjuvant (Steblay & Rudofsky, 1983). The pathogenicity of the resulting antibodies is clearly demonstrated by cross-circulation and serum transfer experiments. There is evidence that a proportion of these antibodies do recognise the same epitope as human anti-GBM antibodies (Jeraj, Michael & Fish, 1982). A similar disease with probably the same pathogenesis as Steblay nephritis can be induced in a number of species (Pusey, Venning & Peters, 1988). In some strains of rat it is possible to induce anti-GBM antibodies by immunisa-tion with isologous (Sado & Naito, 1987) or autologous GBM (Pusey et al., 1984). The pathogenetic processes following the binding of autologous anti-GBM antibodies are likely to be much the same as those operating in nephrotoxic nephritis, although, in at least one model, polymorphs do not seem to be involved (Naito & Sado, 1989).

One interesting exception to the general pathogenetic mechanism is the nephritis induced in chickens by immunisation with heterologous or hom-ologous GBM. This is clearly a T cell-mediated disease: such cells trans-ferred alone result in nephritis, whereas transferred antibody, although it binds to the GBM, does not (Bolton et al., 1988). This model is perhaps more relevant to human glomerulonephritides which are not associated with antibody deposition within the glomerulus (see Chapter 8).

Anti-GBM disease without specific immunisation

Models in the third group represent the development of autoantibodies without deliberate immunisation with GBM, and therefore are potentially the most relevant with respect to the human disease. Unfortunately, the degree of this relevance is far from clear. Spontaneous occurrence of anti-GBM antibodies has been documented in a few species in addition to man. One study of horses found linear immunoglobulin staining of the GBM in three out of 53 animals examined; anti-GBM antibody could be eluted from one of these (Banks & Henson, 1972). However, by light microscopy, two of the kidneys showed normal glomeruli and there were only minimal changes in the third. These antibodies therefore did not appear to be pathogenic. Anti-GBM antibodies have apparently been eluted from the kidneys of certain mouse strains (Wilson & Dixon, 1986), and linear immunofluor-escence on the GBM has been noted in some dogs, although no antibodies could be eluted (Center et al., 1987).

Anti-GBM antibodies are induced by mercuric chloride ($HgCl_2$) treat-ment in Brown Norway rats. This model, introduced by Druet (Sapin, Druet & Druet, 1977), has been extensively studied. $HgCl_2$ acts as a T cell-dependent polyclonal B cell activator and, in addition to anti-GBM antibodies, a wide range of other autoantibodies are produced. There is also a marked increase in total serum IgE concentration. All of these phenomena are self-limiting and return to baseline levels within 4–5 weeks of the start of $HgCl_2$ treatment. Thereafter, the animals are relatively resistant to further challenges with $HgCl_2$. The anti-GBM antibodies are poorly nephrotoxic, resulting in proteinuria but no nephritis or renal impairment. Although the majority of circulating anti-GBM antibodies in this model have anti-laminin specificity (Guéry et al., 1990), there is some evidence that a proportion (those that can be eluted from the kidney) recognise the same GBM components as human anti-GBM antibodies (Makker & Kanalas, 1990). Following the linear deposition of antibody along the GBM in the initial phases, there is a subsequent redistribution and the histological picture comes to resemble membranous nephropathy (see Chapter 3). Of the three phases of this model, the initiation phase is associated with the development of T cells with anti-self MHC activity (Rossert et al., 1988); these are presumably capable of stimulating practically any B cell. The ability to produce these autoantibodies is under genetic control, with the MHC being one of the approximately four loci involved (Sapin et al., 1984). The resistance phase appears to be due to the presence of CD8$^+$ cells that can transfer suppression of anti-GBM antibody production (Bowman et al., 1984). These cells apparently do not mediate the spontaneous resolution of autoantibody production (Pelletier et al., 1990), and the factors involved in this phase remain unclear. Antiidiotypic antibodies are present (Guéry & Druet, 1990) and there is some indirect evidence that they may be involved in immunoregulation (Chalopin & Lockwood, 1984). Alternatively, as in the analogous model of experimental allergic encephalomyelitis (MacPhee, Antoni & Mason, 1989), increased adrenal steroid production may play a role.

Human studies

The similarities in renal immunofluorescent patterns between experimental nephrotoxic nephritis and the nephritis occurring in man in association with pulmonary haemorrhage were noted in 1964 (Scheer & Grossman, 1964). Subsequently, a key experiment demonstrated that antibody eluted from such a human kidney and transferred to squirrel monkeys produced similar linear staining of the GBM and nephritis (Lerner, Glassock & Dixon, 1967). The information now available on this autoantibody will be considered under the broad headings of initiation of antibody production, properties of the antibody, and possible regulation of antibody production.

Initiation of anti-GBM antibody production

The environmental factors that act on genetically predisposed individuals to initiate anti-GBM antibody production are largely unknown. There are numerous reports of respiratory infections or exposure to hydrocarbon fumes preceding the development of anti-GBM disease, and analysis of the latter association in particular suggests that this is not due to chance (Daniell, Couser & Rosenstock, 1988). A major problem in interpreting these observations arises from the fact that low levels of anti-GBM antibody may be present in the absence of clinical manifestations. As intercurrent infection is known to exacerbate renal injury in experimental nephrotoxic nephritis (see above), and a respiratory tract insult in the form of smoking is known to trigger pulmonary haemorrhage in human anti-GBM disease (Donaghy & Rees, 1983), these putative environmental factors could simply be acting to allow expression of disease, without playing a more fundamental role in pathogenesis. However, the postulated mechanism, lung damage leading to the release of alveolar basement membrane and the initiation of an autoimmune response cross-reacting with the GBM (see below), is plausible. A similar process may explain the development of anti-GBM disease on the background of other forms of renal damage, such as membranous nephropathy (Coggins, 1988), in which there is considerable distortion and disruption of the GBM in advanced cases (see Chapter 3). There are also single case reports of the disease developing after traumatic cortical necrosis (Hume et al., 1970), renal obstruction (Weber, Pullig & Boesken, 1990), and extracorporeal shock-wave lithotripsy, which is known to cause the release of some renal antigens into the circulation (Guerin et al., 1990). Perhaps the clearest example of a precipitating factor is provided by renal transplantation in Alport's syndrome. This is an X-linked hereditary nephritis associated with deafness (Flinter et al., 1988) characterised, on electron microscopy, by thickening and splitting of the GBM. Anti-GBM antibodies do not bind to the GBM in cases of Alport's syndrome (McCoy et al., 1976), a finding subsequently confirmed using a monoclonal antibody that shares the same specificity (Savage et al., 1986c). It seems likely that patients with this syndrome lack, or have a modified version of (Savage et al., 1989), the epitope recognised by anti-GBM antibodies and, as a result, do not develop self-tolerance to this epitope. It is therefore perhaps not surprising that a significant proportion of such patients develop anti-GBM antibodies (although not necessarily nephritis) when transplanted with a normal kidney that does display the epitope (Savige, Mavrova & Kincaid-Smith, 1989; Goldman et al., 1990). Although in the case of Alport's syndrome this is not strictly an autoimmune response, patients with spontaneous anti-GBM disease will occasionally experience a similar triggering of antibody production following transplantation, presumably due to fresh exposure to antigen (Almkuist *et al.*, 1981; Beleil *et al.*, 1973).

Properties of anti-GBM antibodies

In contrast to our ignorance concerning the production of anti-GBM antibodies, there is considerable data available on the properties of such antibodies once formed. As mentioned above, these are nearly always IgG and, furthermore, mainly restricted to the IgG_1 and IgG_4 subclasses (Bowman, Ambrus & Lockwood, 1987). This is probably relevant to their pathogenicity as IgG_1 antibodies can fix complement and bind to macrophages. This point is illustrated by the two recurrences in a series of 49 patients (Bowman, Ambrus & Lockwood, 1987). One of these was as an IgG_1 antibody and was associated with nephritis, whereas the other was as an IgG_4 antibody and was not. Further evidence of the pathogenicity of the antibody is provided by the transfer experiment mentioned above, the recurrence in transplants if performed while antibody is still present (Briggs *et al.*, 1979), the almost complete association between the antibody and the disease, and the correlation between titre of antibody and severity of nephritis (Savage *et al.*, 1986a). As with certain of the animal models, it is known that intercurrent infection can exacerbate target organ damage (kidney, lung) without a change in antibody titre (Rees, Lockwood & Peters, 1977). In addition to the environmental factors that might be involved in the precipitation of pulmonary haemorrhage, variations in the pattern of reactivity of anti-GBM sera with the alveolar basement membrane (ABM), and differences between individuals in the composition of the ABM, may also be important (Yoshioka *et al.*, 1988).

The precise nature of the antigen recognised by anti-GBM antibodies (the Goodpasture antigen) is still unclear. The fact that a mouse monoclonal antibody raised against human GBM will inhibit the binding of most, if not all, anti-GBM antibodies (Pusey *et al.*, 1987) demonstrates that these antibodies recognise a very restricted epitope. There is general agreement that this epitope resides on the noncollagenous-1 (NC-1) domain of type IV collagen (Rees & Lockwood, 1988). Although type IV collagen is found in all basement membranes, and there is some evidence that the Goodpasture antigen may be similarly distributed (Weber, Pullig & Köhler, 1990), anti-GBM antibodies only bind with high affinity to the GBM, the alveolar basement membrane, and certain other basement membranes in the eye, ear, choroid plexus and endocrine organs (Cashman, Pusey & Evans, 1988). One possible explanation is that the ubiquitous type IV collagen, consisting of two α1 and one α2 chains, is supplemented by, or enriched for, additional types of chain in specialised locations such as the GBM. Two such candidate chains have been reported. One, the α3 chain, does appear to possess the necessary restricted distribution. This chain has been isolated from bovine (Saus et al., 1988) and, probably, human material (Butkowski et al., 1990) and only a partial protein sequence is available at the moment. However, the gene for the other chain, termed $\alpha5$, has been partially cloned and sequenced (Hostikka et al., 1990). The gene maps to the X chromosome, and there is now convincing evidence that mutations in this gene are the cause of some, if not all, cases of Alport's syndrome (Barker et al., 1990).

Immunoregulation of anti-GBM antibodies

The evidence for spontaneous immunoregulation of anti-GBM antibody production in man is entirely indirect. The possibility is suggested by the spontaneous disappearance of the antibody in the absence of treatment, usually within one to two years, and by the rarity of recurrence following transplantation if this is performed once the antibody has disappeared (Dahlberg et al., 1978). Furthermore, recurrences of antibody production, although well documented in some cases (Dahlberg et al., 1978), are rare (Bowman, Ambrus & Lockwood, 1987). These features are somewhat unusual, as autoimmune diseases in which there is persistence of the autoantigen tend to be characterised by a long-term course with many relapses and remissions. Analogies with the self-limiting production of anti-GBM antibodies in the Brown Norway rat model (see above) have prompted a search for evidence of similar immunoregulatory mechanisms in man. At least with respect to the presence of antiidiotypic antibodies, these investigations have proved negative (Savage, 1986b). There do not appear to have been any studies of defects of GBM-specific suppression, and its re-establishment as a possible mechanism for the regulation of autoantibody synthesis.

Cellular immunity in anti-GBM disease

Although studies on human anti-GBM disease have concentrated on the autoantibody there is some information available on the contribution of the cellular compartment. Assessment of intra-glomerular macrophages and T cells has shown that these are most prominent in anti-GBM disease as compared to other proliferative nephritides (Bolton et al., 1987), and that this is the only condition with a significant increase of CD4[+] T cells (Nolasco et al., 1987). This non-specific observation is supplemented by a number of studies that have examined specific reactivity of T cells against GBM extracts (for review see Fillit & Zabriskie, 1982). In general, T cells from most patients with anti-GBM disease do show such reactivity, usually as assessed by a migration inhibition factor production assay. Interpretation is complicated by the occurrence of similar reactivity in patients with acute tubular necrosis (Macanovic, Evans & Peters, 1972), renal cortical necrosis (Mahieu, Dardenne & Bach, 1972), and other forms of glomerulonephritis, raising the possibility that it is simply a reflection of an immune response to antigens released by renal damage and not of more fundamental importance in initiation of disease.

Anti-GBM disease and anti-neutrophil cytoplasm antibodies (ANCA)

Recently, a subgroup of patients with anti-GBM antibodies who also have anti-neutrophil cytoplasm antibodies (ANCA; see Chapter 8) has been recognised (Jayne et al., 1990). Some of these patients appear to have an ANCA-positive systemic vasculitis as their primary illness; the anti-GBM antibodies may not be directed against the classical Goodpasture antigen (Bygren et al., 1989), but against other GBM components such as entactin (Saxena et al., 1990), and could perhaps reflect an immune response directed against antigens released from damaged glomeruli. Other patients, however, clearly have classical anti-GBM disease. At present, the contribution, if any, of ANCA to pathogenesis in this latter group is unclear, but there are hints that patients of this type may respond to intensive treatment even if dialysis dependent (Jayne et al., 1990).

Therapeutic aspects

The evidence for the pathogenicity of anti-GBM antibodies in man and the ability to measure these conveniently with a radioimmunoassay (Mahieu, Lambert & Miescher, 1974; Bowman & Lockwood, 1985), provide a logical basis for the approach to therapy and a means of monitoring the efficacy of such treatment. This is a unique situation in renal autoimmunity. Current treatment strategies consist of measures to reduce tissue inflammation and damage (corticosteroids) combined with inhibition of autoantibody synthesis (cytotoxic drugs) and rapid removal of the autoantibody, usually by plasma exchange. The rationale for the addition of plasma exchange rests on the considerable delay that would result if cytotoxic therapy alone was used to suppress anti-GBM antibody production.

Comparison with historical controls suggests that this approach, and, in particular, plasma exchange, has greatly improved the prognosis of the disease (Rees & Lockwood, 1988). However, there are well-known problems in the use of historical controls, and the one controlled trial of plasma exchange reported is therefore of particular interest (Johnson et al., 1985). This did indeed demonstrate a quicker disappearance of autoantibody in the group receiving plasma exchange in addition to steroids and cytotoxic therapy as compared to the group given drugs alone. The plasma exchange group also did better with respect to recovery of renal function. The problem with interpreting these results arises from the small numbers involved, a consequence of the rarity of the disease. In particular, despite randomisation, the groups were not well matched for the major prognostic variable (Savage *et al.*, 1986*a*), namely severity of renal damage at presentation; once patients have become anuric or dialysis dependent then recovery is very rare even with intensive treatment. The plasma exchange group happened to contain a greater proportion of patients with milder disease, and indeed the severity of renal damage at presentation correlated better with outcome than did the treatment regime. Another prospective study of plasma exchange also involved small numbers, but again suggested a possible additional benefit of plasma exchange (Simpson *et al.*, 1982).

Despite these reservations the historical data and knowledge of immunopathogenesis provide a strong case for rapid autoantibody removal, and there is uncontrolled data demonstrating immediate improvement in renal function in the majority of patients with the start of plasma exchange (Rees & Lockwood, 1988). The difficulties in performing a controlled trial mean that this is unlikely to be formally tested again. The regime outlined at the beginning of this section, or variants, will therefore remain the standard therapy, at least for patients with pulmonary haemorrhage or who are not dialysis-dependent at presentation. Future modifications may involve more selective removal of autoantibody, as has been achieved, for instance, with the use of a protein A column to remove only IgG (Bygren *et al.*, 1985).

Concluding remarks

This chapter began with the comment that anti-GBM disease had the best understood immunopathogenesis of human autoimmune renal disease. Although true, this understanding applies principally to the events following the production of the autoantibody. The data from animal models allow a good understanding of the pathogenetic processes that result from the binding of the antibody to the GBM. There are a number of details that are still uncertain, such as the contribution, if any, of effector T cells to glomerular damage, but the main elements seem reasonably clear. By contrast, there is very little understanding of the factors involved in initiation and regulation of autoantibody production.

The one situation in which initiation of anti-GBM antibody production is probably understood is following transplantation for Alport's syndrome. Such patients, lacking the Goodpasture antigen, are presumably not tolerant to it and there is no reason why they should not mount an immune response. Furthermore, antibodies in a range of species (sheep, Brown

Norway rat) appear to recognise a similar epitope, suggesting that it is particularly immunogenic; perhaps without the post-transplant immunosuppression, many more Alport's patients would develop anti-GBM antibodies.

Spontaneous anti-GBM disease is analogous to animal models employing immunisation with autologous GBM. Immunisation with an autologous antigen very rarely results in autoantibody production. Similarly in man, only rare genetically predisposed individuals can experience a breakdown in tolerance to GBM. Quite how the known genetic associations are linked to this breakdown is a matter of speculation, but they may well relate to the T cell compartment. The presence of an autoreactive T cell can be inferred from the MHC associations and the nature of the autoantibody response, which has the characteristics of a T cell-dependent response (IgG, high affinity, memory). The DR2 (and possibly DR4) molecule may be particularly efficient at binding and presenting the (unknown) T cell epitope to this autoreactive T cell. Another (and not mutually exclusive) possibility is that the DR2 molecule, via the process of positive selection during thymic ontogeny, shapes the T cell repertoire in such a way that an autoreactive response against the GBM is possible. DR2 negative individuals therefore do not have T cells that possess receptors with the necessary specificity for mounting such a response. The B8 association may reflect the involvement of an MHC class I-restricted cytotoxic T cell in mediating glomerular injury once tolerance has been broken.

The initiation of an autoantibody response to such a restricted (possibly single) epitope is also interesting. Tolerance is probably less complete in the B cell compartment as compared to the T cell compartment (Mackay, 1983). This implies that there might be a number of different B cell clones, recognising different epitopes on a structure, that could be helped by a single autoreactive T cell recognising the same structure. Certainly in other autoimmune diseases, autoantibodies are produced that recognise multiple epitopes on an autoantigen (Doble *et al.*, 1988). The fact that this does not occur in anti-GBM disease may be due to a degree of tolerance in the B cell compartment. Another possibility is that the epitope recognised on the Goodpasture antigen is immunodominant: antibodies to this epitope are of such high affinity that B cells secreting such antibodies successfully compete with other B cell clones recognising the same antigen, sequestering the antigen and preventing presentation by these other clones. Whatever the explanation, the restricted autoantibody repertoire may have therapeutic implications (see below).

The role of immunoregulation in the control of human anti-GBM antibodies is similarly speculative. The evidence for this is indirect and weak; the one attempt to find direct evidence for antiidiotypic antibodies was unsuccessful. Immunoregulation undoubtedly occurs in the $HgCl_2$-induced anti-

GBM antibody model in the Brown Norway rat, but this may bear little relationship to the human disease. Although there are similarities, such as the immunogenetic control (including a major contribution from the MHC) and the probable identity of some GBM components recognised by antibodies from rat and man, there are also important differences. The polyclonal activation produced by $HgCl_2$, and the resulting array of autoantibodies, are not features of human anti-GBM disease. This reflects a fundamental difference in initiation of antibody production, with the generation of self MHC-reactive T cells capable of activating a wide range of B cells in the rat compared to a much more discrete breakdown in tolerance to the NC-1 domain of GBM type IV collagen in man. It would be somewhat surprising if such different processes shared much similarity in their regulation.

The attraction of attempting to identify immunoregulation of human anti-GBM antibodies is that it may be possible to exploit it for therapeutic purposes. In some experimental systems it is possible to induce specific suppression to a particular autoantigen (see Chapter 9); a disease already subject to a degree of endogenous regulation may be particularly susceptible to this approach. Availability of the autoantigen in large quantities would also allow the construction of specific affinity columns for extracorporeal immunoadsorption. It may be possible to circumvent difficulties in obtaining the necessary amounts of antigen by exploiting the limited heterogeneity of the autoantibody. A suitable monoclonal antiidiotypic antibody might therefore be an efficient immunoadsorbent, and would be much easier to produce in bulk.

References

Almkuist, R. D., Buckalew, V. M. Jr., Hirszel, P., Maher, J. F., James, P. M. & Wilson, C. B. (1981). Recurrence of anti-glomerular basement membrane antibody mediated glomerulonephritis in an isograft. *Clinical Immunology and Immunopathology*, **18**, 54–60.

Banks, K. L. & Henson, J. B. (1972). Immunologically mediated glomerulonephritis of horses. II. Antiglomerular basement membrane antibody and other mechanisms in spontaneous disease. *Laboratory Investigation*, **26**, 708–15.

Barker, D. F., Hostikka, S. L., Zhou, J. *et al.* (1990). Identification of mutations in the COL4A5 collagen gene in Alport syndrome. *Science*, **248**, 1224–7.

Beirne, G. J., Wagnild, J. P., Zimmerman, S. W., Macken, P. D. & Burkholder, P. M. (1977). Idiopathic crescentic glomerulonephritis. *Medicine*, **56**, 349–81.

Beleil, O. M., Coburn, J. W., Shinaberger, J. H. & Glassock, R. J. (1973). Recurrent glomerulonephritis due to anti-glomerular basement membrane antibodies in two successive allografts. *Clinical Nephrology*, **1**, 377–80.

Bhan, A. K., Schneeberger, E. E., Collins, A. B. & McClusky, R. T. (1978). Evidence for a pathogenic role of a cell-mediated immune mechanism in experimental glomerulonephritis. *Journal of Experimental Medicine*, **148**, 246–60.

Bolton, W. K., Innes, D. J., Sturgill, B. C. & Kaiser, D. L. (1987). T-cells and macrophages in rapidly progressive glomerulonephritis: clinicopathologic correlations. *Kidney International*, **32**, 869–76.

Bolton, W. K., Chandra, M., Tyson, T. M., Kirkpatrick, P. R., Sadovnic, M. J. & Sturgill, B. C. (1988). Transfer of experimental glomerulonephritis in chickens by mononuclear cells. *Kidney International*, **34**, 598–610.

Bowman, C. & Lockwood, C. M. (1985). Clinical application of a radio-immunoassay for auto-antibodies to glomerular basement membrane. *Journal of Clinical and Laboratory Immunology*, **17**, 197–202.

Bowman, C., Mason, D. W., Pusey, C. D. & Lockwood, C. M. (1984). Autoregulation of autoantibody synthesis in mercuric chloride nephritis in the Brown Norway rat. I. A role for T suppressor cells. *European Journal of Immunology*, **14**, 464–70.

Bowman, C., Ambrus, K. & Lockwood, C. M. (1987). Restriction of human IgG subclass expression in the population of auto-antibodies to glomerular basement membrane. *Clinical and Experimental Immunology*, **69**, 341–9.

Briggs, W. A., Johnson, J. P., Teichman, S., Yeager, H. C. & Wilson, C. B. (1979). Antiglomerular basement membrane antibody-mediated glomerulonephritis and Goodpasture's syndrome. *Medicine*, **58**, 348–61.

Burns, A., So, A., Pusey, C. D. & Rees, A. J. (1990). The susceptibility to Goodpasture's syndrome. *Quarterly Journal of Medicine*, **77**, 1094–5.(Abstract).

Butkowski, R. J., Shen, G-Q., Wieslander, J., Michael, A. F. & Fish, A. J. (1990). Characterization of type IV collagen NC1 monomers and Goodpasture antigen in human renal basement membranes. *Journal of Laboratory and Clinical Medicine*, **115**, 365–73.

Bygren, P., Freiburghaus, C., Lindholm, T., Simonsen, O., Thysell, H. & Wieslander, J. (1985). Goodpasture's syndrome treated with staphylococcal protein A immunoadsorption. *Lancet*, **ii**, 1295–6.

Bygren, P., Cederholm, B., Heinegard, D. & Wieslander, J. (1989). Non-Goodpasture anti-GBM antibodies in patients with glomerulonephritis. *Nephrology Dialysis and Transplantation*, **4**, 254–61.

Cashman, S. J., Pusey, C. D. & Evans, D. J. (1988). Extraglomerular distribution of immunoreactive Goodpasture antigen. *Journal of Pathology*, **155**, 61–70.

Center, S. A., Smith, C. A., Wilkinson, E., Erb, H. N. & Lewis, R. M. (1987). Clinicopathologic, renal immunofluorescent, and light microscopic features of glomerulonephritis in the dog: 41 cases (1975–1985). *Journal of the American Veterinary Medical Association*, **190**, 81–90.

Chalopin, J. M. & Lockwood, C. M. (1984). Autoregulation of autoantibody synthesis in mercuric chloride nephritis in the Brown Norway rat. II. Presence of antigen-augmentable plaque-forming cells in the spleen is associated with humoral factors behaving as auto-anti-idiotypic antibodies. *European Journal of Immunology*, **14**, 470–5.

Coggins, C. H. (1988). Membranous nephropathy. In *Diseases of the Kidney*, 4th edn, ed. R. W. Schrier & C. W. Gottschalk, pp. 2005–33. Boston/Toronto: Little, Brown and Company.

d'Apice, A. J., Kincaid-Smith, P., Becker, G. H., Loughead, M. G., Freeman, J. W. & Sands, J. M. (1978). Goodpasture's syndrome in identical twins. *Annals of Internal Medicine*, **88**, 61–2.

Dahlberg, P. J., Kurtz, S. B., Donadio, J. V. *et al.* (1978). Recurrent Goodpasture's syndrome. *Mayo Clinic Proceedings*, **53**, 533–7.

Daniell, W. E., Couser, W. G. & Rosenstock, L. (1988). Occupational solvent exposure and glomerulonephritis. A case report and review of the literature. *Journal of the American Medical Association*, **259**, 2280–3.

Diabetes Epidemiology Research International. (1987). Preventing insulin dependent diabetes mellitus: the environmental challenge. *British Medical Journal*, **295**, 479–81.

Disney, A. P. S. (1986). *Ninth Report of the Australian and New Zealand Combined Dialysis and Transplantation Registry*. Woodville, South Australia: Queen Elizabeth Hospital.

Doble, N. D., Banga, J. P., Pope, R., Lalor, E., Kilduff, P. & McGregor, A. M. (1988). Autoantibodies to the thyroid microsomal/thyroid peroxidase antigen are polyclonal and directed to several distinct antigenic sites. *Immunology*, **64**, 23–9.

Donaghy, M. & Rees, A. J. (1983). Cigarette smoking and lung haemorrhage in glomerulonephritis caused by autoantibodies to glomerular basement membrane. *Lancet*, **ii**, 1390–3.

Fillit, H. M. & Zabriskie, J. B. (1982). Cellular immunity in glomerulonephritis. *American Journal of Pathology*, **109**, 227–43.

Fish, A. J., Carmody, K. M. & Michael, A. F. (1979). Spatial orientation and distribution of antigens within human glomerular basement membrane. *Journal of Laboratory and Clinical Medicine*, **94**, 447–57.

Flinter, F. A., Cameron, J. S., Chantler, C., Houston, I. & Bobrow, M. (1988). Genetics of classic Alport's syndrome. *Lancet*, **ii**, 1005–7.

Garovoy, M. R. (1982). Immunogenetic associations in nephrotic states. *Contemporary Issues in Nephrology*, **9**, 259–82.

Goldman, M., Depierreux, M., De Pauw, L. *et al.* (1990). Failure of two subsequent renal grafts by anti-GBM glomerulonephritis in Alport's syndrome: case report and review of the literature. *Transplant International*, **3**, 82–5.

Guerin, V., Rabian, C., Noel, L. H. *et al.* (1990). Anti-glomerular-basement-membrane disease after lithotripsy. *Lancet*, **335**, 856–7.

Guéry, J. C. & Druet, P. (1990). A spontaneous hybridoma producing autoanti-idiotypic antibodies that recognize a V kappa-associated idiotope in mercury-induced autoimmunity. *European Journal of Immunology*, **20**, 1027–31.

Guéry, J. C., Druet, E., Glotz, D. *et al.* (1990). Specificity and cross-reactive idiotypes of anti-glomerular basement membrane autoantibodies in HgCl$_2$-induced autoimmune glomerulonephritis. *European Journal of Immunology*, **20**, 93–100.

Holdsworth, S. R., Neale, T. J. & Wilson, C. B. (1981). Abrogation of macrophage-dependent injury in experimental glomerulonephritis in the rabbit. *Journal of Clinical Investigation*, **68**, 686–98.

Hostikka, S. L., Eddy, R. L., Byers, M. G., Höyhtyä, M., Shows, T. B. & Tryggvason, K. (1990). Identification of a distinct type IV collagen α chain with restricted kidney distribution and assignment of its gene to the locus of X chromosome-linked Alport syndrome. *Proceedings of the National Academy of Sciences, USA*, **87**, 1606–10.

Hume, D. M., Sterling, W. A., Weymouth, R. J., Siebel, H. R., Madge, G. E. & Lee, H. M. (1970). Glomerulonephritis in human renal homotransplants. *Transplantation Proceedings*, **2**, 361–412.

Jayne, D. R. W., Marshall, P. D., Jones, S. J. & Lockwood, C. M. (1990). Autoantibodies to GBM and neutrophil cytoplasm in rapidly progressive glomerulonephritis. *Kidney International*, **37**, 965–70.

Jeraj, K., Michael, A. F. & Fish, A. J. (1982). Immunologic similarities between Goodpasture's and Steblay's antibodies. *Clinical Immunology and Immunopathology*, **23**, 408–13.

Johnson, J. P., Moore, J. Jr., Austin, H. A., Balow, J. E., Antonovych, T. T. & Wilson, C. B. (1985). Therapy of antiglomerular basement membrane antibody mediated disease: analysis of prognostic significance of clinical, pathologic and treatment factors. *Medicine*, **64**, 219–27.

Johnson, R. J., Klebanoff, S. J. & Couser, W. G. (1988). Oxidants in glomerular injury. In *Immunopathology of Renal Disease. Contemporary Issues in Nephrology. 18*, ed. C. B. Wilson, B. M. Brenner & J. H. Stein, pp. 87–110. New York, Edinburgh, London, Melbourne: Churchill Livingstone.

Lerner, R. A., Glassock, R. J. & Dixon, F. J. (1967). The role of anti-glomerular basement membrane antibody in the pathogenesis of human glomerulonephritis. *Journal of Experimental Medicine*, **126**, 989–1004.

Macanovic, M., Evans, D. J. & Peters, D. K. (1972). Allergic response to glomerular basement membrane in patients with glomerulonephritis. *Lancet*, **ii**, 207–10.

Mackay, I. R. (1983). Natural autoantibodies to the fore – forbidden clones to the rear? *Immunology Today*, **4**, 340–2.

MacPhee, I. A. M., Antoni, F. A. & Mason, D. W. (1989). Spontaneous recovery of rats from experimental allergic encephalomyelitis is dependent on regulation of the immune system by endogenous adrenal corticosteroids. *Journal of Experimental Medicine*, **169**, 431–45.

Mahieu, P., Dardenne, M. & Bach, J. F. (1972). Detection of humoral and cell-mediated immunity to kidney basement membranes in human renal disease. *American Journal of Medicine*, **53**, 185–92.

Mahieu, P., Lambert, P. H. & Miescher, P. A. (1974). Detection of anti-glomerular basement membrane antibodies by a radioimmunological technique. Clinical application in human nephropathies. *Journal of Clinical Investigation*, **54**, 128–37.

Makker, S. P. & Kanalas, J. J. (1990). Renal antigens in mercuric chloride induced, anti-GBM autoantibody glomerular disease. *Kidney International*, **37**, 64–71.

McCoy, R. C., Johnson, H. K., Stone, W. J. & Wilson, C. B. (1976). Variations in glomerular basement membrane antigens in hereditary nephritis. *Laboratory Investigation*, **34**, 325–6. (Abstract).

Naito, I. & Sado, Y. (1989). Early changes of rat experimental autoimmune glomerulonephritis induced with nephritogenic antigen from bovine renal basement membranes. *Journal of Clinical and Laboratory Immunology*, **28**, 187–93.

Neale, T. J. & Wilson, C. B. (1982). Glomerular antigens in glomerulonephritis. *Springer Seminars in Immunopathology*, **5**, 221–49.

Nolasco, F. E. B., Cameron, J. S., Hartley, B., Coelho, A., Hildreth, G. & Reuben, R. (1987). Intraglomerular T cells and macrophages in nephritis: study with monoclonal antibodies. *Kidney International*, **31**, 1160–6.

Pelletier, L., Rossert, J., Pasquier, R., Vial, M-C. & Druet, P. (1990). Role of CD8$^+$ cells in mercury-induced autoimmunity or immunosuppression in the rat. *Scandinavian Journal of Immunology*, **31**, 65–74.

Perl, S. I., Pussell, B. A., Charlesworth, J. A., Macdonald, G. J. & Wolnizer, M. (1981). Goodpasture's (anti-GBM) disease and HLA-DRW2. *New England Journal of Medicine*, **305**, 463–4.

Pusey, C. D., Sinico, R. A., Peters, D. K. & Lockwood, C. M. (1984). Auto-immunity induced by homologous glomerular basement membrane alone in the Brown Norway rat. *Clinical Science*, **67** suppl. 9, 38 (Abstract).

Pusey, C. D., Dash, A., Kershaw, M. J. *et al.* (1987). A single autoantigen in Goodpasture's syndrome identified by a monoclonal antibody to human glomerular basement membrane. *Laboratory Investigation*, **56**, 23–31.

Pusey, C. D., Venning, M. C. & Peters, D. K. (1988). Immunopathology of glomerular and interstitial disease. In *Diseases of the Kidney*, 4th edn, ed. R. W. Schrier & C. W. Gottschalk, pp. 1827–83. Boston/Toronto: Little, Brown and Company.

Queluz, T. H., Pawlowski, I., Brunda, M. J., Brentjens, J. R., Vladutiu, A. O. & Andres, G. (1990). Pathogenesis of an experimental model of Goodpasture's hemorrhagic pneumonitis. *Journal of Clinical Investigation*, **85**, 1507–15.

Rees, A. J., Peters, D. K., Compston, D. A. S. & Batchelor, J. R. (1978). Strong association between HLA DRw2 and antibody mediated Goodpasture's syndrome. *Lancet*, **i**, 966–8.

Rees, A. J., Amos, N. & Peters, D. K. (1981). Infection and heterologous phase proteinuria in nephrotoxic nephritis. *Kidney International*, **20**, 687 (Abstract).

Rees, A. J., Demaine, A. G. & Welsh, K. I. (1984). Association of immunoglobulin Gm allotypes with antiglomerular basement membrane antibodies and their titer. *Human Immunology*, **10**, 213–20.

Rees, A. J. & Lockwood, C. M. (1988). Antiglomerular basement membrane antibody-mediated nephritis. In *Diseases of the Kidney*, 4th edn, ed. R. W. Schrier & C. W. Gottschalk, pp. 2091–126. Boston/Toronto: Little, Brown and Company.

Rees, A. J., Lockwood, C. M. & Peters, D. K. (1977). Enhanced allergic tissue injury in Goodpasture's syndrome by intercurrent bacterial infection. *British Medical Journal*, 2, 723–6.

Rees, A. J., Peters, D. K., Amos, N., Welsh, K. I. & Batchelor, J. R. (1984). The influence of HLA-linked genes on the severity of anti-GBM antibody-mediated nephritis. *Kidney International*, 26, 444–50.

Rossert, J., Pelletier, L., Pasquier, R. & Druet, P. (1988). Autoreactive T cells in mercury-induced autoimmunity. Demonstration by limiting dilution analysis. *European Journal of Immunology*, 18, 1761–6.

Sado, Y. & Naito, I. (1987). Experimental autoimmune glomerulonephritis in rats by soluble isologous or homologous antigens from glomerular and tubular basement membranes. *British Journal of Experimental Pathology*, 68, 695–704.

Sapin, C., Druet, E. & Druet, P. (1977). Induction of anti-glomerular basement membrane antibodies in the Brown-Norway rat by mercuric chloride. *Clinical and Experimental Immunology*, 28, 173–9.

Sapin, C., Hirsch, F., Delaporte, J-P., Bazin, H. & Druet, P. (1984). Polyclonal IgE increase after $HgCl_2$ injections in BN and LEW rats: a genetic analysis. *Immunogenetics*, 20, 227–36.

Saus, J., Wieslander, J., Langeveld, J. P. M., Quinones, S. & Hudson, B. G. (1988). Identification of the Goodpasture antigen as the $\alpha3(IV)$ chain of collagen IV. *Journal of Biological Chemistry*, 263, 13374–80.

Savage, C. O. S., Pusey, C. D., Bowman, C., Rees, A. J. & Lockwood, C. M. (1986a). Antiglomerular basement membrane antibody mediated disease in the British Isles 1980–4. *British Medical Journal*, 292, 301–4.

Savage, C. O. S. (1986b). Regulation of autoantibody production in man. The role of idiotype-antiidiotype network interactions in anti-glomerular basement membrane antibody mediated disease. University of London: PhD Thesis.

Savage, C. O. S., Pusey, C. D., Kershaw, M. J. *et al.* (1986c). The Goodpasture antigen in Alport's syndrome: studies with a monoclonal antibody. *Kidney International*, 30, 107–12.

Savage, C. O. S., Noel, L. H., Crutcher, E., Price, S. R. & Grunfeld, J. P. (1989). Hereditary nephritis: immunoblotting studies of the glomerular basement membrane. *Laboratory Investigation*, 60, 613–18.

Savige, J. A., Mavrova, L. & Kincaid-Smith, P. (1989). Inhibitable anti-GBM antibody activity after renal transplantation in Alport's syndrome. *Transplantation*, 48, 704–5.

Saxena, R., Bygren, P., Butkowski, R. & Wieslander, J. (1990). Entactin: a possible auto-antigen in the pathogenesis of non-Goodpasture anti-GBM nephritis. *Kidney International*, 38, 263–72.

Scheer, R. L. & Grossman, M. A. (1964). Immune aspects of the glomerulonephritis associated with pulmonary haemorrhage. *Annals of Internal Medicine*, 60, 1009–21.

Schrijver, G., Schalkwijk, J., Robben, J. C. M., Assman, K. J. M. & Koene, R. A. P. (1989). Antiglomerular basement membrane nephritis in beige mice. Deficiency of leukocytic neutral proteinases prevents the induction of albuminuria in the heterologous phase. *Journal of Experimental Medicine*, 169, 1435–48.

Schrijver, G., Bogman, M. J. J. T., Assman, K. J. M. *et al.* (1990). Anti-GBM nephritis in the mouse: role of granulocytes in the heterologous phase. *Kidney International*, 38, 86–95.

Simonsen, H., Brun, C., Thomsen, O. F., Larsen, S. & Ladefoged, J. (1982). Goodpasture's syndrome in twins. *Acta Medica Scandinavica*, 212, 425–8.

Simpson, I. J., Amos, N., Evans, D. J., Thomson, N. M. & Peters, D. K. (1975). Guinea-pig nephrotoxic nephritis. I. The role of complement and polymorphonuclear leucocytes and the effect of antibody subclass and fragments in the heterologous phase. *Clinical and Experimental Immunology*, **19**, 499–511.

Simpson, I. J., Doak, P. B., Williams, L. C. *et al.* (1982). Plasma exchange in Goodpasture's syndrome. *American Journal of Nephrology*, **2**, 301–11.

Steblay, R. W. & Rudofsky, U. M. (1983). Experimental autoimmune glomerulonephritis induced by anti-glomerular basement membrane antibody. II. Effects of injecting heterologous, homologous, or autologous glomerular basement membranes and complete Freund's adjuvant into sheep. *American Journal of Pathology*, **113**, 125–33.

Thomson, N. M., Moran, J., Simpson, I. J. & Peters, D. K. (1976). Defibrination with ancrod in nephrotoxic nephritis in rabbits. *Kidney International*, **10**, 343–7.

Tipping, P. G., Boyce, N. W. & Holdsworth, S. R. (1989). Relative contributions of chemo-attractant and terminal components of complement to anti-glomerular basement membrane (GBM) glomerulonephritis. *Clinical and Experimental Immunology*, **78**, 444–8.

Tipping, P. G., Neale, T. J. & Holdsworth, S. R. (1985). T lymphocyte participation in antibody-induced experimental glomerulonephritis. *Kidney International*, **27**, 530–7.

Tomosugi, N. I., Cashman, S. J., Hay, H. *et al.* (1989). Modulation of antibody-mediated glomerular injury *in vivo* by bacterial lipopolysaccharide, tumour necrosis factor, and interleukin-1. *Journal of Immunology*, **142**, 3083–90.

Unanue, E. R. & Dixon, F. J. (1964). Experimental glomerulonephritis. IV. Participation of complement in nephrotoxic nephritis. *Journal of Experimental Medicine*, **119**, 965–82.

Unanue, E. R. & Dixon, F. J. (1965). Experimental glomerulonephritis. V. Studies on the interactions of nephrotoxic antibodies with tissues of the rat. *Journal of Experimental Medicine*, **121**, 697–714.

Unanue, E. R., Dixon, F. J. & Lees, S. (1966). Experimental glomerulonephritis. VIII. The *in vivo* fixation of heterologous nephrotoxic antibodies to, and their exchange among, tissues of the rat. *International Archives of Allergy and Applied Immunology*, **29**, 140–50.

van Zyl Smit, R., Rees, A. J. & Peters, D. K. (1983). Factors affecting severity of injury during nephrotoxic nephritis in rabbits. *Clinical and Experimental Immunology*, **54**, 366–72.

Weber, M., Pullig, O. & Boesken, W. H. (1990). Anti-glomerular basement membrane disease after renal obstruction (letter). *Lancet*, **336**, 512–13.

Weber, M., Pullig, O. & Köhler, H. (1990). Distribution of Goodpasture antigens within various human basement membranes. *Nephrology Dialysis and Transplantation*, **5**, 87–93.

Wilson, C. B. & Dixon, F. J. (1974). Diagnosis of immunopathologic renal disease. *Kidney International*, **5**, 389–401.

Wilson, C. B. & Dixon, F. J. (1986). The renal response to immunological injury. In *The Kidney*, 3rd edn, ed. B. M. Brenner & F. C. Rector, pp. 800–89. Philadelphia: W.B.Saunders Company.

Yoshioka, K., Iseki, T., Okada, M., Morimoto, Y., Eryu, N. & Maki, S. (1988). Identification of Goodpasture antigens in human alveolar basement membrane. *Clinical and Experimental Immunology*, **74**, 419–24.

–3–
Membranous nephropathy

Membranous nephropathy, a term first used by Bell (Bell, 1950), is characterised by diffuse, uniform thickening of the glomerular capillary wall. Clinically the main feature is proteinuria, often of nephrotic proportions, with occasional haematuria, hypertension and, in an important subgroup, impairment of renal function which is usually progressive. Membranous nephropathy is probably the commonest primary cause of the adult nephrotic syndrome, occurring in approximately 25% of renal biopsies in that condition (Coggins, Frommer & Glassock, 1982). It is found in about 10% of all renal biopsies performed for glomerular disease (Central Commitee of the Toronto Glomerulonephritis Registry, 1981) and in about 8% of cases of end stage renal failure due to primary glomerular disease for which histology is available (Jacobs et al., 1977).

Although membranous nephropathy is a distinctive histopathological entity, this does not imply that there is necessarily a uniform cause and it is possible that a number of disease processes can lead to the same histological features. It is worth considering these features in more detail because of the possible insight that they offer into aspects of the underlying immunopathology.

As defined by Ehrenreich and Churg (Ehrenreich & Churg, 1968) the glomerular morphology can be divided into a number of stages. In stage I, small electron dense deposits appear on the subepithelial aspect of the basement membrane. There is little distortion of the basement membrane itself and the light microscopic appearances may be indistinguishable from minimal change nephropathy. Stage II, the commonest at presentation (Donadio et al., 1988), is characterised by the outgrowth of basement membrane material between numerous subepithelial deposits. With silver stains, these projections have the appearance of spikes projecting outward from the basement membrane towards the urinary space. Further outgrowth of basement membrane material results in encirclement of the deposits and incorporation into the basement membrane (stage III). This is associated with a variable loss of density by the deposits. Finally, the basement membrane assumes a greatly thickened, vacuolated appearance (stage IV) associated with collapse of capillary loops and sclerosis. Except in certain

41

secondary cases, e.g. SLE and infections (see below), there are few, if any, mesangial deposits. There is usually no proliferation of any of the cellular elements of the glomerulus. The appearances on immunofluorescence reflect the changes in the deposits visible on electron microscopy. IgG is initially deposited in a diffuse granular pattern along the capillary loops. With progression these IgG deposits coalesce and become larger and ultimately there may be some loss of staining corresponding to the loss of electron density. Again, there is little staining of mesangial regions.

It is not clear that the histological stages actually represent the evolution in time of this disease. Some studies have found no relationship between the stage and either clinical severity or prognosis (Franklin, Jennings & Earle, 1973; Row *et al.*, 1975; Collaborative Study of the Adult Idiopathic Nephrotic Syndrome, 1979; Ramzy *et al.*, 1981; Latham *et al.*, 1982; Donadio *et al.*, 1988). In other cases, however, the earlier stages do appear to be associated with a good prognosis and/or disease of short duration (Beregi & Varga, 1974; Noel *et al.*, 1979; Ramirez *et al.*, 1982; Tu *et al.*, 1983; Zucchelli *et al.*, 1987*b*). One serial study with repeated biopsies has provided a possible explanation for these discrepancies (Törnroth, Honkanen & Pettersson, 1987). This showed a close relationship between the presence of electron-dense deposits and the initial presentation; subsequent remission was associated with the development of lucent deposits, interpreted as healing. A relapse was characterised by a fresh collection of electron-dense deposits. Light microscopic changes were rather more variable. Continuing disease activity was associated with continuing deposition with simultaneous resolution, producing a complex picture the nature of which was thought to depend on the speed of deposition. If these ideas are correct, then the classical Ehrenreich and Churg staging only reflects the evolution of a particular subset of membranous lesions, and the rather variable findings in the studies mentioned above are not surprising.

The appearances outlined above may occur in isolation (idiopathic membranous nephropathy) or in the context of a number of underlying diseases (Table 3.1). Except where qualified, membranous nephropathy will be used to refer to the idiopathic disease; some of the secondary causes, and their possible pathogenetic mechanisms, are considered further later.

Immunogenetics

The MHC

As is usual, the dominant immunogenetic associations are with the MHC. Membranous nephropathy was one of the earliest diseases to be studied from this viewpoint and the initial report of an association with DR3

Table 3.1. *Secondary causes of membranous nephropathy*

Drugs (penicillamine, gold)
Neoplasia (particularly carcinoma)
Autoimmunity (lupus, autoimmune thyroid disease)
Infections: bacterial (e.g. syphilis)   viral (e.g. hepatitis B)   protozoal (e.g. malaria)
Diabetes

(Klouda *et al.*, 1979) has subsequently been confirmed in other studies (Garovoy, 1980; Müller *et al.*, 1981; Le Petit, Laurent & Berthoux, 1982; Rashid *et al.*, 1983; Cameron, Healy & Adu, 1990). There are differences between the various subpopulations in that, for example, the association appears stronger in the United Kingdom (relative risk 12; Klouda *et al.*, 1979) and France (relative risk 7.4; Le Petit, Laurent & Berthoux, 1982) than in the United States, where no significant association was found, although the numbers studied were small (Garovoy, Braun & Duquesnoy, 1980*b*). This variation between populations is a common feature in immunogenetics and often reflects the different frequencies of particular alleles. The point is made particularly by data from Japan where DR3 is comparatively rare (approximately 1–3% versus 20% in Caucasians). In the Japanese, membranous nephropathy is associated with DR2 with a relative risk of approximately seven and there is no association with DR3 (Hiki *et al.*, 1984; Tomura *et al.*, 1984). The DR3 allele found in patients with membranous nephropathy appears to be the same as the DR3 allele in normal controls, at least as judged by RFLP analysis (Sacks *et al.*, 1987).

It is intriguing that several of the secondary causes of membranous nephropathy also have links with DR3: membranous nephropathy as a result of gold or penicillamine treatment is most likely to occur in DR3 positive individuals (Speerstra *et al.*, 1983); both SLE (Woodrow, 1988) and diabetes mellitus (Sheehy *et al.*, 1989) are associated with DR3, as is autoimmune thyroid disease (Farid & Bear, 1981).

Other class II specificities that have been examined are MT1 (now DQw1) and MT2 (now DRw52). In the Japanese population, DQw1 was significantly increased in the patient population (Tomura *et al.*, 1984); the association was not as strong as that with DR2 and, as DQw1 is in linkage disequilibrium with DR2, was probably secondary to the DR2 association. Another study, however, found that a DQA1 allele was more strongly associated than DR3 (Vaughan, Demaine & Welsh, 1989). The association with DRw52 has been noted in both American and German populations (Garovoy, Braun & Duquesnoy, 1980b; Müller *et al.*, 1981). Of note in the American data is the fact that there was a significant association with DRw52 (relative risk 14, $p_c < 0.001$) in the absence of an association with DR3. The DRw52 specificity is determined by the DR $\beta 3$ chain found in association with haplotypes bearing DR3, DR5, DRw6(w13) and DRw8. Although part of the DRw52 association may again be secondary to the DR3 linkage, it is possible that DRw52 has an independent association of its own.

A number of MHC class I alleles have also been linked to membranous nephropathy. The original report found an increased frequency of B8 and B18 although only the latter was significant (Klouda *et al.*, 1979). This association with B18 has not been confirmed in other studies, but significant associations have been found with B8 (Le Petit, Laurent & Berthoux, 1982; Hassan, Le Petit & Berthoux, 1987) and A1 (Cameron, Healy & Adu, 1990), and with Aw33 in a Chinese population (together with DR3) (Huang, 1989). All of these class I alleles are in linkage disequilibrium with DR3 (Bodmer & Bodmer, 1978) and the associations are almost certainly a reflection of the DR3 association.

Of the complement components coded for within the MHC, associations have been described with Bf and C4. Again, the initial association with a particular Bf allele, BfF1 (Dyer *et al.*, 1980), has not been found in subsequent studies (Müller *et al.*, 1981; Le Petit, Laurent & Berthoux, 1982; Cameron, Healy & Adu, 1990); because of the rarity of BfF1 in these studies it has not been possible to test the claim that the B18-BfF1-DR3 haplotype is associated with a particularly bad prognosis (Short *et al.*, 1983). More generally, most (but not all, e.g. Zucchelli *et al.*, 1987a) other studies have found no link between MHC alleles and prognosis, e.g. Cameron, Healy & Adu, 1990. Returning to complement alleles, a non-significant increased incidence of a rare C4B allele, C4B*2.9, has been noted (Wank *et al.*, 1984); this may be artefactual, as there is evidence that this variant is acquired in the presence of uraemia (Welch & Beischel, 1985). In another study there was an excess of null (non-coding) alleles at the C4 loci (both A and B), and a decrease in the BfS allele (Berthoux *et al.*, 1990). Null C4 alleles are found particularly on DR3-bearing haplotypes (Woodrow, 1988), and it is unclear which is the primary association; the decrease in the BfS allele contrasts with an increase in BfSS homozygotes in combination with B8-DR3 noted elsewhere (Papiha *et al.*, 1987).

Other loci

An association with IgG Gm allotypes as been found by one group (Demaine *et al.*, 1984) but not by another (Brenchley *et al.*, 1983). Other associations reported include a decrease in a heterozygous RFLP phenotype defined by a probe for the IgM switch region (Sμ), no significant associations with an analogous Sα probe, and an increase in a heterozygous phenotype defined by a probe for the T cell receptor Cβ region (Demaine *et al.*, 1988); neither the association with the T cell receptor gene (Niven *et al.*, 1990) nor that with the Sμ locus (Moore *et al.*, 1990) has been confirmed. A possible association with an allele of the complement component C7 is of interest (Nishimukai *et al.*, 1989), given the role of the membrane attack complex in pathogenesis (see below).

Immunopathology

Animal studies

The study of animal models of membranous nephropathy is dominated by Heymann nephritis. This condition, first described in 1959 (Heymann *et al.*, 1959), is produced by immunising susceptible strains of rat with an extract of homologous kidney in complete Freund's adjuvant; as in man, this susceptibility is linked to the MHC (Stenglen, Thoenes & Günther, 1978). A condition very similar to membranous nephropathy results: the rats develop the nephrotic syndrome and histology demonstrates subepithelial deposits with corresponding granular immunofluorescence, exactly as found in the human lesion. The immunopathology of Heymann nephritis is now reasonably well understood, and it is instructive to follow the way in which thinking about this model has evolved as it illustrates a more general point concerning the importance of circulating immune complexes in the immunopathogenesis of renal disease (see Chapter 1).

The antigen used initially to elicit Heymann nephritis was a crude tubular extract known as Fx1A. Subsequent purification demonstrated that a preparation from the membrane of brush border cells (RTEα5) was nephritogenic (Edgington, Glassock & Dixon, 1968). The suggested mechanism for the production of glomerular deposits by immunisation with a tubular antigen was the release of antigen from damaged tubules leading to the formation of circulating immune complexes, followed by trapping within the glomerulus (Edgington, Glassock & Dixon, 1968). Doubts about this mechanism were raised by the observation that the disease could be induced by injection of heterologous anti-brush border antibodies (passive Heymann nephritis) (Barabas & Lannigan, 1974; Feenstra *et al.*, 1975). Even more convincingly, such antibodies would produce deposits in the isolated perfused kidney, i.e. in the absence of any circulating antigen (Couser, Steinmuller & Stilmant, 1978; van Damme *et al.*, 1978). The solution to this puzzle was provided by further characterisation of the key nephritogenic antigen (Kerjaschki & Farquhar, 1982, 1983). This is a glycoprotein of molecular weight 330 kD known as gp330. Immunocytochemical studies show that not only is gp330 found in the brush border of the proximal convoluted tubule but that it is also present on glomerular epithelial cells, principally in association with the clathrin-coated pits that are involved in endocytosis (Brown, McCluskey & Ausiello, 1987). The current view of the pathogenesis of Heymann nephritis (Verroust, 1989) is that anti-gp330 antibodies, induced by immunisation with tubular extracts or infused directly, bind *in situ* to gp330 already present on the glomerular epithelial cell. Cross-linking of the target antigen leads to redistribution of the complexes with shedding into the subepithelial space. They then attach firmly to the glomerular basement membrane and presumably initiate the sequence of changes in the basement membrane described at the beginning of this chapter.

There are a number of aspects of the pathogenesis that are still unclear. Antigens apart from gp330 may be involved in the pathogenesis, possibly in the form of circulating immune complexes (Hori & Abrass, 1990), and the relative contributions of the various antigen-antibody systems are uncertain; this may be of particular significance in man, given the lack of evidence for involvement of the gp330 homologue in human membranous nephropathy (see below). The process by which gp330-containing immune deposits attach to the basement membrane, which can occur within minutes (Kerjaschki, Miettinen & Farquhar, 1987), is not understood, but the affinity of gp330 for various matrix proteins may well be relevant (Mendrick, Chung & Rennke, 1990). The cellular immune system is involved in pathogenesis, and treatment directed at this compartment is effective (Gronhagen-Riska *et al.*, 1990); however, the relative importance of T cells is unclear. The initial production of proteinuria in passive (and probably active) Heymann nephritis, and other models of membranous nephropathy, is dependent on assembly of the membrane attack complex (C5b-9) of the complement cascade (de Heer *et al.*, 1985; Baker *et al.*, 1989). How this leads to proteinuria is uncertain, although intermediate steps are being defined (Cybulsky *et al.*, 1989); it is probably distinct from the more chronic changes dependent on the resulting disruption in the basement membrane. This is illustrated by the transplantation of a kidney undergoing active Heymann nephritis to a normal host (Lewis *et al.*, 1972; Makker & Kanalas, 1989). There is reasonably rapid resolution of heavy proteinuria, which may reflect cessation of ongoing immune deposit formation, but a degree of long term proteinuria remains, presumably due to the induced basement membrane abnormalities.

Despite these remaining questions the general pathogenetic mechanism involved, reaction of a circulating antibody with an antigen present *in situ* within the glomerulus, is clear and could also be the basis for other animal models of membranous nephropathy. This is illustrated by the model produced by infusing cationic human immunoglobulin into rats. The cationic protein binds to anionic sites within the glomerular basement membrane and acts as the target for subsequently infused rabbit anti-human immunoglobulin antibodies (Oite *et al.*, 1982). The same process may well underlie the membranous nephropathy produced in some forms of chronic serum sickness in the rabbit: there is evidence that the initial event is the binding of cationic bovine serum albumin to the glomerular capillary wall (Border *et al.*, 1982; Adler *et al.*, 1983). Similarly, DNA has a particular affinity for the glomerular basement membrane and may play a role, together with anti-DNA antibodies, in the membranous nephropathy of SLE (Izui, Lambert & Miescher, 1976). A very similar mechanism appears to be involved in the production of membranous nephropathy in the mouse, although an antigen (gp90) distinct from gp330 is involved (Assman *et al.*, 1989).

The central role of this type of mechanism in animal models of membranous nephropathy does not exclude some contribution from the classical process of deposition of circulating immune complexes. Indeed, once immune aggregates are deposited, they will tend to grow by the capture of further circulating antigen or antigen–antibody complexes (see Chapter 1). There is evidence for the presence of such circulating complexes and free antigen in a number of models, including Heymann nephritis (Singh & Makker, 1985). In addition, a study employing preformed immune complexes of defined composition showed that complexes composed of low affinity antibody would produce subepithelial deposits when infused into mice (Lew, Staines & Steward, 1984). Infusion of antigen alone followed later by antibody did not lead to such deposits, suggesting that *in vivo* dissociation, followed by initial planting of antigen prior to *in situ* reassociation of the complex, was not the mechanism.

The extent to which immunoregulation is involved in any of these models is unclear (Cornish *et al.*, 1989). There is some evidence that resistance to Heymann nephritis can be induced by prior immunisation with Fx1A (Harmon, Grupe & Parkman, 1980) or antibody eluted from diseased kidneys (Ebert *et al.*, 1981), and antigen-specific suppressor cells are present in the spleen late in the disease (de Heer *et al.*, 1986). The model of anti-glomerular basement membrane (GBM) disease produced by mercuric chloride ($HgCl_2$) in Brown Norway rats (see Chapter 2) has a membranous-like phase. This disease is clearly subject to immunoregulatory control, both by suppressor cells (Bowman *et al.*, 1984) and possibly by antiidiotypic antibodies (Chalopin & Lockwood, 1984). Interestingly, Lewis rats, although they do not develop anti-GBM antibodies following treatment with $HgCl_2$, are rendered partially resistant to the induction of Heymann nephritis (Pelletier *et al.*, 1987), suggesting that HgCl$_2$ produces a generalised increase in suppression.

Human studies

As with Heymann nephritis, human membranous nephropathy was for some time thought to be due to the deposition of circulating immune complexes (Dixon, 1968). The difficulty in identifying such complexes (Coggins, 1988) and the compelling analogies with Heymann nephritis have led to the current view that human membranous nephropathy has a similar pathogenesis (Verroust, 1989), and to attempts to identify the corresponding antigen. It is not gp330, or a human brush border antigen that cross-reacts with this (Kerjaschki *et al.*, 1987), as these antigens are not expressed in human glomerular epithelial cells (Goodyer, Mills & Kaplan, 1986). Some initial reports that a renal tubular antigen was present in diseased glomeruli (Naruse *et al.*, 1973) have not been confirmed (Whitworth *et al.*, 1976; Thorpe & Cavallo, 1980; Collins, Andres & McClusky, 1981; Gilboa, 1981). Similarly, although antibody with specificity for brush border antigens has been identified in the glomeruli in some cases of secondary membranous nephropathy (Pusey, Venning & Peters, 1988), this finding has not been generalisable (Zager *et al.*, 1979). Two more recent reports of possible target antigens await confirmation (Niles *et al.*, 1987; Kerjaschki, 1989). The description of membranous nephropathy in a neonate which was probably induced by transplacental passage of antibodies to an unidentified antigen(s) present in tubular brush borders and glomeruli is intriguing (Nauta *et al.*, 1990), as is another report of anti-brush border antibodies in association with membranous nephropathy (Douglas *et al.*, 1981). The characterisation of the antigen(s) involved, and a search for similar antibodies in other cases of membranous nephropathy, would be of considerable interest.

In more general terms, one study attempted to test the hypothesis that human membranous nephropathy has a similar pathogenesis to Heymann nephritis by perfusing human kidneys *ex vivo* with polyclonal and monoclonal antibodies raised against human brush border and glomerular epithelial cell preparations (Fukatsu *et al.*, 1989). One such monoclonal antibody to a 60 kD protein with a distribution on human glomerular epithelial cells analogous to that of gp330 on rat epithelial cells could induce redistribution of the antigen and the formation of deposits. However, these were much less severe than the corresponding changes induced by anti-gp330 antibodies in the rat. Despite a number of intriguing reports, there is therefore, at present, no consensus as to the nature of the antigen in idiopathic human membranous nephropathy.

A variety of immunological abnormalities, most of questionable specificity, have been described in idiopathic membranous nephropathy. These
include changes in ratios of lymphocyte subsets (Rothschild & Chatenoud,
1984), an increase in concanavalin induced suppression (Matsumoto, Osakabe & Hatano, 1983) and a reduced splenic uptake of sensitised red cells
(Berthoux *et al.*, 1984). These abnormalities are not found universally and in
particular it may be that they are the result of the nephrotic state (Taube,
Brown & Williams, 1984), and have no significance with respect to pathogenesis. Whether the subclass restriction of glomerular IgG represents a
clonally restricted response to a particular antigen is uncertain (Noël *et al.*,
1988). The extent to which the cellular immune system is involved in
pathogenesis is unknown. It has been reported that there is a correlation
between increased interstitial mononuclear cells and progressive renal
impairment, which has led to the suggestion that progression to renal
impairment is determined by cellular immunity (Alexopoulos *et al.*, 1989).

There are a number of instances in which membranous nephropathy has
occurred together with other renal pathology, either sequentially or simul-
taneously (Coggins, 1988). The development of a crescentic nephritis,
occasionally with anti-glomerular basement membrane antibodies, is perhaps the commonest of these associations. This is considered further in
Chapter 8. In several instances, a proliferative nephritis has transformed
into membranous nephropathy (Richet *et al.*, 1974), in some cases in the
context of SLE (Lentz, Michael & Friend, 1981; Hall-Craggs & Ramos,
1981; see below).

Secondary membranous nephropathy

Consideration of some of the conditions that may be associated with
membranous nephropathy (Table 3.1) is of interest because of the possible
links with the pathogenesis of the idiopathic condition.

Gold and penicillamine can both cause a renal lesion indistinguishable
from idiopathic membranous nephropathy (Hall *et al.*, 1987, 1988). Furthermore, there are similarities in the immunogenetics in that individuals with
DR3 appear more susceptible (Speerstra *et al.*, 1983). Major differences
from the idiopathic condition are that withdrawal of either drug usually
leads to rapid resolution of proteinuria and that progressive renal impairment is exceedingly rare (Hall *et al.*, 1987, 1988). The pathogenesis is
obscure. The hypothesis that gold damages renal tubules, leading to the
release of tubular antigens and a Heymann-like nephropathy (Skrifvars,
1979), lacks support for the reasons discussed in the previous section.
Although it has been suggested that penicillamine might be acting as a
hapten (Jaffe, 1979), there is no evidence of an anti-penicillamine response.

This agent is also a polyclonal activator in animals (Goodman & Weigle, 1981), but other conditions associated with such activation do not produce membranous nephropathy. A possible clue is given by the inhibitory effects of penicillamine on the C4 component of the classical pathway of complement (Sim, Dodds & Goldin, 1989). This inhibition occurs at concentrations of the drug easily achieved *in vivo* and might be expected to interfere with the normal disposal of immune complexes (see Chapters 1 and 4). Furthermore, haplotypes carrying the DR3 allele contain a high proportion of C4 null alleles. DR3 positive individuals, with an already subnormal level of C4, may be particularly susceptible to this effect of penicillamine.

A number of secondary causes of membranous nephropathy are associated with the deposition of exogenous antigens within the glomerulus. These include autoimmune thyroid disease (thyroglobulin) (Jordan *et al.*, 1981), tumours (tumour-specific antigens) (Lewis, Loughridge & Phillips, 1971; Costanza *et al.*, 1973; Couser *et al.*, 1974) and a number of different infections, notably hepatitis B (HBsAg, HBcAg and HBeAg) (Lai, Mac-Moune & Tam, 1989; Venkataseshan *et al.*, 1990). In the past, such cases have been used to support the pathogenetic role of circulating immune complexes. However, the interpretation of the presence of these antigens is complicated by the known ability of pre-existing deposits to trap circulating proteins (Bellon *et al.*, 1982), raising the possibility that they might be quite unconnected with the membranous nephropathy. Despite this fact, there is considerable circumstantial evidence for a causal link. This is exemplified by hepatitis B: in series from endemic areas there is a very high incidence of hepatitis B virus infection in patients with membranous nephropathy, particularly in children (Hirose *et al.*, 1984). Initial claims that HBsAg could be demonstrated in the glomeruli of such patients (referenced in Maggiore *et al.*, 1981) were probably incorrect and due to non-specific capture of the fluorescinated reagents by deposited immune complexes (Maggiore *et al.*, 1981). There is much better evidence for the pathogenetic role of HBeAg: this antigen is certainly present along the capillary wall, usually in patients negative for anti-HBeAg (Maggiore *et al.*, 1981). Even more convincingly, there is evidence that development of an anti-HBeAg response can lead to resolution of the nephropathy with a corresponding change of the deposits on electron microscopy from electron dense to lucent (Ito *et al.*, 1981), although in other cases additional factors appear to be involved (Lin, 1990). It remains possible that other hepatitis B antigens may be involved in the pathogenesis of the associated nephropathy (Venkataseshan *et al.*, 1990).

Rather similar findings have been reported in at least one case of tumour-associated membranous nephropathy (Couser *et al.*, 1974). An antibody with reactivity for glomerular deposits, specifically absorbable by a tumour homogenate, was transiently present following removal of the tumour. A repeat renal biopsy four months later showed absence of the tumour-associated antigen and clearing of the complexes on electron microscopy. Examples such as hepatitis and tumour-associated membranous nephropathy, although providing evidence for involvement of the respective antigens in pathogenesis, do not discriminate between deposition of circulating immune complexes and *in situ* formation of such complexes following antigen planting.

The possible role in lupus nephritis of DNA fixed to the glomerular basement membrane has been mentioned above. It has been suggested that a membranous pattern is associated particularly with anti-DNA antibodies of relatively low affinity that are non-precipitating (Friend, 1978). This was particularly well illustrated by a case that initially exhibited a proliferative pattern but which subsequently transformed to a membranous nephropathy (Lentz, Michael & Friend, 1981). This transformation was associated with a change of DNA antibodies from high titre and precipitating to low titre and non-precipitating.

Membranous nephropathy occurring in a renal allograft is particularly complex (Truong et al., 1989). In approximately one third of cases this is a recurrence of the original disease (uncommon with idiopathic membranous nephropathy), with the remainder representing *de novo* membranous nephropathy (Coggins, 1988). Possible factors in the aetiology of the *de novo* cases include an immune response to alloantigens on the transplanted kidney, including MHC antigens, and a response to viral antigens, the presence of which is favoured by the immunosuppressed state (Cameron, 1982).

Therapeutic aspects

The treatment of membranous nephropathy has recently been reviewed (Mathieson & Rees, 1990). From an immunological viewpoint there are two main points to consider. First, is membranous nephropathy amenable to immunological manipulation, and secondly, if so, what is the best form of such intervention? It is also important to decide which subset of patients should be so treated, as many patients will have a relatively benign course; it has been argued that patients with deteriorating renal function should have particular consideration (Mathieson & Rees, 1990).

There is now a body of evidence suggesting that various treatments with immunomodulatory properties can affect aspects of the natural history of membranous nephropathy. Corticosteroids can undoubtedly reduce proteinuria in some patients (Mathieson & Rees, 1990). However, it is now reasonably clear that steroids do not prevent the deterioration in renal function seen in a subgroup of patients (Black, Rose & Brewer, 1970;

Collaborative Study of the Adult Idiopathic Nephrotic Syndrome, 1979; Cattran *et al.*, 1989; Cameron, Healy & Adu, 1990), although not all agree (Hopper, 1989). This suggests that steroids do not influence the underlying immunopathogenesis, but because of the many effects of steroids and our ignorance of the mechanism of proteinuria it is impossible to be certain. There is better evidence, however, that the addition of cytotoxic agents can favourably influence the prognosis. Thus the controlled trial by Ponticelli *et al.* of a regime alternating steroids with chlorambucil demonstrated a significant difference in serum creatinine in favour of the treatment group, as well as a much higher incidence of remissions of proteinuria (Ponticelli *et al.*, 1984, 1989). Small, uncontrolled studies of the subgroup with deteriorating renal function have also suggested that the Ponticelli regime (Mathieson *et al.*, 1988), a combination of steroids and azathioprine (Williams & Bone, 1989) or steroids and cyclophosphamide (Bruns *et al.*, 1991) can halt or reverse the decline in function. Other groups have not reported such favourable results using various modifications of the Ponticelli regime (Warwick & Boulton-Jones, 1988; Wetzels, Hoitsma & Koene, 1989), but the outcome may still have been better than the untreated state which tends to be relentlessly progressive. This is clearly an area where controlled trials are needed.

A variety of other potentially immunomodulatory treatments have been tried including non-steroidal anti-inflammatory agents (Velosa *et al.*, 1985), cyclosporin A (De Santo, Capodicasa & Giordano, 1987; Zietse *et al.*, 1989; Rostoker *et al.*, 1989) and intravenous pooled normal human immunoglobulin (Palla, Bionda & Marchitiello, 1986). The numbers involved in these studies were small, and no definite conclusions can be drawn.

On balance, it therefore seems likely that immunomodulatory treatment can influence the natural history of membranous nephropathy. However, more controlled evidence is required, and the question as to which is the best form of therapy, beyond the fact that steroids on their own are relatively ineffective, remains open.

Concluding remarks

It seems very likely that idiopathic membranous nephropathy has an autoimmune basis in man. A powerful (albeit indirect) case for this is provided by the presence of immune deposits, the immunogenetic associations, the analogies with Heymann nephritis, the mechanisms involved in the secondary causes, and the response to immunosuppressive treatment. What is far less clear is the immunopathogenesis. The available evidence does not support a role for the deposition of circulating immune complexes, at least in the idiopathic condition. Of the other possibilities, analogies with

Heymann nephritis would suggest an autoimmune response to an intrinsic glomerular antigen. The failure, despite an intensive search, to identify such an antigen is weak evidence favouring a response to an extrinsic planted antigen; this is certainly likely to be the mechanism in some types of secondary membranous nephropathy. These last two possibilities are not mutually exclusive, and idiopathic membranous nephropathy may have a heterogeneous aetiology.

The range of glomerular pathology that can include membranous nephropathy, both in animal models such as chronic serum sickness and in human diseases such as SLE, and the transformation of other pathology into membranous nephropathy, and vice versa, suggests that membranous nephropathy is only one possible pattern that can result from a given antigen/antibody system. The variables involved in determining the pathological pattern may include the nature of the antigen, affinity and concentration of the antibody, and the site, rate of formation and handling of the immune complexes. A membranous pattern appears to be favoured when the antigen has a particular affinity for the basement membrane; the antibody is of low affinity and concentration; and the complexes, usually formed *in situ*, accumulate relatively slowly and do not incite an inflammatory response. The possible role of null C4 alleles on DR3 positive haplotypes in penicillamine nephropathy (see above) may hint at a more general involvement of abnormal handling of immune complexes in the pathogenesis of idiopathic membranous nephropathy, a DR3 associated disease.

References

Adler, S. G., Wang, H., Ward, H. J., Cohen, A. H. & Border, W. A. (1983). Electrical charge: its role in the pathogenesis and prevention of experimental membranous nephropathy in the rabbit. *Journal of Clinical Investigation*, **71**, 487–99.

Alexopoulos, E., Seron, D., Hartley, R. B., Nolasco, F. & Cameron, J. S. (1989). Immune mechanisms in idiopathic membranous nephropathy: the role of the interstitial infiltrates. *American Journal of Kidney Disease*, **13**, 404–12.

Assman, K. J., Ronco, P., Tangelder, M. M., Lange, W. P., Verroust, P. & Koene, R. A. (1989). Involvement of an antigen distinct from the Heymann antigen in membranous glomerulonephritis in the mouse. *Laboratory Investigation*, **60**, 138–46.

Baker, P. J., Ochi, R. F., Schulze, M., Johnson, R. J., Campbell, C. & Couser, W. G. (1989). Depletion of C6 prevents development of proteinuria in experimental membranous nephropathy in rats. *American Journal of Pathology*, **135**, 185–94.

Barabas, A. Z. & Lannigan, R. (1974). Induction of an autologous immune-complex glomerulonephritis in the rat by intravenous injection of heterologous anti-rat kidney tubular antibody. I. Production of chronic progressive immune-complex glomerulonephritis. *British Journal of Experimental Pathology*, **55**, 47–55.

Bell, E. T. (1950). *Renal Disease*. 2nd edn, Philadelphia: Lea & Febiger.

Bellon, B., Belair, M. F., Kuhn, J., Druet, P. & Bariety, J. (1982). Trapping of circulating proteins in immune deposits of Heymann nephritis. *Laboratory Investigation*, **46**, 306–12.

Beregi, E. & Varga, I. (1974). Analysis of 260 cases of membranous glomerulonephritis in renal biopsy material. *Clinical Nephrology*, 2, 215–21.

Berthoux, F. C., Laurent, B., Le Petit, J-C. *et al.* (1984). Immunogenetics and immunopathology of human primary membranous nephropathy: HLA-A,B,DR antigens; functional activity of splenic macrophage Fc-receptors and peripheral blood T-lymphocyte subpopulations. *Clinical Nephrology*, 22, 15–20.

Berthoux, F. C., Berthoux, P., Hassan, A. A. *et al.* (1990). Immunogenetique des glomerulonephrites extra membraneuses primitives. *Presse Medicale*, 19, 990–3.

Black, D. A. K., Rose, G. & Brewer, D. B. (1970). Controlled trial of prednisone in adult patients with the nephrotic syndrome. *British Medical Journal*, 3, 421–6.

Bodmer, W. F. & Bodmer, J. G. (1978). Evolution and function of the HLA-system. *British Medical Bulletin*, 34, 309–16.

Border, W. A., Ward, H. J., Kamis, E. S. & Cohen, A. H. (1982). Induction of membranous nephropathy in rabbits by administration of an exogenous cationic antigen: demonstration of a pathogenic role for electrical charge. *Journal of Clinical Investigation*, 69, 451–61.

Bowman, C., Mason, D. W., Pusey, C. D. & Lockwood, C. M. (1984). Autoregulation of autoantibody synthesis in mercuric chloride nephritis in the Brown Norway rat. I. A role for T suppressor cells. *European Journal of Immunology*, 14, 464–70.

Brenchley, P., Feehally, J., Doré, P. *et al.* (1983). Gm allotypes in membranous nephropathy (letter). *New England Journal of Medicine*, 309, 556–57.

Brown, D., McCluskey, R. T. & Ausiello, D. A. (1987). The cell biology of Heymann nephritis: a model of human membranous glomerulonephritis. *American Journal of Kidney Disease*, 10, 74–6.

Bruns, F. J., Adler, S., Fraley, D. S. & Segel, D. P. (1991). Sustained remission of membranous glomerulonephritis after cyclophosphamide and prednisone. *Annals of Internal Medicine*, 114, 725–30.

Cameron, J. S. (1982). Glomerulonephritis in renal transplants. *Transplantation*, 34, 237–45.

Cameron, J. S., Healy, M. J. R. & Adu, D. (1990). The Medical Research Council trial of short-term high dose alternate day prednisolone in idiopathic membranous nephropathy with nephrotic syndrome in adults. *Quarterly Journal of Medicine*, 74, 133–56.

Cattran, D. C., Delmore, T., Roscoe, J. *et al.* (1989). A randomized controlled trial of prednisone in patients with idiopathic membranous nephropathy. *New England Journal of Medicine*, 320, 210–15.

Central Commitee of the Toronto Glomerulonephritis Registry. (1981). Regional program for the study of glomerulonephritis. *Canadian Medical Association Journal*, 124, 158–61.

Chalopin, J. M. & Lockwood, C. M. (1984). Autoregulation of autoantibody synthesis in mercuric chloride nephritis in the Brown Norway rat. II. Presence of antigen-augmentable plaque-forming cells in the spleen is associated with humoral factors behaving as auto-anti-idiotypic antibodies. *European Journal of Immunology*, 14, 470–5.

Coggins, C. H. (1988). Membranous nephropathy. In *Diseases of the Kidney*, 4th edn, ed. R. W. Schrier & C. W. Gottschalk, pp. 2005–33. Boston/Toronto: Little, Brown and Company.

Coggins, C. H., Frommer, J. P. & Glassock, R. J. (1982). Membranous nephropathy. *Seminars in Nephrology*, 2, 264–73.

Collaborative Study of the Adult Idiopathic Nephrotic Syndrome. (1979). A controlled study of short-term prednisone treatment in adults with membranous nephropathy. *New England Journal of Medicine*, 301, 1301–6.

Collins, A. B., Andres, G. A. & McClusky, R. T. (1981). Lack of evidence for a role of renal tubular antigen in human membranous glomerulonephritis. *Nephron*, 27, 297–301.

Cornish, J., Barabas, A. Z., Lannigan, R. & Rozin, G. J. (1989). Immunoregulation in Heymann nephritis. II. Functional studies. *British Journal of Experimental Pathology*, 70, 505–13.

Costanza, M. E., Pinn, V., Schwartz, R. S. & Nathanson, L. (1973). Carcinoembryonic antigen–antibody complexes in a patient with colonic carcinoma and nephrotic syndrome. *New England Journal of Medicine*, **289**, 520–2.

Couser, W. G., Steinmuller, D. R. & Stilmant, M. M. (1978). Experimental glomerulonephritis in the isolated perfused rat kidney. *Journal of Clinical Investigation*, **62**, 1275–87.

Couser, W. G., Wagonfeld, J. B., Spargo, B. H. & Lewis, E. J. (1974). Glomerular deposition of tumor antigen in membranous nephropathy associated with colonic carcinoma. *American Journal of Medicine*, **57**, 962–70.

Cybulsky, A. U., Salant, D. J., Quigg, R. J., Badalamenti, J. & Bonventre, J. V. (1989). Complement C5b-9 complex activates phospholipases in glomerular epithelial cells. *American Journal of Physiology*, **257**, F826-36.

de Heer, E., Daha, M. R., Bhakdi, S., Bazin, H. & Van Es, L. A. (1985). Possible involvement of terminal complement complex in active Heymann nephritis. *Kidney International*, **27**, 388–93.

de Heer, E., Daha, M. R., Burgers, J. & Van Es, L. A. (1986). Reestablishment of self tolerance by suppressor T-cells after active Heymann's nephritis. *Cellular Immunology*, **98**, 28–33.

De Santo, N. G., Capodicasa, G. & Giordano, C. (1987). Treatment of idiopathic membranous nephropathy unresponsive to methylprednisolone and chlorambucil with cyclosporin (letter). *American Journal of Nephrology*, **7**, 74–6.

Demaine, A. G., Cameron, J. S., Taube, D. T., Vaughan, R. W. & Welsh, K. I. (1984). Immunoglobulin (Gm) allotype frequencies in idiopathic membranous nephropathy and minimal change nephropathy. *Transplantation*, **37**, 507–8.

Demaine, A. G., Vaughan, R. W., Taube, D. H. & Welsh, K. I. (1988). Association of membranous nephropathy with T-cell receptor constant beta chain and immunoglobulin heavy chain switch region polymorphisms. *Immunogenetics*, **27**, 19–23.

Dixon, F. J. (1968). The pathogenesis of glomerulonephritis. *American Journal of Medicine*, **44**, 493–8.

Donadio, J. V. Jr., Torres, V. E., Velosa, J. A. *et al.* (1988). Idiopathic membranous nephropathy: the natural history of untreated patients. *Kidney International*, **33**, 708–15.

Douglas, M. F. S., Rabideau, D. P., Schwartz, M. M. & Lewis, E. J. (1981). Evidence of autologous immune-complex nephritis. *New England Journal of Medicine*, **305**, 1326–9.

Dyer, P. A., Klouda, P. T., Harris, R. & Mallick, N. P. (1980). Properdin factor B alleles in patients with idiopathic membranous nephropathy. *Tissue Antigens*, **15**, 505–7.

Ebert, T. H., McClusky, R. T., Collins, A. B. & Colvin, R. B. (1981). Modulation of autologous immune complex nephritis (AIC) by pre-immunization with autoantibodies or sensitized cells. *Kidney International*, **19**, 181.(Abstract)

Edgington, T. S., Glassock, R. J. & Dixon, F. J. (1968). Autologous immune complex nephritis induced with renal tubular antigen. I. Identification and isolation of the pathogenetic antigen. *Journal of Experimental Medicine*, **127**, 555–72.

Ehrenreich, T. & Churg, J. (1968). Pathology of membranous nephropathy. In *Pathology Annual*, ed. S. C. Sommers, pp. 145–86. New York: Appleton-Century-Crofts.

Farid, N. R. & Bear, J. C. (1981). The human major histocompatibility complex and endocrine disease. *Endocrine Reviews*, **2**, 50–86.

Feenstra, K., van de Lee, R., Greben, H. A., Arends, A. & Hoedemaeker, P. H. J. (1975). Experimental glomerulonephritis in the rat induced by antibodies directed against tubular antigen. I. The natural history: a histologic and immunohistologic study at the light microscopic and ultrastructural level. *Laboratory Investigation*, **32**, 235–42.

Franklin, W. A., Jennings, R. B. & Earle, D. P. (1973). Membranous glomerulonephritis: long-term serial observations on clinical course and morphology. *Kidney International*, **4**, 36–56.

Friend, P. S. (1978). A unique antibody response associated with the development of membranous nephropathy in systemic lupus erythematosus. *American Heart Journal*, 95, 672–3.

Fukatsu, A., Yuzawa, Y., Olson, L. *et al.* (1989). Interaction of antibodies with human glomerular epithelial cells. *Laboratory Investigation*, 61, 389–403.

Garovoy, M. R. (1980). Idiopathic membranous glomerulonephritis: an HLA-associated disease. In *Histocompatibility Testing 1980*, ed. P. I. Terasaki, pp. 673–680. Los Angeles: UCLA.

Garovoy, M. R., Braun, W. B. & Duquesnoy, R. (1980). Idiopathic membranous glomerulonephritis (IMGN): association with a new B cell antigen (MT) system in the major histocompatibility complex. *Clinical Research*, 28, 445A.(Abstract).

Gilboa, N. (1981). Membranous nephropathy: further evidence against the involvement of renal tubular epithelial antigens (letter). *Nephron*, 27, 323.

Goodman, M. G. & Weigle, W. O. (1981). Nonspecific activation of murine lymphocytes. VIII. Effects of D-penicillamine. *Cellular Immunology*, 65, 337–51.

Goodyer, P. R., Mills, M. & Kaplan, B. S. (1986). Analysis of the Heymann nephritogenic glycoprotein in rat, mouse, and human kidney. *Biochemistry and Cell Biology*, 64, 441–7.

Gronhagen-Riska, C., von Willebrand, E., Tikkanen, T. *et al.* (1990). The effect of cyclosporin A on the interstitial mononuclear cell infiltration and the induction of Heymann's nephritis. *Clinical and Experimental Immunology*, 79, 266–72.

Hall, C. L., Fothergill, N. J., Blackwell, M. M., Harrison, P. R., MacKenzie, J. C. & MacIver, A. G. (1987). The natural course of gold nephropathy: long term study of 21 patients. *British Medical Journal*, 295, 745–8.

Hall, C. L., Jawad, S., Harrison, P. R. *et al.* (1988). Natural course of penicillamine nephropathy: a long term study of 33 patients. *British Medical Journal*, 296, 1083–6.

Hall-Craggs, M. & Ramos, E. (1981). Transformation of diffuse proliferative glomerulonephritis to membranous nephritis in a patient with systemic lupus erythematosus. *Nephron*, 28, 42–5.

Harmon, W. E., Grupe, W. E. & Parkman, R. (1980). Control of autologous immune complex nephritis. I. Suppression of the disease in the presence of T cell sensitization. *Journal of Immunology*, 124, 1034–8.

Hassan, A. A., Le Petit, J. C. & Berthoux, F. C. (1987). Immunogenetics of membranous glomerulonephritis. *Kidney International*, 32, 606.(Abstract).

Heymann, W., Hackel, D. B., Harwood, S., Wilson, S. G. F. & Hunter, J. L. P. (1959). Production of nephrotic syndrome in rats by Freund's adjuvant and rat kidney suspensions. *Proceedings of the Society for Experimental Biology and Medicine*, 100, 660–4.

Hiki, Y., Kobayashi, Y., Itoh, I. & Kashiwagi, N. (1984). Strong association of HLA-DR2 and MT1 with idiopathic membranous nephropathy in Japan. *Kidney International*, 25, 953–67.

Hirose, H., Udo, K., Kojima, M. *et al.* (1984). Deposits of hepatitis B e antigen in membranous glomerulonephritis: identification by F(ab')₂ fragments of monoclonal antibody. *Kidney International*, 26, 338–41.

Hopper, J. (1989). Prednisone in the treatment of idiopathic membranous nephropathy (letter). *New England Journal of Medicine*, 321, 260–1.

Hori, M. T. & Abrass, C. K. (1990). Isolation and characterization of circulating immune complexes from rats with experimental membranous nephropathy. *Journal of Immunology*, 144, 3849–55.

Huang, C. C. (1989). Strong association of HLA-DR3 in Chinese patients with idiopathic membranous nephropathy. *Tissue Antigens*, 33, 425–6.

Ito, H., Hattori, S., Matusda, I. *et al.* (1981). Hepatitis B e antigen-mediated membranous glomerulonephritis. Correlation of ultrastructural changes with HBeAg in the serum and glomeruli. *Laboratory Investigation*, 44, 214–20.

Izui, S., Lambert, P-H. & Miescher, P. A. (1976). In vitro demonstration of a particular affinity of glomerular basement membrane and collagen for DNA. A possible basis for a local formation of DNA–anti-DNA complexes in systemic lupus erythematosus. *Journal of Experimental Medicine*, **144**, 428–43.

Jacobs, C., Brunner, F. P., Chantler, C. *et al.* (1977). Combined report on regular dialysis and transplantation in Europe, VII, 1976. *Proceedings of the European Dialysis and Transplantation Association*, **14**, 3–69.

Jaffe, I. A. (1979). Penicillamine in rheumatoid arthritis: clinical pharmacology and biochemical properties. *Scandinavian Journal of Rheumatology*, Suppl **28**, 58–64.

Jordan, S. C., Buckingham, B., Sakai, R. & Olson, D. (1981). Studies of immune-complex glomerulonephritis mediated by human thyroglobulin. *New England Journal of Medicine*, **304**, 1212–15.

Kerjaschki, D. & Farquhar, M. G. (1982). The pathogenic antigen of Heymann nephritis is a membrane glycoprotein of the renal proximal tubule brush border. *Proceedings of the National Academy of Sciences, USA*, **79**, 5557–61.

Kerjaschki, D. & Farquhar, M. G. (1983). Immunocytochemical localization of the Heymann nephritis antigen (GP330) in glomerular epithelial cells of normal Lewis rats. *Journal of Experimental Medicine*, **157**, 667–86.

Kerjaschki, D., Miettinen, A. & Farquhar, M. G. (1987). Initial events in the formation of immune deposits in passive Heymann nephritis. *Journal of Experimental Medicine*, **166**, 109–28.

Kerjaschki, D., Horvat, R., Binder, S. *et al.* (1987). Identification of a 400-kD protein in the brush border of human kidney tubules that is similar to gp330, the nephritogenic antigen of rat Heymann nephritis. *American Journal of Pathology*, **129**, 183–91.

Kerjaschki, D. (1989). In Nephrology Forum: kinetics of immune deposits in membranous nephropathy. *Kidney International*, **35**, 1418–28.

Klouda, P. T., Manos, J., Acheson, E. J. *et al.* (1979). Strong association between idiopathic membranous nephropathy and HLA-DRw3. *Lancet*, **ii**, 770–1.

Lai, K. N., Mac-Moune, F. & Tam, J. S. (1989). Comparison of polyclonal and monoclonal antibodies in determination of glomerular deposits of hepatitis B virus antigen in hepatitis B virus-associated glomerulonephritis. *American Journal of Clinical Pathology*, **92**, 159–65.

Latham, P., Poucell, S., Koresaar, A., Arbus, G. & Baumal, R. (1982). Idiopathic membranous glomerulopathy in Canadian children: a clinicopathologic study. *Journal of Pediatrics*, **101**, 682–5.

Le Petit, J. C., Laurent, B. & Berthoux, F. C. (1982). HLA-DR3 and idiopathic membranous nephritis (IMN) association. *Tissue Antigens*, **20**, 227–8.

Lentz, R. D., Michael, A. F. & Friend, P. S. (1981). Membranous transformation of lupus nephritis. *Clinical Immunology and Immunopathology*, **19**, 131–8.

Lew, A. M., Staines, N. A. & Steward, M. W. (1984). Glomerulonephritis induced by preformed immune complexes containing monoclonal antibodies of defined affinity and isotype. *Clinical and Experimental Immunology*, **57**, 413–22.

Lewis, E. J., Bolton, W. K., Spargo, B. A. & Stuart, F. P. (1972). Persistent proteinuria in the rat with Heymann (autologous immune complex) nephritis. *Clinical Research*, **20**, 763.(Abstract).

Lewis, M. G., Loughridge, L. W. & Phillips, T. M. (1971). Immunological studies in nephrotic syndrome associated with extrarenal malignant disease. *Lancet*, **ii**, 134–5.

Lin, C. Y. (1990). Hepatitis B virus-associated membranous nephropathy: clinical features, immunological profile and outcome. *Nephron*, **55**, 37–44.

Maggiore, Q., Bartolomeo, F., L'Abbate, A. & Misefari, V. (1981). HBsAg glomerular deposits in glomerulonephritis: fact or artifact? *Kidney International*, **19**, 579–86.

Makker, S. P. & Kanalas, J. J. (1989). Course of transplanted Heymann nephritis kidney in normal host. Implications for mechanism of proteinuria in membranous glomerulonephropathy. *Journal of Immunology*, 142, 3406–10.

Mathieson, P. W. & Rees, A. J. (1990). A critical review of treatment for membranous nephropathy. In *Advances in Nephrology vol. 19*, ed. J-P. Grunfeld, J. F. Bach, J-L. Funck-Brentano & M. H. Maxwell, pp. 145–67. Chicago, London, Boca Raton: Year Book Medical Publishers, Inc.

Mathieson, P. W., Turner, A. N., Maidment, C. G. H., Evans, D. J. & Rees, A. J. (1988). Prednisolone and chlorambucil treatment in idiopathic membranous nephropathy with deteriorating renal function. *Lancet*, ii, 869–72.

Matsumoto, K., Osakabe, K. & Hatano, M. (1983). Impaired cell-mediated immunity in idiopathic membranous nephropathy mediated by suppressor cells. *Clinical Nephrology*, 19, 213–14.

Mendrick, D. L., Chung, D. C. & Rennke, H. G. (1990). Heymann antigen GP330 demonstrates affinity for fibronectin, laminin, and type I collagen and mediates proximal tubule epithelial adherence to such matrices *in vitro*. *Experimental Cell Research*, 188, 23–35.

Moore, R. H., Hitman, G. A., Sinico, R. A. *et al.* (1990). Immunoglobulin heavy chain switch gene polymorphisms in glomerulonephritis. *Kidney International*, 38, 332–6.

Müller, G. A,, Müller, C., Liebau, G., Kömpf, J., Ising, H. & Wernet, P. (1981). Strong association of idiopathic membranous nephropathy (IMN) with HLA-DR3 and MT-2 without involvement of HLA-B18 and no association to BfF1. *Tissue Antigens*, 17, 332–7.

Naruse, T., Kitamura, K., Miyakawa, Y. & Shibata, S. (1973). Deposition of renal tubular epithelial antigen along the glomerular capillary walls of patients with membranous nephropathy. *Journal of Immunology*, 110, 1163–6.

Nauta, J., de Heer, E., Baldwin, W. M., ten Kate, F. J., van den Heijden, A. J. & Wolff, E. D. (1990). Transplacental induction of membranous nephropathy in a neonate. *Paediatric Nephrology*, 4, 111–16.

Niles, J., Collins, B., Baird, L. *et al.* (1987). Antibodies reactive with a renal glycoprotein and with deposits in membranous nephritis. *Kidney International*, 31, 338.(Abstract).

Nishimukai, H., Nakanishi, I., Takeuch, Y. *et al.* (1989). Complement C6 and C7 polymorphisms in Japanese patients with chronic glomerulonephritis. *Human Heredity*, 39, 150–5.

Niven, M. J., Caffrey, C., Moore, R. H. *et al.* (1990). T-cell receptor beta-subunit gene polymorphisms and autoimmune disease. *Human Immunology*, 27, 360–7.

Noel, L. H., Zanetti, M., Droz, D. & Barbanel, C. (1979). Long-term prognosis of idiopathic membranous glomerulonephritis. Study of 116 untreated patients. *American Journal of Medicine*, 66, 82–90.

Noël, L-H., Aucouturier, P., Monteiro, R. C., Preud'homme, J-L. & Lesavre, P. (1988). Glomerular and serum immunoglobulin G subclasses in membranous nephropathy and antiglomerular basement membrane nephritis. *Clinical Immunology and Immunopathology*, 46, 186–94.

Oite, T., Batsford, S. R., Mihatsch, M. J., Takamiya, H. & Vogt, A. (1982). Quantitative study of *in situ* immune complex glomerulonephritis in the rat induced by planted, cationized antigen. *Journal of Experimental Medicine*, 155, 460–74.

Palla, R., Bionda, A. & Marchitiello, M. (1986). High-dose intravenous gammaglobulin for membranous nephropathy (letter). *Clinical Nephrology*, 26, 314.

Papiha, S. S., Pareek, S. K., Rodger, R. S. C. *et al.* (1987). HLA-A, B, DR and Bf allotypes in patients with idiopathic membranous nephropathy (IMN). *Kidney International*, 31, 130–4.

Pelletier, L., Galceran, M., Pasquier, R. *et al.* (1987). Down modulation of Heymann's nephritis by mercuric chloride. *Kidney International*, 32, 227–32.

Ponticelli, C., Zucchelli, P., Imbasciati, E. *et al.* (1984). Controlled trial of methylprednisolone and chlorambucil in idiopathic membranous nephropathy. *New England Journal of Medicine*, 310, 946–50.

Ponticelli, C., Zucchelli, P., Passerini, P. *et al.* (1989). A randomized trial of methylpredniso-lone and chlorambucil in idiopathic membranous nephropathy. *New England Journal of Medicine*, **320**, 8–13.

Pusey, C. D., Venning, M. C. & Peters, D. K. (1988). Immunopathology of glomerular and interstitial disease. In *Diseases of the Kidney*, 4th edn, ed. R. W. Schrier & C. W. Gottschalk, pp. 1827–83. Boston/Toronto: Little, Brown and Company.

Ramirez, F., Brouhard, B. H., Travis, L. B. & Ellis, E. N. (1982). Idiopathic membranous nephropathy in children. *Journal of Pediatrics*, **101**, 677–81.

Ramzy, M. H., Cameron, J. S., Turner, D. R., Neild, G. H., Ogg, C. S. & Hicks, J. (1981). The long-term outcome of idiopathic membranous nephropathy. *Clinical Nephrology*, **16**, 13–19.

Rashid, H. U., Papiha, S. S., Agroyannis, B. *et al.* (1983). The association of HLA and other genetic markers with glomerulonephritis. *Human Genetics*, **63**, 38–44.

Richet, G., Fillastre, J-P., Morel-Maroger, L. & Bariety, J. (1974). Change from diffuse proliferative to membranous glomerulonephritis: serial biopsies in four cases. *Kidney International*, **5**, 57–71.

Rostoker, G., Toro, L., Ben Maadi, A. *et al.* (1989). Cyclosporin in idiopathic steroid-resistant membranous glomerulonephritis (letter). *Lancet*, **ii**, 975–6.

Rothschild, E. & Chatenoud, L. (1984). T cell subset modulation of immunoglobulin pro-duction in IgA nephropathy and membranous glomerulonephritis. *Kidney International*, **25**, 557–64.

Row, P. G., Cameron, J. S., Turner, D. R. *et al.* (1975). Membranous nephropathy: long-term follow-up and association with neoplasia. *Quarterly Journal of Medicine*, **44**, 207–39.

Sacks, S. H., Bushell, A., Rust, N. A. *et al.* (1987). Functional and biochemical subtypes of the haplotype HLA-DR3 in patients with coeliac disease or idiopathic membranous nephro-pathy. *Human Immunology*, **20**, 175–87.

Sheehy, M. J., Scharf, S. J., Rowe, J. R. *et al.* (1989). A diabetes-susceptible HLA haplotype is best defined by a combination of HLA-DR and -DQ alleles. *Journal of Clinical Investigation*, **83**, 830–5.

Short, C. D., Dyer, P. A., Cairns, S. A. *et al.* (1983). A major histocompatibility system haplotype associated with poor prognosis in idiopathic membranous nephropathy. *Disease Markers*, **1**, 189–96.

Sim, E., Dodds, A. W. & Goldin, A. (1989). Inhibition of the covalent binding reaction of complement component C4 by penicillamine, an anti-rheumatic agent. *Biochemical Journal*, **259**, 415–19.

Singh, A. K. & Makker, S. P. (1985). Isolation and characterization of antigens in normal rat serum which cross react with the nephritogenic GP60-antigen of Heymann nephritis. *Kidney International*, **27**, 223.(Abstract).

Skrifvars, B. (1979). Hypothesis for the pathogenesis of sodium aurothiomalate induced immune complex nephritis. *Scandinavian Journal of Rheumatology*, **8**, 113–18.

Speerstra, R., Reekers, P., van der Putte, L. B., van den Brouche, J. R., Rasker, J. J. & de Rooi, D. J. (1983). HLA-DR antigens and proteinuria induced by aurothioglucose and D-penicillamine in patients with rheumatoid arthritis. *Journal of Rheumatology*, **10**, 448–53.

Stenglen, B., Thoenes, G. H. & Günther, E. (1978). Genetic control of susceptibility to autologous immune complex glomerulonephritis in inbred rat strains. *Clinical and Experi-mental Immunology*, **33**, 88–94.

Taube, D., Brown, Z. & Williams, D. G. (1984). Impaired lymphocyte and suppressor cell function in minimal change nephropathy, membranous nephropathy and focal glomerulo-sclerosis. *Clinical Nephrology*, **22**, 176–82.

Thorpe, L. W. & Cavallo, T. (1980). Renal tubule brush border antigens: failure to confirm a pathogenic role in human membranous glomerulonephritis. *Journal of Clinical and Labora-tory Immunology*, **3**, 125–7.

Tomura, S., Kashiwabara, H., Tuchida, H. *et al.* (1984). Strong association of idiopathic membranous nephropathy with HLA-DR2 and MT1 in Japanese. *Nephron*, **36**, 242–5.

Truong, L., Gelfand, J., D'Agati, V. *et al.* (1989). De novo membranous glomerulonephropathy in renal allografts: a report of ten cases and review of the literature. *American Journal of Kidney Disease*, **14**, 131–44.

Tu, W-H., Petitti, D. B., Biava, C. G., Tulunay, Ö. & Hopper, J. (1983). Membranous nephropathy: predictors of terminal renal failure. *Nephron*, **36**, 118–24.

Törnroth, T., Honkanen, E. & Pettersson, E. (1987). The evolution of membranous glomerulonephritis reconsidered: new insights from a study on relapsing disease. *Clinical Nephrology*, **28**, 107–17.

van Damme, B. J. C., Fleuren, G. J., Bakker, W. W., Vernier, R. L. & Hoedemaeker, Ph. J. (1978). Experimental glomerulonephritis in the rat induced by antibodies directed against tubular antigens. V. Fixed glomerular antigens in the pathogenesis of heterologous immune complex glomerulonephritis. *Laboratory Investigation*, **38**, 502–10.

Vaughan, R. W., Demaine, A. G. & Welsh, K. I. (1989). A DQA1 allele is stongly associated with idiopathic membranous nephropathy. *Tissue Antigens*, **34**, 261–9.

Velosa, J. A., Torres, V. E., Donadio, J. V., Wagoner, R. D., Holley, K. E. & Offord, K. P. (1985). Treatment of severe nephrotic syndrome with meclofenamate: an uncontrolled pilot study. *Mayo Clinic Proceedings*, **60**, 586–92.

Venkataseshan, V. S., Lieberman, K., Kim, D. U. *et al.* (1990). Hepatitis-B-associated glomerulonephritis: pathology, pathogenesis, and clinical course. *Medicine*, **69**, 200–16.

Verroust, P. J. (1989). Kinetics of immune deposits in membranous nephropathy. *Kidney International*, **35**, 1418–28.

Wank, R., Schendel, D. J., O'Neil, G. J., Riethmüller, G., Held, E. & Feucht, H. E. (1984). Rare variant of complement C4 is seen in high frequency in patients with primary glomerulonephritis. *Lancet*, **i**, 872–4.

Warwick, G. & Boulton-Jones, J. M. (1988). Immunosuppression for membranous nephropathy (letter). *Lancet*, **ii**, 1361.

Welch, T. R. & Beischel, L. (1985). C4 uremic variant: an acquired C4 allotype. *Immunogenetics*, **22**, 553–62.

Wetzels, J. F. M., Hoitsma, A. J. & Koene, R. A. P. (1989). Immunosuppression for membranous nephropathy (letter). *Lancet*, **i**, 211.

Whitworth, J. A., Leibowitz, S., Kennedy, M. C. *et al.* (1976). Absence of glomerular renal tubular epithelial antigen in membranous glomerulonephritis. *Clinical Nephrology*, **5**, 159–62.

Williams, P. S. & Bone, J. M. (1989). Immunosuppression can arrest progressive renal failure due to idiopathic membranous glomerulonephritis. *Nephrology Dialysis and Transplantation*, **4**, 181–6.

Woodrow, J. C. (1988). Immunogenetics of systemic lupus erythematosus. *Journal of Rheumatology*, **15**, 197–9.

Zager, R. A., Couser, W. G., Andrews, B. S., Bolton, W. K. & Pohl, M. A. (1979). Membranous nephropathy: a radioimmunologic search for anti-renal tubular epithelial antibodies and circulating immune complexes. *Nephron*, **24**, 10–16.

Zietse, R., Wenting, G. J., Kramer, P., Mulder, P., Schalekamp, M. A. & Weimar, W. (1989). Contrasting response to cyclosporin in refractory nephrotic syndrome. *Clinical Nephrology*, **31**, 22–5.

Zucchelli, P., Ponticelli, C., Cagnoli, L., Aroldi, A. & Tabacchi, P. (1987*a*). Genetic factors in the outcome of idiopathic membranous nephropathy (letter). *Nephrology Dialysis and Transplantation*, **1**, 265–6.

Zucchelli, P., Ponticelli, C., Cagnoli, L. & Passerini, P. (1987*b*). Long-term outcome of idiopathic membranous nephropathy with nephrotic syndrome. *Nephrology Dialysis and Transplantation*, **2**, 73–8.

–4–
Lupus nephritis

Systemic lupus erythematosus (SLE) is a multi-system disease characterised by the production of a wide range of autoantibodies, particularly anti-nuclear antibodies. It is a relatively common disease, with a prevalence in caucasian populations of approximately 1 in 2000–3000 adult females (sex ratio 9 female:1 male); this rises to approximately 1 in 200–300 American black females (Fessel, 1974). Criteria for the classification of SLE based on the diverse clinical manifestations and laboratory investigations have been published (Tan *et al.*, 1982). There is a large literature on SLE, much of which is outside the scope of this chapter, which will attempt to concentrate on the renal manifestations. More general aspects will be dealt with in another volume in this series. This chapter will also concentrate on glomerular involvement; interstitial nephritis in the context of SLE is considered further in Chapter 9.

The incidence of renal involvement in SLE depends on how vigorously it is sought. Using simple clinical criteria (proteinuria, urine sediment, renal function) such involvement is present in approximately two thirds of patients at diagnosis; this rises to 90% if a renal biopsy is included in the investigations, and almost 100% if electron microscopy and immunofluor-escence are used to examine the biopsy (Glassock *et al.*, 1986). Renal involvement is responsible for a significant proportion of the morbidity and mortality associated with SLE. In one series ten year survival was 76% when nephritis was present but 93% when absent (Wallace *et al.*, 1981); these figures, however, are not particularly useful in an individual case as the renal prognosis varies considerably depending on the type of renal involvement (see below).

The clinical manifestations of lupus nephritis cover a wide range of presentations, including hypertension, trivial proteinuria or haematuria, the nephrotic syndrome, acute crescentic nephritis and end-stage renal failure. There is some correlation (see below) between these clinical features and the appearances on renal biopsy, which can be classified on the basis of general glomerular morphology (light and electron microscopy, immunoflu-orescence) and in terms of an activity and chronicity index. The principal morphological classification in use is that of the World Health Organisation (Glassock *et al.*, 1986; Hayslett & Kashgarian, 1988), which has five principal patterns, with some workers recognising a sixth. Class I comprises normal glomeruli, with no evidence of immune deposits by electron microscopy or immunofluorescence; as mentioned above, this is very rare. In Class II, changes are confined to the mesangium; in IIa immunofluorescence and electron microscopy reveal mesangial deposits with normal light microscopy, whilst in IIb there is evidence of uniform mesangial hypercellularity as well. In all classes, immune deposits often contain a 'full house' of IgG, IgM, IgA and complement components. Classes III and IV (proliferative glomerulonephritis) probably represent a continuum, and are distinguished from each other by the extent of involvement. Both have light microscopic changes of a focal and segmental glomerulonephritis superimposed on the mesangial changes noted above; the changes may be proliferative, necrotising or sclerosing. Electron microscopy reveals deposits in the capillary walls, usually in a subendothelial position. Crescents may also be present. By definition, less than 50% of glomeruli are involved in Class III, and greater than 50% in Class IV. Class V (membranous) is very similar in appearance to idiopathic membranous nephropathy (see Chapter 3), except that mesangial deposits are usually present. The Class VI distinguished by some is characterised by sclerosing changes; it is unclear whether this can be a primary response to immunological injury (Baldwin *et al.*, 1977), or whether it simply represents the end-stage of the abnormalities found in other classes.

There are some approximate clinical correlates with these classes (Baldwin *et al.*, 1977; Gladman *et al.*, 1989): a membranous pattern is often associated with the nephrotic syndrome, as is the diffuse proliferative type; the latter, however, is associated with impaired renal function in approximately 50% of cases and may present with the clinical picture of rapidly progressive glomerulonephritis. There are many exceptions to these generalisations, e.g. some patients with severe diffuse proliferative changes may have minimal clinical evidence of renal involvement. There is more uniformity with respect to the significance of a particular pattern for long-term renal prognosis. The individual patterns tend to be stable over time (Appel *et al.*, 1987), although transformations are well recognised (Baldwin *et al.*, 1977), particularly class III evolving to class IV, and the proliferative forms transforming into a membranous pattern with treatment (Hecht *et al.*, 1976). It is rare for class II to transform into a more severe lesion, and this pattern has a good long-term prognosis (Appel *et al.*, 1987). The proliferative patterns, particularly class IV, carry the worst prognosis. The prognostic significance of a membranous (class V) pattern is uncertain. Initial reports suggested that this was a relatively benign lesion, but a recent study found a relatively high rate of progression to renal failure (Appel *et al.*, 1987).

Subgroups within this category, particularly those with superimposed proliferative features, may carry a particularly poor prognosis (Adler *et al.*, 1990).

Apart from the WHO class, other features that may be of prognostic importance are the chronicity index (see below) and electron-dense subendothelial deposits. The presence of such deposits, irrespective of whether a focal or diffuse proliferative lesion was present, was correlated with heavy proteinuria and renal insufficiency (Tateno *et al.*, 1983). Their significance is perhaps emphasised by the disappearance of deposits with a successful response to treatment, and their persistence otherwise (Hecht *et al.*, 1976).

Histological assessment may also include activity and chronicity indices (Austin *et al.*, 1983). An activity index incorporates features such as cellular proliferation, crescents, fibrinoid necrosis and mononuclear cell infiltration, whilst a chronicity index emphasises glomerular sclerosis, interstitial fibrosis and tubular atrophy. The suggestion is that the activity index may indicate the potential for reversibility with treatment, whereas the chronicity index predicts long-term renal prognosis. Another study, however, found no relationship between the chronicity index and renal prognosis (Appel *et al.*, 1987). This may reflect a difference in the populations studied, as there was a much higher proportion of patients with proliferative lesions in the study by Austin *et al.* However, even in the subgroup of patients with diffuse proliferative lupus nephritis other work suggests that the sensitivity and specificity of the chronicity index as a predictor of renal failure are too low for it to be a useful measure (Schwartz *et al.*, 1989), although not all agree (Nossent *et al.*, 1990). It has been suggested that an index of tubulointerstitial damage is a better predictor of renal outcome than the activity or chronicity indices (Esdaile *et al.*, 1989).

Immunogenetics

Much of the following discussion applies to the immunogenetics of SLE in general, but where available data relating specifically to lupus nephritis are included. An idea of the genetic contribution to the aetiology of SLE can be gained from the increased incidence in first degree relatives of patients (approximately 1–2% versus 0.05% in the general population; Siegel & Lee, 1973). That this is mainly due to shared genetic rather than environmental factors is shown by the concordance rates in monozygotic twins of 60%–70% (Block *et al.*, 1975).

The MHC

Following the familiar pattern, initial associations with SLE were described with a number of class I alleles (for review see Walport, Black & Batchelor,

1982). These associations were almost certainly secondary to associations with other MHC loci, as subsequent studies have consistently shown stronger links with DR2 and DR3 (for review see Woodrow, 1988). A pooled analysis of these studies has shown that in caucasian populations DR2 and DR3 are associated with relative risks of 2 and 2.4 respectively, with no evidence of significant heterogeneity between studies (Woodrow, 1988). Non-significant associations with DR2, but not DR3, have been found in Japanese populations (Kameda et al., 1982; Hashimoto et al., 1985), and a significant association with DR2 in southern China (Hawkins et al., 1987), where there is a low incidence of DR3. The situation for American black patients is less clear, as with some exceptions (Alarif et al., 1983 showing a link with DR3), most studies have shown no significant associations with alleles at either DR (Gladman et al., 1979; Howard et al., 1986) or DQ (Reveille et al., 1989). One study looked at a number of ethnic groups and compared patients with and without renal involvement (Fronek et al., 1988). This showed that the clinical subset with lupus nephritis were more genetically homogeneous despite ethnic differences, and that a particular DR2 allele, DR2-DQw1.AZH, was increased in the nephritic versus non-nephritic subgroups with a relative risk of 8.3 in all ethnic groups. The serologically defined DQw1 allele (which is linked to DR2) was also increased in the nephritic subgroup (relative risk 4.4), whereas DR4 was decreased (relative risk 0.3). Further analysis has demonstrated that at least one of three particular DQβ alleles (DQβ1.AZH, DQβ1.1 or DQβ1.9) is found in 50% of cases of lupus nephritis (Fronek et al., 1990). These alleles share polymorphic residues in the first and third hypervariable regions, and these residues could therefore be of particular importance in the predisposition to nephritis in lupus.

Of the complement components coded for within the MHC, genetically determined deficiencies of C2 (Glass et al., 1976) and C4 are associated with immune complex diseases in general and lupus-like syndromes in particular. This association is particularly striking for C4A in that 11–14% of patients with SLE are homozygous for the C4A*Q0 null allele compared to 1% of controls (Fielder et al., 1983; Howard et al., 1986), and there is a correspondingly increased incidence of heterozygotes for C4A*Q0. The linkage disequilibrium between the C4A*Q0 null allele and DR3 in Caucasian populations, particularly in the context of the A1 B8 C4A*Q0 C4B1 DR3 haplotype, raises the question as to whether the associations between SLE and these two alleles are independent, or whether one is secondary to the other. The evidence suggests that it is, in fact, the association with C4A*Q0 that is the primary association. First, a re-analysis of the data from (Fielder et al., 1983) suggests that the DR3 association is secondary (Green, Montasser & Woodrow, 1986). Secondly, when only DR3 negative patients and controls are studied, the incidence of C4A*Q0 is still increased in patients (Woodrow, 1988). Finally, in populations with a low incidence of DR3 (Hawkins et al., 1987), or in which there are no recognised class II associations (Goldstein et al., 1988), an increased incidence of C4A null alleles is still observed. The evidence suggests that homozygous C4A deficiency has a relative risk for the development of SLE of 24, and the heterozygous state a relative risk of 3 (Woodrow, 1988). By contrast, whether C4B deficiency alone is associated with an increased incidence of SLE is less certain, and it may be relevant in this context that C4A is almost twice as efficient as C4B at preventing immune complex precipitation (Schifferli et al., 1986). One piece of indirect evidence that C4B deficiency may be important is the finding of a DR4 association with hydralazine-induced lupus (Speirs et al., 1989). This study showed an increased incidence of null complement alleles for both C4A and C4B, just as in idiopathic SLE. However, it is only the C4B null allele that is in linkage disequilibrium with DR4, and the association with this class II allele may therefore imply a specific role for C4B deficiency.

Recent data suggest that some of the above studies demonstrating a link between C4 null alleles and lupus must be interpreted with caution. It may be that this link is particularly important in English/Irish populations, and it has, in fact, not been found in other ethnic groups (Fronek et al., 1990; Schur et al., 1990).

Complement deficiencies may also be involved in the DR2 association: although C4A null alleles are linked to DR3, an abnormal C4A protein appears to be DR2 associated (Fronek et al., 1988). The C2 deficiencies mentioned above as predisposing to SLE are also DR2 linked (Agnello, 1978). These consistent links between abnormalities of complement components (see also non-MHC complement genes below) and SLE has led to the proposal that they are causal, and that acquired deficiencies of complement may be involved in the aetiology of SLE not associated with genetic deficiencies (Lachmann, 1987). This hypothesis is considered further in the final section of this chapter.

In addition to the complement genes, other linked loci may also contribute to the MHC class II gene associations. Thus DR2 and DQw1 individuals frequently exhibit low production of tumour necrosis factor (TNF) alpha by their mitogen-stimulated peripheral blood lymphocytes (Jacob et al., 1990). This is of particular interest given that the DR2, DQw1-positive genotype is associated with a relatively high incidence of nephritis (Fronek et al., 1990), and that decreased production of TNF is linked to an increase in the severity of nephritis in a mouse model (see below).

Finally in the context of the MHC, some of the autoantibodies found in SLE and certain other rheumatological diseases (mixed connective tissue disease, primary Sjögren's syndrome), have closer associations with MHC alleles than do their parent diseases (Arnett et al., 1988). Thus patients with anti-Ro and/or anti-La antibodies are mostly DR2 or DR3 positive; lupus patients who develop epidermolysis bullosa acquisita, caused by an autoantibody to type VII collagen, are almost all DR2 positive. This link does not extend to some of the autoantibody idiotypes that appear closely associated with lupus nephritis (Hahn et al., 1990; idiotypes discussed further below).

Other loci

As mentioned above, hereditary deficiencies of complement components coded for outside the MHC are also associated with a high incidence of SLE-like diseases, as are deficiencies of complement control proteins (for review see Rynes, 1982). The CR1 receptor for breakdown products of C3 and C4, found principally on erythrocytes (Siegel, Liu & Gleicher, 1981), is subject to allelic variation in density (Wilson et al., 1982). Because of the reduced levels of CR1 on erythrocytes from patients with SLE and their relatives, but not spouses (Wilson et al., 1982), an hereditary contribution was suspected. However, genotyping shows no difference in the frequency of the alleles in patients versus controls (Moldenhaur et al., 1987), suggesting that this deficiency is acquired.

Studies of T cell receptor β chain gene RFLPs have given variable results, with one study finding no differences between patients and controls (Fronek et al., 1986), whilst another found an increase in a particular RFLP pattern in DR3 positive SLE patients versus DR3 positive controls (Goldstein et al., 1987). Certain Gm allotypes appear to be linked to SLE in a number of racial groups, including Japanese (Nakao et al., 1980), Black Americans (Fedrick et al., 1983), and Caucasians (Whittingham et al., 1983; Schur, Pandey & Fedrick, 1985). A study of a Km light chain allotype found no difference between patients and controls (Schur, Pandey & Fedrick, 1985).

Any of the factors considered above could contribute to the increased incidence of lupus in relatives of patients. In addition, relatives have a higher incidence of raised immune complexes (Elkon et al., 1983), autoantibodies and hypergammaglobulinaemia (for review see Walport, Black & Batchelor, 1982), and share certain idiotypes found on anti-DNA antibodies (Isenberg et al., 1985; Halpern et al., 1985; Dudeney et al., 1986); some of these idiotypes, such as the 16/6 idiotype (see below), are probably germline encoded, as opposed to being derived via somatic mutation (Chen et al., 1988). Family members also exhibit defects in non-specific suppressor cell activity (Miller & Schwartz, 1979); the genetic substrate for this, if any, and its significance are unknown.

Immunopathology

Animal studies

Although an SLE-like disease has been found in a number of species, e.g. the dog (Lewis & Schwartz, 1971), the most extensively studied is the mouse, in which a number of SLE-prone strains exist (MRL/lpr, BXSB, (NZBxNZW)F$_1$). The following discussion will therefore be confined to murine lupus, and it should be noted that, even with this restriction, different factors are probably involved in each of the susceptible strains. Because of the vast literature on this topic, the discussion will necessarily be selective and focused on the pathogenesis of nephritis; more comprehensive reviews are available (see, for instance, Theofilopoulos et al., 1983a,b)

Autoantibodies

There is abundant evidence for polyclonal B cell activation (which may in part be T cell dependent; see next section) in these mouse models (see reviews referenced above), which is closely linked to the development of autoimmunity (Klinman, 1990). Although many autoantibodies are produced, particular interest has centred on anti-DNA antibodies, and to a lesser extent anti-retroviral antibodies (anti-gp70). Together, anti-nuclear and anti-retroviral antibodies make up the majority of the immunoglobulin eluted from the glomeruli of diseased mice (Dixon, Oldstone & Tonietti, 1971), and anti-nuclear antibodies, but not anti-gp70 antibodies, are concentrated in the glomerulus relative to serum (Andrews et al., 1978). The corresponding nuclear antigens can also be identified within the glomeruli (Lambert & Dixon, 1968), strengthening the case for an immune complex-mediated pathogenesis. Present evidence suggests that the DNA–anti-DNA system is involved in pathogenesis (Parker, Hahn & Osterland, 1974), whereas the anti-viral system is not (Andrews et al., 1978). In certain of the models, notably chronic graft-versus-host disease, there is also good evidence for the pathogenicity of autoantibodies directed against laminin and dipeptidyl peptidase IV (Bruijn et al., 1990).

The initial assumption was that pathogenic immune complexes were formed in the circulation and subsequently deposited within the glomerulus (Dixon, 1979). This may indeed be an important mechanism, but it is unlikely that pure DNA is involved in such complexes. Free DNA has a very short half-life within the circulation and is relatively non-immunogenic; it may be that DNA complexed to proteins in the form of chromatin represents the relevant immunogen (Fournié, 1988). More recently a number of other possible pathogenic mechanisms have been suggested. DNA has a particular affinity for the glomerular basement membrane and could act as a planted antigen at this site, leading to *in situ* immune complex formation (Izui, Lambert & Miescher, 1976). An experimental model involving the injection of lipopolysaccharide into mice is consistent with this (Izui *et al.*, 1977): large amounts of circulating DNA are found first, followed by the appearance of anti-DNA antibodies, and then by the deposition of complexes within the glomerulus. At no stage are circulating DNA–anti-DNA complexes detectable. However, other attempts to obtain indirect evidence for such local formation have been unsuccessful (Jones, Pisetsky & Kurlander, 1986). Finally, anti-DNA antibodies may cause damage by binding to molecules other than DNA. This possibility is suggested by the observation that monoclonal anti-DNA antibodies are also capable of binding to phospholipids (Lafer *et al.*, 1981), cell surface molecules (Tron, Jacob & Bach, 1984), and a variety of other structures. Support for this mechanism is provided by the observation that infusion of anti-DNA antibodies into an isolated perfused kidney causes proteinuria (Raz *et al.*, 1989); cross-reactivity with other glomerular components could explain this finding, but reactivity to DNA already bound *in situ* is not excluded. A further variation on this theme is provided by the very high affinity that histones manifest for the glomerular basement membrane (Schmiedeke *et al.*, 1989); it has been shown that the apparent cross-reactivity of some monoclonal anti-DNA antibodies for heparan sulphate (a major constituent of the glomerular basement membrane) is mediated via bound complexes of DNA and histones (Termaat *et al.*, 1990).

Common cross-reactive idiotypes are present on a high proportion of anti-DNA antibodies in NZB/W mice, and immunisation with such an idiotype (Hahn & Ebling, 1983), or administration of a monoclonal antiidiotypic antibody (Hahn & Ebling, 1984), suppresses the development of nephritis in NZB/W mice. Administration of other anti-DNA antibodies to MRL/lpr mice produces a protective antiidiotypic response, and furthermore this antiidiotype appears to define nephritogenic anti-DNA antibodies in man as well (Weisbart *et al.*, 1990). Even more remarkably, immunisation of non-lupus prone mice with a human monoclonal antibody bearing an important idiotype found in human SLE (the 16/6 id; see below) induces a lupus-like disease (Mendlovic *et al.*, 1988). This disease involves the production of a wide range of autoantibodies and immune complex deposition within the glomerular mesangium; these complexes contain the 16/6 id. Studies with a range of monoclonal antibodies with diverse reactivities suggest that it is the 16/6 idiotype which is crucial for the induction of this disease (Blank *et al.*, 1990). Immunisation with a murine anti-16/6 id monoclonal antibody produces a similar syndrome (Mendlovic *et al.*, 1989). All these observations serve to highlight the potential importance of idiotypic–antiidiotypic interactions in the immunoregulation of murine lupus.

These observations on the pathogenetic properties of idiotypes raise the wider question of whether particular subsets of anti-DNA antibodies are particularly pathogenic. In addition to anti-DNA antibodies with pathogenic idiotypes, other possibilities include crossreactive anti-DNA antibodies (Pankewycz, Migliorini & Madaio, 1987), although this has been questioned (Brinkman et al., 1990), antibodies of high avidity (Asano & Nakamoto, 1978), and possibly cationic anti-DNA antibodies (Ebling & Hahn, 1980), although more recently the relevance of charge to pathogenicity has been challenged (Yoshida et al., 1985; Pankewycz, Migliorini & Madaio, 1987).

Cellular immunology

There is increasing evidence that the cellular immune system is also involved in the pathogenesis of lupus nephritis. Treatment with anti-T cell antibodies is of benefit in MRL/lpr mice but not in NZB/W mice (Wofsey et al., 1985). This lack of effect in NZB/W mice may in part be due to the non-selective nature of the treatment: potentially protective T cell subsets are depleted as well as pathogenic ones. Some evidence for this is provided by the fact that anti-CD4 antibodies are effective in ameliorating nephritis in NZB/W mice (Wofsey & Seaman, 1987). Although attempts to demonstrate a role for T cells by studying the effects of thymectomy on the development of nephritis have produced conflicting results, the point was elegantly made by producing NZB/W mice that were also homozygous for the nu gene, i.e. congenitally athymic (Mihara et al., 1988). Such mice retain the B cell hyperactivity of normal NZB/W mice but do not develop circulating antibodies to single stranded DNA and do not develop nephritis. A similar dissociation between autoantibody production and immunopathology is produced by treatment with cyclosporin (Mountz et al., 1987). Because of this evidence for T cell involvement it is not surprising that antibodies to MHC class II antigens, the ligands for CD4[+] T cells, are also of benefit (McDevitt, Perry & Steinman, 1987). All of these results are consistent with either a direct pathogenic effect of T cells on the kidney, or a critical role in helping the production of pathogenic autoantibodies. There is direct evidence for this latter possibility (Datta, Patel & Berry, 1987), but the two are not mutually inconsistent.

It has been suggested that defects in suppressor cell function have a role in the pathogenesis of murine lupus, and there is some experimental support for this (Krakauer, Waldmann & Strober, 1976). However, it is far from clear that the reported abnormalities are causal, as opposed to being a consequence of the abnormal immunological milieu. Furthermore, attempts to accelerate disease by depletion of a putative CD8[+] suppressor cell population have been unsuccessful (Wofsey, 1988).

Inflammatory mediators

It is unlikely that any particular mediator of glomerular damage is unique to
lupus nephritis, but because of the availability of the animal models such
mediators have been well studied in this context, often via the effect of
therapeutic manoeuvres aimed at particular pathogenic processes.

Prostacyclin and prostaglandin E1 will both produce considerable amelioration of nephritis in NZB/W mice (Clark *et al.*, 1987). The similarly
dramatic beneficial effect of a diet rich in omega-3 fatty acids is presumably
mediated via an alteration in the balance of these or similar compounds
(Alexander, Smythe & Jokinen, 1987).

The role of tumour necrosis factor (TNF) is unclear. Although it might be
expected to exacerbate tissue damage in autoimmunity (Old, 1987), a
deficiency of TNF is associated with a more severe lesion in a murine lupus
model (Jacob & McDevitt, 1988). Furthermore, in this latter model,
administration of recombinant TNF was beneficial. Other work has, however, found that TNF (and IL1) may indeed exacerbate renal injury; the
discrepancies in these studies may be related to the dose and timing of TNF
administration (Brennan *et al.*, 1989). Another cytokine that appears to be
important is gamma interferon: specific monoclonal antibodies ameliorate
murine lupus, whereas administration of excess gamma interferon acceler-
ates the disease (Border *et al.*, 1982).

The coagulation system is involved in the mediation of glomerular
damage in a number of experimental systems (see Cole *et al.*, 1990 for
references). Induction of monocyte procoagulant activity occurs with increasing age in BXSB mice (Cole, Sweet & Levy, 1986), and defibrination of
such animals with ancrod significantly improves survival, almost certainly as
a result of amelioration of the renal lesion (Cole *et al.*, 1990). Of note,
circulating anti-DNA antibody concentrations and deposition of IgG in the
kidney were unaffected, indicating that ancrod was not affecting the underlying autoimmune response.

Human studies

Autoantibodies

As in the mouse, although there is evidence in human SLE for polyclonal B
cell activation (Fauci & Moutsopoulos, 1981), much interest has centred on
anti-DNA antibodies. Antibodies with anti-nuclear activity are present in
the glomeruli, and concentrated with respect to serum, which most other
antibodies are not (Koffler, Schur & Kunkel, 1967). Glomerular deposits of
single stranded (ss) DNA are found in most patients with active lupus
nephritis, but not in patients with other forms of proliferative nephritis

(Andres *et al.*, 1970), supporting the case for an immune complex-mediated pathogenesis. Further evidence is provided by the rough correlation (with many individual exceptions) that exists between the concentration of anti-DNA antibodies, circulating immune complexes and evidence of complement activation (low C3 and C4 concentrations) on the one hand and activity of lupus nephritis on the other (Glassock *et al.*, 1986; Hayslett & Kashgarian, 1988; ter Borg *et al.*, 1990). Again, it seems likely that the DNA involved in the formation of immune complexes is associated with histones (Rumore & Steinman, 1990). However, DNA–anti-DNA immune complexes represent only a minority of the circulating complexes found in lupus (Fournié, 1988), and the other pathogenic mechanisms discussed above in the context of murine lupus may also be relevant here; in particular, there is direct evidence for the polyspecificity of human polyclonal (Sabbaga *et al.*, 1990) and monoclonal (André-Schwartz *et al.*, 1984; Shoenfeld *et al.*, 1985) anti-DNA antibodies. Other antibody systems may also be involved, both in probable immune complex deposition (e.g. Maddison & Reichlin, 1979) and in direct binding to other target antigens, e.g. the anti-endothelial antibodies found in up to 74% of patients (Rosenbaum *et al.*, 1988). Although reactivity with myeloperoxidase may be found in a small number of cases, classical antineutrophil cytoplasm antibodies (ANCA; see Chapter 8) are not found (Nässberger *et al.*, 1990).

In addition to the correlation between disease activity and anti-DNA antibodies mentioned above, there have been numerous attempts to document correlations between antibodies (and other serological parameters) and the particular histological pattern of lupus nephritis (Glassock *et al.*, 1986). In some cases, high avidity (precipitating) anti-DNA antibodies appear to be associated with a subendothelial or mesangial location of immune deposits (Asano & Nakamoto, 1978) and a proliferative nephritis (Hill *et al.*, 1978), whereas non-precipitating antibodies are associated with subepithelial deposits and a membranous pattern (Friend *et al.*, 1977; see also Chapter 3). Work with experimental models (see Chapter 1) provides further examples of relationships between properties of antibodies and patterns of immune deposition and nephritis, but in the clinical context there is such variation that prediction of histology from serological findings is very inexact.

Although approximately 20 different idiotypes on human anti-DNA antibodies have been described, it is apparent that close correlations exist between many of these, suggesting that they are related (Isenberg *et al.*, 1990). The 16/6 idiotype (for review see Isenberg, 1990), has already been mentioned above in the context of induction of murine lupus. This idiotype is found in normal individuals on antibodies of unknown specificity and on a separate population of anti-DNA antibodies associated with lupus (Datta, Naparstek & Schwartz, 1986). There is indirect evidence that this latter group of antibodies is pathogenic: the concentration of the 16/6 id correlates with disease activity, in some cases more closely than the DNA binding (Isenberg et al., 1984), and the 16/6 id has been found in 42% of renal biopsies from lupus patients (Isenberg & Collins, 1985). Another idiotype, IdGN2, is also closely associated with the development of nephritis (Kalunian et al., 1989; Hahn et al., 1990).

Cellular immunology

Little is known of the role of T cells in human lupus. Many of the autoantibodies have the characteristics typical of a T cell-dependent response, e.g. IgG, high affinity, and recent reports describe the identification of T cells that could be involved in helping this response (Shivakumar, Tsokos & Datta, 1989; Rajagopalan et al., 1990); further study of these cells will be of great interest. The ability to transfer some of the manifestations of human lupus to severe combined immunodeficient (SCID) mice with peripheral blood lymphocytes (Duchosal et al., 1990) should also aid in the dissection of the various cell populations involved in pathogenesis.

There is a large literature on defects of non-specific suppression in SLE (for review see Tomer & Shoenfeld, 1989) but as with the mouse it is not clear whether this is cause or effect. Similarly, a defect of a particular subset of $CD4^+$ cells that under some circumstances can behave as suppressor-inducer cells (Morimoto et al., 1986) has been reported to be linked to relapses of lupus nephritis (Morimoto et al., 1987). However, this may simply represent the non-specific loss of the subset-defining cell marker, which is known to occur upon activation of the cell (Akbar et al., 1988), or the production of anti-lymphocyte antibodies specific for this subset (Tanaka et al., 1989). Possibly of more relevance is a report describing difficulty in the generation of DNA-specific suppressor cells from patients with SLE as opposed to normal controls (Liebling et al., 1988).

Lupus variants

It is beyond the scope of this chapter to discuss overlap syndromes such as mixed connective tissue disease (MCTD) in any detail, but it is worth noting that a lower incidence of renal involvement (Nimelstein et al., 1980), and a predisposition to a membranous or mesangial pattern (Kitridou et al., 1980), have been claimed in MCTD as compared to SLE. However, there is no doubt that more severe renal involvement can occur, and indeed there is controversy as to whether MCTD is a distinct clinical entity at all (LeRoy, 1982).

Drug-induced lupus, although it does not usually lead to severe renal involvement, is of interest because of the possible clues that it offers to the pathogenesis of the idiopathic disease. Many of the drugs that can induce lupus are also capable of reacting with the activated form of C4 (Sim, Gill & Sim, 1984), leading to a functional deficiency of this protein. This could clearly be related to the known predisposition to lupus-like disease in individuals genetically deficient in C4 (see section on immunogenetics). The implications of this are discussed further at the end of this chapter.

Therapeutic aspects

The prognosis of SLE in general, and of lupus nephritis in particular, has improved considerably over the past few decades. No doubt this is in part due to improvements in diagnostic techniques allowing the detection of many milder cases, but there have been therapeutic advances as well. In broad terms, treatment of lupus nephritis can be considered under the headings of therapy designed to modulate the autoimmune response (generally immunosuppression of one form or another), and therapy designed to interfere with the mediators of renal injury that are engaged by the autoimmune response. As discussed above, mild forms of lupus nephritis (WHO class I and II) have a relatively good prognosis; the long-term outlook for membranous lupus nephritis (WHO class V) is uncertain, and it is even less clear that aggressive treatment is of benefit. Therefore most of the succeeding discussion applies particularly to the proliferative forms of lupus nephritis (WHO class III and IV).

The first form of immunosuppression to be used in SLE was corticosteroids. Whilst these undoubtedly had a dramatic effect on the extra-renal manifestations their effect on lupus nephritis was less clear. Some uncontrolled studies concluded that steroids were effective (Pollack, Pirani & Kark, 1961; Rothfield, McClusky & Baldwin, 1963), but that more severe cases of nephritis were unaffected by their use (Rothfield, McClusky & Baldwin, 1963). A review of the evaluable published data up to the end of the 1970s concluded that the introduction of corticosteroids had made no difference to the steady improvement in mortality seen with time (Albert, Hadler & Ropes, 1979). Closer analysis of a large series from one institution suggested that steroids did not affect survival in lupus nephritis *per se*, but probably were of benefit when the nephritis was part of a severe case in terms of other organ systems (Albert, Hadler & Ropes, 1979).

Initial results of uncontrolled and controlled studies of the addition of azathioprine and/or cyclophosphamide (for review see Felson & Anderson, 1984) to steroids were also inconclusive, leading some authorities to the conclusion that there was no evidence at that stage supporting the use of immunosuppression in the treatment of lupus nephritis (Wagner, 1976; Donadio, 1977). Then, in 1984, an analysis of histological changes on repeat

renal biopsies on 62 patients demonstrated that the group receiving azathioprine and/or cyclophosphamide did not, on average, experience progressive
renal scarring, whereas the group receiving steroids alone did; after adjust-
ment for prognostic factors this difference was highly significant (Balow *et
al.*, 1984). As was pointed out in an accompanying editorial (Donadio,
1984), these differences were not at the time accompanied by a corresponding difference in renal function. The probable reason for this was provided
by a pooled analysis of randomised trials which showed, first, a significant
advantage in favour of steroids plus azathioprine and/or cyclophosphamide
versus steroids alone, and secondly that previous trials had probably been
too small to detect this difference (Felson & Anderson, 1984). The authors
used a power analysis to show that at least 100 high risk patients (50%
chance of developing renal failure) would be needed to demonstrate a 50%
superiority of cytotoxic drugs plus steroids over steroids alone, and that
previous studies had therefore reached false negative conclusions. Finally,
continuing analysis of 107 patients, a subset of which had been reported in
the histological study mentioned above (Balow *et al.*, 1984), showed
improved preservation of renal function in all patients receiving various
cytotoxic drug combinations versus those receiving steroids alone (Austin *et
al.*, 1986). Although this improvement was only significant for intravenous
cyclophosphamide plus low dose steroids versus high dose steroids alone, it
was particularly apparent in the high risk subgroup with chronic changes on
the initial renal biopsy. Given that intravenous pulses of cyclophosphamide
are not associated with haemorrhagic cystitis or an undue increase in major
infections or malignancies (Austin *et al.*, 1986), this form of therapy can
probably be regarded as the present treatment of choice for severe lupus
nephritis, and possibly for other serious manifestations of SLE (McCune *et
al.*, 1988).

Plasma exchange has been studied intensively as a further possible means
of modulating the autoimmune response in SLE. It would appear logical to
attempt the removal of circulating autoantibodies and immune complexes
and there is, indeed, ample evidence that plasma exchange can achieve this
(Jones, 1982). Plasma exchange is also able to improve reticulo-endothelial
function and therefore enhance endogenous clearance of immune complexes (Lockwood *et al.*, 1979). Given these findings it is perhaps not
surprising that plasma exchange, when added to other immunosuppressive
treatment, has been reported to be of benefit in uncontrolled studies (e.g.
Jones *et al.*, 1979; Leaker *et al.*, 1986). However, when used alone plasma
exchange can be associated with an increase in disease activity (Jones, 1982).
This may represent the human equivalent of animal work demonstrating
enhanced synthesis of specific antibody following its removal by exchange
transfusion (Bystryn, Graf & Uhr, 1970). In view of this potentially
deleterious effect, it is again perhaps not surprising that controlled trials of

plasma exchange added to conventional immunosuppressive treatment have failed to demonstrate any useful benefit (Wei *et al.*, 1983; Derksen *et al.*, 1988). However, in spite of the negative findings to date, it may be possible to exploit the proliferation of autoreactive B cell clones induced by plasma exchange, as dividing cells are particularly vulnerable to treatment with cyclophosphamide (Bruce, Meeker & Valeriote, 1966). Uncontrolled observations, using a variety of protocols, have found encouraging results when pulse cyclophosphamide is synchronised with plasma exchange, e.g. Schroeder, Euler & Löffler, 1987. A standardised protocol testing this combination is the subject of a current multicenter trial (Lupus Plasmapheresis Study Group, Clinical Co-Ordinating Centre, University of Kiel, Germany).

A number of other more or less specific immunomodulatory treatments have been used in uncontrolled studies in SLE, e.g. total lymphoid irradiation (Strober *et al.*, 1985), extra-corporeal protein A absorption of anti-DNA antibodies (Palmer *et al.*, 1988), and intravenous immunoglobulin (Lin, Hsu & Chiang, 1989; Akashi *et al.*, 1990). Further information is required before their role relative to standard forms of treatment can be assessed. Lastly, it is worth noting that continuing activity of lupus nephritis once end stage renal failure is reached is unusual, and recurrence in transplants very rare (Cheigh *et al.*, 1990); this presumably reflects the immunosuppression associated with these states.

Turning to therapy designed to interfere with the mediators of renal damage, experimental work discussed above has suggested that vasoactive eicosanoids are involved in modulating renal haemodynamics in lupus nephritis. Direct administration of prostaglandin E1 may be beneficial in some cases (Nagayama *et al.*, 1988; Lin, 1990). Short-term treatment with a selective antagonist of the vasoconstrictor thromboxane A_2 leads to improvement in glomerular filtration rate (Pierucci *et al.*, 1989); whether this is of long-term benefit will require trials with long-lasting thromboxane antagonists. A more indirect approach to the manipulation of intra-renal eicosanoids is to alter dietary lipids. This is certainly of benefit in murine lupus nephritis (see above) and a short-term study in man has demonstrated favourable effects on lipids, platelets and rheology (Clark *et al.*, 1989); there was no effect on immunological measures and proteinuria, but longer term trials are clearly required. Another important mediator system is the coagulation cascade, and intra-glomerular thrombi may play a particularly significant role in the more severe forms of lupus nephritis (Kant *et al.*, 1981): the presence of glomerular thrombi appears uniquely predictive of subsequent glomerulosclerosis. The defibrinating agent ancrod has produced significant improvement in certain patients with marked glomerular thrombosis (Dosekun *et al.*, 1984; Hariharan *et al.*, 1990), and also seems capable of favourably modulating some of the immunopathological abnormalities, perhaps due to the immunosuppressive properties of fibrin degradation products (Kim *et al.*, 1988). However, it seems unlikely that this agent will be of widespread or long-term use, not least because it is a foreign protein and therefore immunogenic. However, endogenous regulators of the coagulation system are now available in recombinant form (e.g. tissue plasminogen activator) and may be more suitable in this context.

Concluding remarks

It is useful to distinguish between, on the one hand, the immunopathogenesis of SLE in general, and, on the other, the pathogenesis of the nephritis and the particular factors that lead to the various forms of renal lesion. With respect to the first issue the association between lupus and complement deficiencies, both inherited and acquired, has led to the suggestion that this is a causal relationship. The hypothesis has been discussed in greater detail elsewhere (Lachmann, 1987) and so will only be outlined here. In normal individuals, the bulk of immune complexes, solubilised by the complement system, are probably carried via the CR1 receptor on red blood cells to the liver for proteolytic disposal. In the presence of abnormalities of the complement system or receptor, either congenital or acquired, complexes are not cleared as efficiently by this route and can deposit in target organs such as the kidney. Here, they set up an inflammatory response, which by the release of cytokines and autoantigens drives the production of autoantibodies. This leads to the formation of further immune complexes and the perpetuation of the cycle. This hypothesis has therapeutic implications, as it predicts that replacement of deficient complement components would be beneficial; there are obvious practical difficulties associated with testing this.

   With respect to the pathogenesis of lupus nephritis, there are close analogies with experimental models of immune complex-mediated glomerulonephritis (see Chapter 1). Although there are undoubtedly additional factors, e.g. involvement of T cells and cross-reactivity of anti-DNA antibodies, it seems probable that most of the glomerular damage is due to the deposition of immune complexes, whether from the circulation or via *in situ* formation. The particular pattern of nephritis that results is no doubt dependent on multiple factors, such as antibody affinity and class, quantity and rate of deposition, state of activation of the various mediator systems, and so on. As a crude generalisation, low affinity antibodies present in relatively low concentration and forming small, unstable complexes result in a membranous pattern (see Chapter 3); binding of DNA to the glomerular basement membrane followed by *in situ* immune complex formation may also play a role, and could indeed be the major mechanism involved. Complexes formed from high affinity antibodies are initially deposited via normal filtration processes in the mesangium, causing mesangial changes. Increasing size or numbers of complexes, as in experimental serum sickness, may be associated with deposition in peripheral locations, particularly in subendothelial sites. Here, they are readily accessible to circulating factors such as the complement and coagulation systems, and a severe lesion results.

References

Adler, S. G., Johnson, K., Louie, J. S., Liebling, M. R. & Cohen, A. H. (1990). Lupus membranous glomerulonephritis: different prognostic subgroups obscured by imprecise histologic classifications. *Modern Pathology*, **3**, 186–91.

Agnello, V. (1978). Complement deficiency states. *Medicine*, **57**, 1–23.

Akashi, K., Nagasawa, K., Mayumi, T., Yokota, E., Oochi, N. & Kusaba, T. (1990). Succesful treatment of refractory systemic lupus erythematosus with intravenous immunoglobulin. *Journal of Rheumatology*, **17**, 375–9.

Akbar, A. N., Terry, L., Timms, A., Beverley, P. C. L. & Janossy, G. (1988). Loss of CD45R and gain of UCHL1 reactivity is a feature of primed T cells. *Journal of Immunology*, **140**, 2171–8.

Alarif, L. I., Ruppert, G. B., Wilson, R. & Barth, W. F. (1983). HLA-DR antigens in blacks with rheumatoid arthritis and systemic lupus erythematosus. *Journal of Rheumatology*, **10**, 297–300.

Albert, D. A., Hadler, N. M. & Ropes, M. W. (1979). Does corticosteroid therapy affect the survival of patients with systemic lupus erythematosus? *Arthritis and Rheumatism*, **22**, 945–53.

Alexander, N. J., Smythe, N. L. & Jokinen, M. P. (1987). The type of dietary fat affects the severity of autoimmune disease in NZB/NZW mice. *American Journal of Pathology*, **127**, 106–21.

Andres, G. A., Accinni, L., Beiser, S. M. *et al.* (1970). Localization of fluorescein-labelled antinucleoside antibodies in glomeruli of patients with active systemic lupus erythematosus. *Journal of Clinical Investigation*, **49**, 2106–18.

Andrews, B. S., Eisenberg, R. A., Theofilopoulos, A. N. *et al.* (1978). Spontaneous murine lupus-like syndromes. Clinical and immunopathological manifestations in several strains. *Journal of Experimental Medicine*, **148**, 1198–215.

André-Schwartz, J., Datta, S. K., Shoenfeld, Y., Isenberg, D. A., Stollar, B. D. & Schwartz, R. S. (1984). Binding of cytoskeletal proteins by monoclonal anti-DNA lupus autoantibodies. *Clinical Immunology and Immunopathology*, **31**, 261–71.

Appel, G. B., Cohen, D. J., Pirani, C. L., Meltzer, J. I. & Estes, D. (1987). Long-term follow-up of patients with lupus nephritis. A study based on the classification of the World Health Organisation. *American Journal of Medicine*, **83**, 877–85.

Arnett, F. C., Goldstein, R., Duvic, M. & Reveille, J. D. (1988). Major histocompatibility complex genes in systemic lupus erythematosus, Sjögren's syndrome, and polymyositis. *American Journal of Medicine*, **85** (suppl 6A), 38–41.

Asano, Y. & Nakamoto, Y. (1978). Avidity of anti-native DNA antibody and glomerular immune complex localization in lupus nephritis. *Clinical Nephrology*, **10**, 134–9.

Austin, H. A., Muenz, L. R., Joyce, K. M. *et al.* (1983). Prognostic factors in lupus nephritis. Contribution of renal histologic data. *American Journal of Medicine*, **75**, 382–91.

Austin, H. A., Klippel, J. H., Barlow, J. E. *et al.* (1986). Therapy of lupus nephritis: controlled trial of prednisone and cytotoxic drugs. *New England Journal of Medicine*, **314**, 614–19.

Baldwin, D. S., Gluck, M. C., Lowenstein, J. & Gallo, G. R. (1977). Lupus nephritis. Clinical course as related to morphologic forms and their transitions. *American Journal of Medicine*, 62, 12–30.

Balow, J. E., Austin, H. A., Muenz, L. R. *et al*. (1984). Effect of treatment on the evolution of renal abnormalities in lupus nephritis. *New England Journal of Medicine*, 311, 491–5.

Blank, M., Krup, M., Mendlovic, S. *et al*. (1990). The importance of the pathogenic 16/6 idiotype in the induction of SLE in naive mice. *Scandinavian Journal of Immunology*, 31, 45–52.

Block, S. R., Winfield, J. B., Lockshin, M. D., D'Angelo, W. A. & Christian, C. L. (1975). Studies of twins with systemic lupus erythematosus. A review of the literature and presentation of 12 additional sets. *American Journal of Medicine*, 59, 533–52.

Border, W. A., Ward, H. J., Kamis, E. S. & Cohen, A. H. (1982). Induction of membranous nephropathy in rabbits by administration of an exogenous cationic antigen. Demonstration of a pathogenic role for electrical charge. *Journal of Clinical Investigation*, 69, 451–61.

Brennan, D. C., Yui, M. A., Wuthrich, R. P. & Kelley, V. E. (1989). Tumor necrosis factor and IL-1 in New Zealand Black/White mice. Enhanced gene expression and acceleration of renal injury. *Journal of Immunology*, 143, 3470–5.

Brinkman, K., Termaat, R., Berden, J. H. M. & Smeenk, R. J. T. (1990). Anti-DNA antibodies and lupus nephritis: the complexity of crossreactivity. *Immunology Today*, 11, 232–4.

Bruce, W. R., Meeker, B. E. & Valeriote, F. A. (1966). Comparison of the sensitivity of normal hematopoietic and transplanted lymphoma colony-forming cells to chemotherapeutic agents administered *in vivo*. *Journal of the National Cancer Institute*, 37, 233–45.

Bruijn, J. A., van Leer, E. H., Baelde, H. J., Corver, W. E., Hogendoorn, P. C. & Fleuren, G. J. (1990). Characterization and *in vivo* transfer of nephritogenic autoantibodies directed against dipeptidyl peptidase IV and laminin in experimental lupus nephritis. *Laboratory Investigation*, 63, 350–9.

Bystryn, J-C., Graf, M. W. & Uhr, J. W. (1970). Regulation of antibody formation by serum antibody. II. Removal of specific antibody by means of exchange transfusion. *Journal of Experimental Medicine*, 132, 1279–87.

Cheigh, J. S., Kim, H., Stenzel, K. H. *et al*. (1990). Systemic lupus erythematosus in patients with end-stage renal disease: long-term follow-up on the prognosis of patients and the evolution of lupus activity. *American Journal of Kidney Disease*, 16, 189–95.

Chen, P. P., Liu, M-F., Sinha, S. & Carson, D. A. (1988). A 16/6 idiotype-positive anti-DNA antibody is encoded by a conserved V_H gene with no somatic mutation. *Arthritis and Rheumatism*, 31, 1429–31.

Clark, W. F., Parbtani, A., McDonald, J. W. D., Taylor, N., Reid, B. D. & Kreeft, J. (1987). The effects of a thromboxane synthase inhibitor, a prostacyclin analog and PGE_1 on the nephritis of the NZB/W F_1 mouse. *Clinical Nephrology*, 28, 288–94.

Clark, W. F., Parbtani, A., Huff, M. W., Reid, B., Holub, B. J. & Falardeau, P. (1989). Omega-3 fatty acid dietary supplementation in systemic lupus erythematosus. *Kidney International*, 36, 653–60.

Cole, E. H., Glynn, M. F. X., Laskin, C. A,, Sweet, J., Mason, N. & Levy, G. A. (1990). Ancrod improves survival in murine systemic lupus erythematosus. *Kidney International*, 37, 29–35.

Cole, E. H., Sweet, J. & Levy, G. A. (1986). Expression of macrophage procoagulant activity in murine systemic lupus erythematosus. *Journal of Clinical Investigation*, 78, 887–93.

Datta, S. K., Naparstek, Y. & Schwartz, R. S. (1986). *In vitro* production of an anti-DNA idiotype by lymphocytes of normal subjects and patients with systemic lupus erythematosus. *Clinical Immunology and Immunopathology*, 38, 302–8.

Datta, S. K., Patel, H. & Berry, D. (1987). Induction of a cationic shift in IgG anti-DNA autoantibodies. Role of T helper cells with classical and novel phenotypes in three murine models of lupus nephritis. *Journal of Experimental Medicine*, **165**, 1252–68.

Derksen, R. H., Hené, R. J., Kallenberg, C. G., Valentijn, R. M. & Kater, L. (1988). Prospective multicentre trial on the short-term effects of plasma exchange versus cytotoxic drugs in steroid-resistant lupus nephritis. *Netherlands Journal of Medicine*, **33**, 168–77.

Dixon, F. J., Oldstone, M. B. A. & Tonietti, G. (1971). Pathogenesis of immune complex glomerulonephritis of New Zealand mice. *Journal of Experimental Medicine*, **134**, 65s–71s.

Dixon, F. J. (1979). The pathogenesis of murine systemic lupus erythematosus. *American Journal of Pathology*, **97**, 10–16.

Donadio, J. V. (1977). Treatment of lupus nephritis. *Nephron*, **19**, 186–9.

Donadio, J. V. (1984). Cytotoxic-drug treatment of lupus nephritis. *New England Journal of Medicine*, **311**, 528–9.

Dosekun, A., Pollack, V. E., Glas-Greenwalt, P. et al. (1984). Ancrod in systemic lupus erythematosus with thrombosis. Clinical and fibrinolysis effects. *Archives of Internal Medicine*, **144**, 37–42.

Duchosal, M. A., McConahey, P. J., Robinson, C. A. & Dixon, F. J. (1990). Transfer of human systemic lupus erythematosus in severe combined immunodeficient (SCID) mice. *Journal of Experimental Medicine*, **172**, 985–8.

Dudeney, C., Shoenfeld, Y., Rauch, J. et al. (1986). A study of anti-poly (ADP-ribose) antibodies and an anti-DNA antibody idiotype and other immunological abnormalities in lupus family members. *Annals of the Rheumatic Diseases*, **45**, 502–7.

Ebling, F. & Hahn, B. H. (1980). Restricted subpopulations of DNA antibodies in kidneys of mice with systemic lupus. Comparison of antibodies in serum and renal eluates. *Arthritis and Rheumatism*, **23**, 392–403.

Elkon, K. B., Walport, M. J., Rynes, R. I., Black, C. M., Batchelor, J. R. & Hughes, G. R. V. (1983). Circulating C1q binding complexes in relatives of patients with systemic lupus erythematosus. *Arthritis and Rheumatism*, **26**, 921–4.

Esdaile, J. M., Levington, C., Federgreen, W., Hayslett, J. P. & Kashgarian, M. (1989). The clinical and renal biopsy predictors of long-term outcome in lupus nephritis: a study of 87 patients and review of the literature. *Quarterly Journal of Medicine*, **72**, 779–833.

Fauci, A. S. & Moutsopoulos, H. M. (1981). Polyclonally triggered B cells in the peripheral blood and bone marrow of normal individuals and in patients with systemic lupus erythematosus and primary Sjögren's syndrome. *Arthritis and Rheumatism*, **24**, 577–84.

Fedrick, J. A., Pandey, J. P., Chen, Z., Fudenberg, H. H., Ainsworth, S. K. & Dobson, R. L. (1983). Gm allotypes in blacks with systemic lupus erythematosus. *Human Immunology*, **8**, 177–81.

Felson, D. T. & Anderson, J. (1984). Evidence for the superiority of immunosuppressive drugs and prednisone over prednisone alone in lupus nephritis. Results of a pooled analysis. *New England Journal of Medicine*, **311**, 1528–33.

Fessel, W. J. (1974). Systemic lupus erythematosus in the community. Incidence, prevalence, outcome, and first symptoms; the high prevalence in black women. *Archives of Internal Medicine*, **134**, 1027–35.

Fielder, A. H. L., Walport, M. J., Batchelor, J. R. et al. (1983). Family study of the major histocompatibility complex in patients with systemic lupus erythematosus; importance of null alleles of C4A and C4B in determining disease susceptibility. *British Medical Journal*, **286**, 425–8.

Fournié, G. J. (1988). Circulating DNA and lupus nephritis. *Kidney International*, **33**, 487–97.

Friend, P. S., Kim, Y., Michael, A. F. & Donadio, J. V. (1977). Pathogenesis of membranous nephropathy in systemic lupus erythematosus: possible role of nonprecipitating DNA antibody. *British Medical Journal*, **I**, 25.

Fronek, Z., Lentz, D., Berliner, N. *et al.* (1986). Systemic lupus erythematosus is not genetically linked to the beta chain of the T cell receptor. *Arthritis and Rheumatism*, **29**, 1023–5.

Fronek, Z., Timmerman, L. A., Alper, C. A. *et al.* (1988). Major histocompatibility complex associations with systemic lupus erythematosus. *American Journal of Medicine*, **85** suppl. 6A, 42–4.

Fronek, Z., Timmerman, L. A., Alper, C. A. *et al.* (1990). Major histocompatibility complex genes and susceptibility to systemic lupus erythematosus. *Arthritis and Rheumatism*, **33**, 1542–53.

Gladman, D. D., Terasaki, P. I., Park, M. S. *et al.* (1979). Increased frequency of HLA-DRw2 in SLE. *Lancet*, **ii**, 902.

Gladman, D. D., Urowitz, M. B., Cole, E., Ritchie, S., Chang, C. H. & Churg, J. (1989). Kidney biopsy in SLE. I. A clinical-morphologic evaluation. *Quarterly Journal of Medicine*, **73**, 1125–33.

Glass, D., Raum, D., Gibson, D., Stillman, J. S. & Schur, P. H. (1976). Inherited deficiency of the second component of complement. Rheumatic disease associations. *Journal of Clinical Investigation*, **58**, 853–61.

Glassock, R. J., Cohen, A. H., Adler, S. G. & Ward, H. J. (1986). Secondary glomerular disease. In *The Kidney*, 3rd edn, ed. B. M. Brenner & F. C. Rector, pp. 1014–84. Philadelphia: W.B.Saunders Company.

Goldstein, R., Krupen, K. I., Crawford, Y. M., Bias, W. B., Duvic, M. & Arnett, F. C. (1987). Interaction of the T cell receptor beta chain gene and HLA-DR in systemic lupus erythematosus. *Arthritis and Rheumatism*, **30**, s22.(Abstract).

Goldstein, R., Olsen, M. L., Arnett, F. C., Duvic, M., Pollack, M. S. & Reveille, J. D. (1988). Deletion of C4A genes in Black Americans with systemic lupus erythematosus. *Arthritis and Rheumatism*, **31**, S22.(Abstract).

Green, J. R., Montasser, M. & Woodrow, J. C. (1986). The association of HLA-linked genes with systemic lupus erythematosus. *Annals of Human Genetics*, **50**, 93–6.

Hahn, B. H. & Ebling, F. M. (1983). Suppression of NZB/NZW murine nephritis by administration of a syngeneic monoclonal antibody to DNA. *Journal of Clinical Investigation*, **71**, 1728–36.

Hahn, B. H. & Ebling, F. M. (1984). Suppression of murine lupus nephritis by administration of an anti-idiotypic antibody to anti-DNA. *Journal of Immunology*, **132**, 187–90.

Hahn, B. H., Kalunian, K. C., Fronek, Z. *et al.* (1990). Idiotype characteristics of immunoglobulins associated with human systemic lupus erythematosus. Association of high levels of IdGN2 with nephritis but not with HLA class II genes predisposing to nephritis. *Arthritis and Rheumatism*, **33**, 978–84.

Halpern, R., Davidson, A., Lazo, A., Solomon, G., Lahita, R. & Diamond, B. (1985). Familial systemic lupus erythematosus. Presence of a cross-reactive idiotype in healthy family members. *Journal of Clinical Investigation*, **76**, 731–6.

Hariharan, S., Pollak, V. E., Kant, K. S., Weiss, M. A. & Wadhwa, N. K. (1990). Diffuse proliferative lupus nephritis: long-term observations in patients treated with ancrod. *Clinical Nephrology*, **34**, 61–9.

Hashimoto, H., Tsuda, H., Matsumoto, T. *et al.* (1985). HLA antigens associated with systemic lupus erythematosus in Japan. *Journal of Rheumatology*, **12**, 919–23.

Hawkins, B. R., Wong, K. L., Wong, R. W. S., Chan, K. H., Dunckley, H. & Serjeantson, S. W. (1987). Strong association between the major histocompatibility complex and systemic lupus erythematosus in Southern Chinese. *Journal of Rheumatology*, **14**, 1128–31.

Hayslett, J. P. & Kashgarian, M. (1988). Nephropathy of systemic lupus erythematosus. In *Diseases of the Kidney*, 4th edn, ed. R. W. Schrier & C. W. Gottschalk, pp. 2253–71. Boston/Toronto: Little,Brown and Company.

Hecht, B., Siegel, N., Adler, M., Kashgarian, M. & Hayslett, J. P. (1976). Prognostic indices in lupus nephritis. *Medicine*, **55**, 163–81.

Hill, G. S., Hinglais, N., Tron, F. & Bach, J-F. (1978). Systemic lupus erythematosus. Morphologic correlations with immunologic and clinical data at the time of biopsy. *American Journal of Medicine*, **64**, 61–79.

Howard, P. F., Hochberg, M. C., Bias, W. B., Arnett, F. C. & McLean, R. H. (1986). Relationship between C4 null genes, HLA-D region antigens, and genetic susceptibility to systemic lupus erythematosus in Caucasion and Black Americans. *American Journal of Medicine*, **81**, 187–93.

Isenberg, D., Williams, W., Axford, J. *et al.* (1990). Comparison of DNA antibody idiotypes in human sera: an international collaborative study of 19 idiotypes from 11 different laboratories. *Journal of Autoimmunity*, **3**, 393–414.

Isenberg, D. A. & Collins, C. (1985). Detection of cross-reactive anti-DNA antibody idiotypes on renal tissue-bound immunoglobulins from lupus patients. *Journal of Clinical Investigation*, **76**, 287–94.

Isenberg, D. A., Shoenfeld, Y., Madaio, M. P. *et al.* (1984). Anti-DNA antibody idiotypes in systemic lupus erythematosus. *Lancet*, **ii**, 417–22.

Isenberg, D. A., Shoenfeld, Y., Walport, M. *et al.* (1985). Detection of cross-reactive anti-DNA antibody idiotypes in the serum of systemic lupus erythematosus patients and of their relatives. *Arthritis and Rheumatism*, **28**, 999–1007.

Isenberg, D. A. (1990). DNA antibody idiotype 16/6. An idiotype system of some importance. *Annales de Medecine Interne*, **141**, 57–63.

Izui, S., Lambert, P-H., Fournié, G. J., Türler, H. & Miescher, P. A. (1977). Features of systemic lupus erythematosus in mice injected with bacterial lipopolysaccharides. Identification of circulating DNA and renal localization of DNA–anti-DNA complexes. *Journal of Experimental Medicine*, **145**, 1115–30.

Izui, S., Lambert, P-H. & Miescher, P. A. (1976). *In vitro* demonstration of a particular affinity of glomerular basement membrane and collagen for DNA. A possible basis for a local formation of DNA–anti-DNA complexes in systemic lupus erythematosus. *Journal of Experimental Medicine*, **144**, 428–43.

Jacob, C. O. & McDevitt, H. O. (1988). Tumour necrosis factor-alpha in murine autoimmune 'lupus' nephritis. *Nature*, **331**, 356–8.

Jacob, C. O., Fronek, Z., Lewis, G. D., Koo, M., Hansen, J. A. & McDevitt, H. O. (1990). Heritable major histocompatibility complex class II-associated differences in production of tumour necrosis factor alpha: relevance to genetic predisposition to systemic lupus erythematosus. *Proceedings of the National Academy of Sciences, USA*, **87**, 1233–7.

Jones, F. S., Pisetsky, D. S. & Kurlander, R. J. (1986). The clearance of a monoclonal anti-DNA antibody following administration of DNA in normal and autoimmune mice. *Clinical Immunology and Immunopathology*, **39**, 49–60.

Jones, J. V., Cummings, R. H., Bacon, P. A. *et al.* (1979). Evidence for a therapeutic effect of plasmapheresis in patients with systemic lupus erythematosus. *Quarterly Journal of Medicine*, **48**, 555–76.

Jones, J. V. (1982). Plasmapheresis in SLE. *Clinics in Rheumatic Diseases*, **8**, 243–60.

Kalunian, K. C., Panosian-Sahakian, N., Ebling, F. M. *et al.* (1989). Idiotypic characteristics of immunoglobulins associated with systemic lupus erythematosus. Studies of antibodies deposited in glomeruli of humans. *Arthritis and Rheumatism*, **32**, 513–22.

Kameda, S., Naito, S., Tanaka, K. *et al.* (1982). HLA antigens of patients with systemic lupus erythematosus in Japan. *Tissue Antigens*, **20**, 221–2.

Kant, K. S., Pollack, V. E., Weiss, M. A., Glueck, H. I., Miller, M. A. & Hess, E. V. (1981). Glomerular thrombosis in systemic lupus erythematosus: prevalence and significance. *Medicine*, **60**, 71–86.

Kim, S., Wadhwa, N. K., Kant, K. S. *et al.* (1988). Fibrinolysis in glomerulonephritis treated with Ancrod: renal functional, immunologic and histopathologic effects. *Quarterly Journal of Medicine*, 69, 879–95.

Kitridou, R. C., Akmal, M., Ehresmann, G. R., Quismorio, F. P. & Massry, S. (1980). Nephropathy in mixed connective tissue disease. *Arthritis and Rheumatism*, 23, 704.(Abstract).

Klinman, D. M. (1990). Polyclonal B cell activation in lupus-prone mice precedes and predicts the development of autoimmune disease. *Journal of Clinical Investigation*, 86, 1249–54.

Koffler, D., Schur, P. H. & Kunkel, H. G. (1967). Immunological studies concerning the nephritis of systemic lupus erythematosus. *Journal of Experimental Medicine*, 126, 607–23.

Krakauer, R. S., Waldmann, T. A. & Strober, W. (1976). Loss of suppressor T cells in adult NZB/NZW mice. *Journal of Experimental Medicine*, 144, 662–73.

Lachmann, P. J. (1987). Complement – friend or foe? *British Journal of Rheumatology*, 26, 409–15.

Lafer, E. M., Rauch, J., Andrzejewski, C. *et al.* (1981). Polyspecific monoclonal lupus autoantibodies reactive with both polynucleotides and phospholipids. *Journal of Experimental Medicine*, 153, 897–909.

Lambert, P. H. & Dixon, F. J. (1968). Pathogenesis of the glomerulonephritis of NZB/W mice. *Journal of Experimental Medicine*, 127, 507–22.

Leaker, B. R., Becker, G. J., Dowling, J. P. & Kincaid-Smith, P. (1986). Rapid improvement in severe lupus glomerular lesions following intensive plasma exchange associated with immunosuppression. *Clinical Nephrology*, 25, 236–44.

LeRoy, E. C. (1982). Overlap features of connective tissue disease. *Arthritis and Rheumatism*, 25, 889–90.

Lewis, R. M. & Schwartz, R. S. (1971). Canine systemic lupus erythematosus. Genetic analysis of an established breeding colony. *Journal of Experimental Medicine*, 134, 417–38.

Liebling, M. R., Wong, C., Radosevich, J. & Louie, J. S. (1988). Specific suppression of anti-DNA production *in vitro*. *Journal of Clinical Immunology*, 8, 362–71.

Lin, C. Y. (1990). Improvement in steroid and immunosuppressive drug resistant lupus nephritis by intravenous prostaglandin E1 therapy. *Nephron*, 55, 258–64.

Lin, C. Y., Hsu, H. C. & Chiang, H. (1989). Improvement of histological and immunological change in steroid and immunosuppressive drug-resistant lupus nephritis by high-dose intravenous gamma globulin. *Nephron*, 53, 303–10.

Lockwood, C. M., Worlledge, S., Nicholas, A., Cotton, C. & Peters, D. K. (1979). Reversal of impaired splenic function in patients with nephritis or vasculitis (or both) by plasma exchange. *New England Journal of Medicine*, 300, 524–30.

Maddison, P. J. & Reichlin, M. (1979). Deposition of antibodies to a soluble cytoplasmic antigen in the kidneys of patients with systemic lupus erythematosus. *Arthritis and Rheumatism*, 22, 858–63.

McCune, W. J., Golbus, J., Zeldes, W., Bohlke, P., Dunne, R. & Fox, D. A. (1988). Clinical and immunologic effects of monthly administration of intravenous cyclophosphamide in severe systemic lupus erythematosus. *New England Journal of Medicine*, 318, 1423–31.

McDevitt, H. O., Perry, R. & Steinman, L. A. (1987). Monoclonal anti-Ia antibody therapy in animal models of autoimmune disease. In *Autoimmunity and Autoimmune Disease (Ciba Foundation Symposium 129)*, ed. D. Evered & J. Whelan, pp. 184–193. Chichester, UK: John Wiley & Sons.

Mendlovic, S., Brocke, S., Shoenfeld, Y. *et al.* (1988). Induction of a systemic lupus erythematosus-like disease in mice by a common human anti-DNA idiotype. *Proceedings of the National Academy of Sciences, USA*, 85, 2260–4.

Mendlovic, S., Fricke, H., Shoenfeld, Y. & Mozes, E. (1989). The role of anti-idiotypic antibodies in the induction of experimental sytemic lupus erythematosus in mice. *European Journal of Immunology*, 19, 729–34.

Mihara, M., Ohsugi, Y., Saito, K. *et al.* (1988). Immunologic abnormality in NZB/NZW F$_1$ mice. Thymus-independent occurrence of B cell abnormality and requirement for T cells in the development of autoimmune disease, as evidenced by an analysis of the athymic nude individuals. *Journal of Immunology*, **141**, 85–90.

Miller, K. B. & Schwartz, R. S. (1979). Familial abnormalities of suppressor-cell function in systemic lupus erythematosus. *New England Journal of Medicine*, **301**, 803–9.

Moldenhaur, F., David, J., Fielder, A. H. L., Lachmann, P. J. & Walport, M. J. (1987). Inherited deficiency of erythrocyte complement receptor type 1 does not cause susceptibility to systemic lupus erythematosus. *Arthritis and Rheumatism*, **30**, 961–6.

Morimoto, C., Letvin, N. L., Distaso, J. A., Brown, H. M. & Schlossman, S. F. (1986). The cellular basis for the induction of antigen-specific T8 suppressor cells. *European Journal of Immunology*, **16**, 198–204.

Morimoto, C., Steinberg, A. D., Letvin, N. L. *et al.* (1987). A defect of immunoregulatory T cell subsets in systemic lupus erythematosus patients demonstrated with anti-2H4 antibody. *Journal of Clinical Investigation*, **79**, 762–8.

Mountz, J. D., Smith, H. R., Wilder, R. L., Reeves, J. P. & Steinberg, A. D. (1987). CS-A therapy in MLR-lpr/lpr mice: amelioration of immunopathology despite autoantibody production. *Journal of Immunology*, **138**, 157–63.

Nagayama, Y., Namura, Y., Tamura, T. & Muso, R. (1988). Beneficial effect of prostaglandin E$_1$ in three cases of lupus nephritis with nephrotic syndrome. *Annals of Allergy*, **61**, 289–95.

Nakao, Y., Matsumoto, H., Miyazaki, T. *et al.* (1980). IgG heavy chain allotypes (Gm) in autoimmune diseases. *Clinical and Experimental Immunology*, **42**, 20–6.

Nimelstein, S. H., Brody, S., Mcshane, D. & Holman, H. R. (1980). Mixed connective tissue disease: a subsequent evaluation of the original 25 patients. *Medicine*, **59**, 239–48.

Nossent, H. C., Henzen-Logmans, S. C., Vroom, T. M., Berden, J. H. M. & Swaak, T. J. G. (1990). Contributions of renal biopsy data in predicting outcome in lupus nephritis. Analysis of 116 patients. *Arthritis and Rheumatism*, **33**, 970–7.

Nässberger, L., Sjöholm, A. G., Jonsson, H., Sturfelt, G. & Akesson, A. (1990). Autoantibodies against neutrophil cytoplasm components in systemic lupus erythematosus and in hydralazine-induced lupus. *Clinical and Experimental Immunology*, **81**, 380–3.

Old, L. J. (1987). Polypeptide mediator network. *Nature*, London, **326**, 330–1.

Palmer, A., Gjorstrup, P., Severn, A., Welsh, K. & Taube, D. (1988). Treatment of systemic lupus erythematosus by extracorporeal immunoadsorption. *Lancet*, **ii**, 272.

Pankewycz, O. G., Migliorini, P. & Madaio, M. P. (1987). Polyreactive autoantibodies are nephritogenic in murine lupus nephritis. *Journal of Immunology*, **139**, 3287–94.

Parker, L. P., Hahn, B. H. & Osterland, C. K. (1974). Modification of NZB/NZW F$_1$ autoimmune disease by development of tolerance to DNA. *Journal of Immunology*, **113**, 292–7.

Pierucci, A., Simonetti, B. M., Pecci, G. *et al.* (1989). Improvement of renal function with selective thromboxane antagonism in lupus nephritis. *New England Journal of Medicine*, **320**, 421–5.

Pollack, V. E., Pirani, C. L. & Kark, R. M. (1961). Effect of large doses of prednisone on the renal lesions and life span of patients with lupus glomerulonephritis. *Journal of Laboratory and Clinical Medicine*, **57**, 495–511.

Rajagopalan, S., Zordan, T., Tsokos, G. C. & Datta, S. K. (1990). Pathogenic anti-DNA autoantibody-inducing T helper cell lines from patients with active lupus nephritis: isolation of CD4$^-$8$^-$ T helper cell lines that express the gamma delta T-cell antigen receptor. *Proceedings of the National Academy of Sciences, USA*, **87**, 7020–4.

Raz, E., Brezis, M., Rosenmann, E. & Eilat, D. (1989). Anti-DNA antibodies bind directly to renal antigens and induce kidney dysfunction in the isolated perfused rat kidney. *Journal of Immunology*, **142**, 3076–82.

Reveille, J. D., Schrohenloher, R. E., Acton, R. T. & Barger, B. O. (1989). DNA analysis of HLA-DR and DQ genes in American blacks with systemic lupus erythematosus. *Arthritis and Rheumatism*, **32**, 1243–51.

Rosenbaum, J., Pottinger, B. E., Woo, P. *et al.* (1988). Measurement and characterisation of circulating anti-endothelial cell IgG in connective tissue diseases. *Clinical and Experimental Immunology*, **72**, 450–6.

Rothfield, N., McClusky, R. T. & Baldwin, D. S. (1963). Renal disease in systemic lupus erythematosus. *New England Journal of Medicine*, **269**, 537–44.

Rumore, P. M. & Steinman, C. R. (1990). Endogenous circulating DNA in systemic lupus erythematosus. Occurrence as multimeric complexes bound to histone. *Journal of Clinical Investigation*, **86**, 69–74.

Rynes, R. I. (1982). Inherited complement deficiency states and SLE. *Clinics in Rheumatic Diseases*, **8**, 29–47.

Sabbaga, J., Pankewycz, O. G., Lufft, V., Schwartz, R. S. & Madaio, M. P. (1990). Cross-reactivity distinguishes serum and nephritogenic anti-DNA antibodies in human lupus from their natural counterparts in normal serum. *Journal of Autoimmunity*, **3**, 215–35.

Schifferli, J. A., Steiger, G., Paccaud, J-P., Sjöholm, A. G. & Hauptmann, G. (1986). Difference in the biological properties of the two forms of the fourth component of human complement (C4). *Clinical and Experimental Immunology*, **63**, 473–7.

Schmiedeke, T. M. J., Stöckl, F. W., Weber, R., Sugisaki, Y., Batsford, S. R. & Vogt, A. (1989). Histones have high affinity for the glomerular basement membrane. Relevance for immune complex formation in lupus nephritis. *Journal of Experimental Medicine*, **169**, 1879–94.

Schroeder, J. O., Euler, H. H. & Löffler, H. (1987). Synchronization of plasmapheresis and pulse cyclophosphamide in severe systemic lupus erythematosus. *Annals of Internal Medicine*, **107**, 344–6.

Schur, P. H., Marcus-Bagley, D., Awdeh, Z., Yunise, J. & Alper, C. A. (1990). The effect of ethnicity on major histocompatibility complex complement allotypes and extended haplotypes in patients with systemic lupus erythematosus. *Arthritis and Rheumatism*, **33**, 985–92.

Schur, P. H., Pandey, J. P. & Fedrick, J. A. (1985). Gm allotypes in white patients with systemic lupus erythematosus. *Arthritis and Rheumatism*, **28**, 828–30.

Schwartz, M. M., Bernstein, J., Hill, G. S., Holley, K. & Phillips, E. A. (1989). Predictive value of renal pathology in diffuse proliferative lupus glomerulonephritis. Lupus Nephritis Collaborative Study Group. *Kidney International*, **36**, 891–6.

Shivakumar, S., Tsokos, G. C. & Datta, S. K. (1989). T cell receptor alpha/beta expressing double-negative (CD4$^-$/CD8$^-$) and CD4$^+$ T helper cells in humans augment the production of pathogenic anti-DNA autoantibodies associated with lupus nephritis. *Journal of Immunology*, **143**, 103–12.

Shoenfeld, Y., Zamir, R., Joshua, H., Lavie, G. & Pinkhas, J. (1985). Human monoclonal anti-DNA antibodies react as lymphocytotoxic antibodies. *Journal of Immunology*, **15**, 1024–8.

Siegel, I., Liu, T. L. & Gleicher, N. (1981). The red-cell immune system. *Lancet*, **ii**, 556–9.

Siegel, M. & Lee, S. L. (1973). The epidemiology of systemic lupus erythematosus. *Seminars in Arthritis and Rheumatism*, **3**, 1–54.

Sim, E., Gill, E. W. & Sim, R. B. (1984). Drugs that induce systemic lupus erythematosus inhibit complement component C4. *Lancet*, **ii**, 422–4.

Speirs, C., Fielder, A. H. L., Chapel, H., Davey, N. J. & Batchelor, J. R. (1989). Complement system protein C4 and susceptibility to hydralazine-induced systemic lupus erythematosus. *Lancet*, **i**, 922–4.

Strober, S., Field, E., Hoppe, R. T. *et al.* (1985). Treatment of intractable lupus nephritis with total lymphoid irradiation. *Annals of Internal Medicine*, **102**, 450–8.

Tan, E. M., Cohen, A. S., Fries, J. F. *et al.* (1982). The 1982 revised criteria for the classification of systemic lupus erythematosus. *Arthritis and Rheumatism*, **25**, 1271–7.

Tanaka, S., Matsuyama, T., Steinberg, A. D., Schlossman, S. F. & Morimoto, C. (1989). Antilymphocyte antibodies against $CD4^+2H4^+$ cell populations in patients with systemic lupus erythematosus. *Arthritis and Rheumatism*, **32**, 398–405.

Tateno, S., Kobayashi, Y., Shigematsu, H. & Hiki, Y. (1983). Study of lupus nephritis: its classification and the significance of subendothelial deposits. *Quarterly Journal of Medicine*, **52**, 311–31.

ter Borg, E. J., Horst, G., Hummel, E. J., Limburg, P. C. & Kallenberg, C. G. M. (1990). Measurement of increases in anti-double stranded DNA antibody levels as a predictor of disease exacerbation in systemic lupus erythematosus. A long-term, prospective study. *Arthritis and Rheumatism*, **33**, 634–43.

Termaat, R-M., Brinkman, K., van Gompel, F. *et al.* (1990). Cross-reactivity of monoclonal anti-DNA antibodies with heparan sulfate is mediated via bound DNA/histone complexes. *Journal of Autoimmunity*, **3**, 531–45.

Theofilopoulos, A. N., Prud'Homme, G., Fieser, T. M. & Dixon, F. J. (1983a). B-cell hyperactivity in murine lupus. II. Defects in response to and production of accessory signals in lupus-prone mice. *Immunology Today*, **4**, 317–19.

Theofilopoulos, A. N., Prud'Homme, G., Fieser, T. M. & Dixon, F. J. (1983b). B-cell hyperactivity in murine lupus. I. Immunological abnormalities in lupus-prone strains and the activation of normal B cells. *Immunology Today*, **4**, 287–91.

Tomer, Y. & Shoenfeld, Y. (1989). The significance of T suppressor cells in the development of autoimmunity. *Journal of Autoimmunity*, **2**, 739–58.

Tron, F., Jacob, L. & Bach, J-F. (1984). Binding of a murine monoclonal anti-DNA antibody to Raji cells. Implications for the interpretation of the Raji cell assay for immune complexes. *European Journal of Immunology*, **14**, 283–6.

Wagner, L. (1976). Immunosuppressive agents in lupus nephritis: a critical analysis. *Medicine*, **55**, 239–50.

Wallace, D. J., Podell, T., Weiner, J., Klinenberg, J. R., Forouzesh, S. & Dubois, E. L. (1981). Systemic lupus erythematosus – survival patterns. *Journal of the American Medical Association*, **245**, 934–8.

Walport, M. J., Black, C. M. & Batchelor, J. R. (1982). The immunogenetics of systemic lupus erythematosus. *Clinics in Rheumatic Diseases*, **8**, 3–21.

Wei, N., Klippel, J. H., Huston, D. P. *et al.* (1983). Randomised trial of plasma exchange in mild systemic lupus erythematosus. *Lancet*, **i**, 17–22.

Weisbart, R. H., Noritake, D. T., Wong, A. L., Chan, G., Kacena, A. & Colburn, K. K. (1990). A conserved anti-DNA antibody idiotype associated with nephritis in murine and human systemic lupus erythematosus. *Journal of Immunology*, **144**, 2653–8.

Whittingham, S., Mathews, J. D., Schanfield, M. S., Tait, B. D. & Mackay, I. R. (1983). HLA and Gm genes in systemic lupus erythematosus. *Tissue Antigens*, **21**, 50–7.

Wilson, J. G., Wong, W. W., Schur, P. H. & Fearon, D. T. (1982). Mode of inheritance of decreased C3b receptors on erythrocytes of patients with systemic lupus erythematosus. *New England Journal of Medicine*, **307**, 981–6.

Wofsey, D., Ledbetter, J. A., Hendler, P. L. & Seaman, W. E. (1985). Treatment of murine lupus with monoclonal anti-T cell antibody. *Journal of Immunology*, **134**, 852–7.

Wofsey, D. & Seaman, W. E. (1987). Reversal of advanced murine lupus in NZB/NZW F1 mice by treatment with monoclonal antibody to L3T4. *Journal of Immunology*, **138**, 3247–53.

Wofsey, D. (1988). The role of Lyt-2$^+$ T cells in the regulation of autoimmunity in murine lupus. *Journal of Autoimmunity*, 1, 207–17.

Woodrow, J. C. (1988). Immunogenetics of systemic lupus erythematosus. *Journal of Rheumatology*, 15, 197–9.

Yoshida, H., Yoshida, M., Izui, S. & Lambert, P. H. (1985). Distinct clonotypes of anti-DNA antibodies in mice with lupus nephritis. *Journal of Clinical Investigation*, 76, 685–94.

–5–
IgA-related glomerulonephropathies

The diseases considered in this chapter are all characterised by mesangial IgA deposition. They have been classified (Woodroffe *et al.*, 1982; Clarkson, Woodroffe & Aarons, 1988) into (a) 'primary' conditions, IgA nephropathy (Berger's disease) and Henoch-Schönlein purpura (HSP), and (b) a miscellaneous group in which these deposits occur in the presence of other diseases ('secondary'; see Table 5.1). The relationship between these various conditions is uncertain, and is discussed further at the end of this chapter.

IgA nephropathy was first described in 1968 (Berger & Hinglais, 1968). The initial series of studies found the condition in approximately 25% of renal biopsies, and subsequent studies from several countries have confirmed that this is indeed a very common lesion (D'Amico, 1987). In fact, although subject to inter-racial differences (Jones *et al.*, 1990), on a worldwide basis IgA nephropathy is probably the commonest form of glomerulonephritis. As approximately 20% of patients will eventually progress to chronic renal failure (Clarkson, Woodroffe & Aarons, 1988), the disease also makes a major contribution to end stage renal failure programs.

Table 5.1. *Conditions associated with mesangial IgA deposition*

Liver disease, especially alcoholic cirrhosis
Coeliac disease and dermatitis herpetiformis
Seronegative spondyloarthropathies (e.g. ankylosing spondylitis)
Neoplasia (carcinoma, mycosis fungoides, IgA paraproteins)
Infection

Clinically, IgA nephropathy is accompanied by haematuria (which may be macroscopic, particularly following an upper respiratory tract infection), proteinuria and hypertension. There is a subgroup of patients that experiences acute renal failure in association with a crescentic nephritis, and another subgroup characterised by steroid-responsive nephrotic syndrome; these are discussed further below. Light microscopy reveals segmental mesangial proliferation, although this is very variable in extent. Occasionally mesangial expansion may lead to peripheral extension into capillary loops and double contouring; this mesangiocapillary pattern tends to be found in more severe forms of HSP (Counahan *et al.*, 1977). The subgroup with more aggressive disease may show all the features of other forms of crescentic nephritis (see Chapter 8). Immunological studies are required for a definitive diagnosis, and demonstrate granular deposition of IgA and usually C3 in the mesangium, variably accompanied by IgG and/or IgM. Electron microscopy reveals electron-dense deposits within the mesangial matrix, often in the paramesangial regions.

HSP is a syndrome characterised by palpable purpura, arthralgia, abdominal pain and glomerulonephritis. The renal lesion is virtually identical to that found in IgA nephropathy, although the changes tend to be more severe, with a greater incidence of necrosis. The extra-renal manifestations are due to a leukocytoclastic vasculitis.

Immunogenetics

The MHC

Initial studies from Australia and France suggested an association between IgA nephropathy and B35 (MacDonald, Dumble & Kincaid-Smith, 1976; Berthoux *et al.*, 1978; Noël *et al.*, 1978). A single report from America, based on only 17 patients, found an increased incidence of B12 in patients (Richman, Mahoney & Fuller, 1979; $P_{corr} < 0.05$). However, subsequent surveys from a number of countries, including France, have shown no association with any class I allele (Brettle, Peters & Batchelor, 1978; Nagy *et al.*, 1979; Savi *et al.*, 1979; Sakai *et al.*, 1979b; Bignon *et al.*, 1980; Chan, Ku & Sinniah, 1981; Mustonen *et al.*, 1981). Despite this, the authors of one of the original reports have recently confirmed the link with B35 (based on data from 259 patients) and furthermore have shown, using multivariate analysis, that the possession of B35 is an independent risk factor for progression to chronic renal failure (Berthoux *et al.*, 1988). No doubt some of the discrepancies between the studies (including the class II associations; see below) are due to the small numbers studied, and to population differences, both ethnic and secondary to renal biopsy policy, but these latter data provide strong support for the reality of the B35 link. There is little information on the immunogenetics of HSP. An apparent association with B35 (Nyulassy *et al.*, 1977) has not been confirmed (Ostergaard, Storm & Lamm, 1990).

Investigation of class II associations has also produced conflicting results. A link with DR4 has been found in both French (Fauchet *et al.*, 1980) and Japanese populations (Hiki *et al.*, 1982; Kasahara *et al.*, 1982; Kashiwabara *et al.*, 1982), but this has not always been confirmed, even within the same populations (Bignon *et al.*, 1980; Berthoux *et al.*, 1988). Other reports describe associations with DR1 (Feehally *et al.*, 1984) and DEn, a class II marker closely related to DR6 (Komori *et al.*, 1979). In patient subgroups, an increased incidence of DR4 has been noted in stable versus progressive disease on the one hand (Hiki *et al.*, 1982), and in more severe disease on the other (Kashiwabara *et al.*, 1982); further analysis suggests that these discrepant findings are probably due to chance, and that DR4 has no significant effect on prognosis (Hiki *et al.*, 1990). DR4 has also been associated with a particular histological subgroup (Kohara *et al.*, 1985), and an increase in DR blanks has been reported in the subgroup with macroscopic haematuria (Beukhoff *et al.*, 1984).

More recent work may help explain some of these conflicting studies. An analysis of RFLPs of the DQβ region in British patients has demonstrated a strong association between IgA nephropathy and the phenotype that possesses both a 2 kb (T2) and a 6 kb (T6) fragment of a Taq 1 digest defined by a DQβ probe (Moore *et al.*, 1990*b*); this association was not, however, found in Italian and Finnish Caucasoid patients (Moore *et al.*, 1990*a*). T2 is probably equivalent to the DQw8 allele, whereas the nature of the T6 fragment is unclear. The T2+/T6+ phenotype is associated with DR4 in patients (although there is no overall link with DR4) but not in controls, suggesting that this phenotype defines a subgroup of DR4$^+$ individuals at higher risk of developing disease. T6 is also linked to DR1, which may be significant with respect to the reported DR1 association. Another study has found a non-significant increase in DR4 and DR5 but a highly significant increase in the DQβ allele DQw7 in patients versus controls (62.6% versus 28%; $p_{corr} < 0.001$; Burns *et al.*, 1991). DQw7 is in linkage disequilibrium with all DR5 haplotypes and some DR4 haplotypes, again emphasising the heterogeneity of the DR4$^+$ population. Further analysis of the DQ sublocus has revealed some associations with DQα polymorphisms (Moore *et al.*, 1990*a*), and some hints that polymorphisms of both DQα and DQβ may be linked with various parameters of the IgA immune response (Moore *et al.*, 1990*c*), suggesting possible pathogenetic mechanisms. There do not appear to be any obvious associations between IgA nephropathy and alleles at the DP sublocus (Moore *et al.*, 1990*b*).

Analysis of the C4 loci (A and B) within the MHC has shown a significant increase of homozygous null phenotypes (at either C4A or C4B) in both IgA nephropathy and HSP (Mclean, Wyatt & Julian, 1984). Other work has emphasised the particular importance of complete C4B deficiency in both IgA nephropathy (Welch, Beischel & Choi, 1989) and HSP (Ault et al., 1990). In one unique case complete C4 deficiency was associated with HSP, and with the recurrence of an identical renal lesion in a subsequent allograft (Lhotta et al., 1990). These associations are almost certainly primary rather than secondary to HLA linkage, as there is no particular associated HLA antigen or extended HLA haplotype (Egido, Julian & Wyatt, 1987). Furthermore, a variety of molecular defects underlie the C4B deficiency found in patients with IgA nephropathy, again suggesting a primary role for the protein deficiency (Welch, Beischel & Choi, 1989). Although total serum C4 concentrations are raised in patients versus controls (Mclean, Wyatt & Julian, 1984), this may conceal the consequences of the functional differences between C4A and C4B (Schifferli et al., 1986). The linkage to C4 may also contribute to the B35 association, as the C4BQ0 null allele is found in an MHC extended haplotype that includes B35 (Welch, Beischel & Choi, 1989). There is, however, doubt about the significance of at least some of the above observations (notably Mclean, Wyatt & Julian, 1984), as re-analysis with appropriate regional control groups, and allowing for bias due to inter-relatedness, has shown no association between IgA nephropathy and C4 deficiency (Wyatt et al., 1990).

Other loci

In addition to C4 deficiency, IgA nephropathy has been reported in association with cases of familial deficiency of complement components H, P, and C2 (Egido, Julian & Wyatt, 1987), and HSP in association with cases of C2 deficiency (for review see Ault et al., 1990). An original claim that the frequency of the C3F allele was increased in patients with IgA nephropathy (Wyatt et al., 1984) has not been confirmed (Welch & Berry, 1987; Rambausek et al., 1987), although there may be an increase in the frequency of C3FF homozygotes (Tomino et al., 1987). There is an apparent association with a particular C7 phenotype (Nishimukai et al., 1989).

Linkage to a number of immunoglobulin gene loci has been examined with variable results. One report did not find any association with Gm gamma heavy chain allotypes, but did note a significant increase in the Kml kappa light chain allotype in the subgroup of patients with chronic renal failure due to IgA nephropathy (Le Petit et al., 1981). This was not confirmed in a subsequent study which did, however, find an association between a Gm allotype and patients without macroscopic haematuria (Beukhoff et al., 1984). More recently, a link between RFLPs of the immunoglobulin α and μ heavy chain switch regions and IgA nephropathy has been observed (Demaine *et al.*, 1988), but a study with larger numbers could not confirm this (Moore *et al.*, 1990a).

More generally, there are a number of accounts of familial IgA nephropathy (for review see Egido, Julian & Wyatt, 1987 and Julian *et al.*, 1988). Although some of the reports of affected siblings have demonstrated sharing of particular HLA antigens, or identity at the MHC, the larger studies have shown no linkage between MHC haplotype and disease expression. The identity of the genetic loci acting in these families remains unknown. Phenotypically, relatives of patients with both sporadic and familial IgA nephropathy have a high incidence of abnormalities of the IgA system and more general immune perturbations (again, for review see Egido, Julian & Wyatt, 1987). These include increased concentrations of serum IgA and IgA-containing immune complexes, increased rates of IgA synthesis, and changes in CD4$^+$/CD8$^+$ T cell ratios. These abnormalities are not always consistently found from study to study, are not associated with overt renal disease, are not inherited in any distinct Mendelian fashion, and are not linked to the MHC.

Immunopathology

Animal studies

These have been reviewed in Rifai, 1987 and Emancipator, 1988. General problems in extrapolating results from these models to man follow from the significant inter-species differences in normal IgA handling (Delacroix *et al.*, 1982) and the fact that none of the models actually reproduces the human disease particularly well.

Administration of preformed complexes

Models involving the administration to mice of preformed IgA immune complexes (IgA-IC), either monoclonal anti-dinitrophenyl (DNP) complexed with DNP-conjugated bovine serum albumin (BSA) (Rifai *et al.*, 1979) or monoclonal anti-dextran complexed with dextrans of varying size and charge (Isaacs & Miller, 1983), have provided useful information on the factors governing the glomerular localisation of such complexes. Only polymeric IgA, as opposed to monomeric, will deposit in the kidney (Rifai *et al.*, 1979). This is probably due to the greater size of IgA-IC possible with polymeric IgA, as covalent crosslinking of monomeric IgA with an affinity labelling antigen to produce larger complexes also resulted in mesangial deposition (Rifai & Millard, 1985). In general IgA–IC have a particular tendency to deposit within the kidney, irrespective of charge or variation in size above a certain threshold (Isaacs & Miller, 1983). This may reflect the unavailability of the erythrocyte CR1-mediated clearance route employed by IgG–IC; such complexes can fix C3b (the CR1 ligand) whereas IgA–IC cannot (Waldo & Cochran, 1989b). Clearance of IgA–IC above a certain size in mice is apparently mediated mainly by the liver (Rifai & Mannik, 1983). Interference with or saturation of this route may be involved in some of the models of secondary IgA nephropathy (see below). Administration of preformed IgA–IC tends to result in rather mild histological changes, although, at least in the case of anti-DNP complexed with DNP-BSA, this is associated with haematuria in a proportion of mice.

Active immunisation

Another group of models involves active immunisation of mice, including systemic immunisation with a variety of dextrans (Isaacs & Miller, 1982) and oral immunisation with protein antigens (Emancipator, Gallo & Lamm, 1983). Repeated systemic immunisation with dextran, although it produces histopathological changes (with normal urine), is of limited relevance to man. Oral immunisation, on the other hand, may well be modelling an important triggering factor for human IgA nephropathy (see below). Such mice develop mesangial IgA deposition together with the immunising antigen but no C3 deposition, glomerular injury or urinary abnormality. However, if they are given an intravenous injection of antigen then IgG and C3 are deposited and haematuria is produced. It is also possible to induce haematuria in such orally immunised mice by the use of cyclophosphamide or estradiol, substances that inhibit the generation of oral tolerance (Gesualdo, Lamm & Emancipator, 1990). Oral tolerance is a mechanism that blunts the IgG and IgM response to antigens chronically presented via the gut, and it is interesting that only the mice treated with cyclophosphamide or estradiol developed mesangial IgG and IgM deposits, whereas all mice (that is including the orally immunised but otherwise untreated controls) had mesangial deposits of antigen and IgA.

Viral diseases

A number of known or suspected viral infections may lead to mesangial IgA deposits in animals. Aleutian disease of mink, a persistent parvovirus infection, is associated with deposition of IgA, together with viral antigens, predominantly in capillary walls and to a lesser extent in the mesangium (Portis & Coe, 1979). Lymphocytic choriomeningitis virus infection of mice *in utero* produces deposits of maternal IgG, and to a lesser extent IgA, in the capillary walls and mesangium (Oldstone & Dixon, 1972). Neither of these diseases, therefore, is similar in terms of histopathology to human IgA nephropathy. However, the glomerulonephritis that develops spontaneously in ageing female ddY mice closely resembles the human disease by light and electron microscopy (Imai *et al.*, 1985). The disease is also associated with proteinuria but not haematuria. The precise aetiology is unclear, but may be related to the retrovirus that ddY mice are known to harbour: there is some evidence that retroviral glycoproteins may participate in immune complex formation (Takeuchi *et al.*, 1989). The condition may therefore have much in common with the glomerulonephritis (usually associated with IgG and IgM deposition) found in ageing mice of many strains, which may well be due to chronic retroviral carriage and resultant immune complex deposition (Markham, Sutherland & Mardiney, 1973).

Liver dysfunction

Lastly, a variety of manoeuvres that induce liver dysfunction lead to mesangial IgA deposition with little if any histological changes. These include carbon tetrachloride induced cirrhosis (Gormly *et al.*, 1981) and bile duct ligation (Melvin *et al.*, 1983) in rats. Saturation of the reticulo-endothelial system in mice with colloidal carbon, together with oral immunisation, produces similar appearances, and inhibition of normal hepatic clearance mechanisms is probably the most important factor involved (Sato, Ideura & Koshikawa, 1986). Of note is the production of mild histological changes and proteinuria in addition to IgA deposition in a model of chronic alcohol abuse (Smith, Yu & Tsukamoto, 1990). Inter-species differences are particularly relevant in the interpretation of this group of models. In rats, transport of polymeric IgA from plasma to bile, mediated by secretory component, is the main mechanism controlling circulating concentrations of polymeric IgA (Lemaître-Coelho, Jackson & Vaerman, 1978). Although secretory component is expressed in human liver, this route is much less important in the control of plasma polymeric IgA in man (Delacroix *et al.*, 1982).

A number of the above models are characterised by mesangial IgA deposition in the absence of significant histological changes, urinary abnormalities or other evidence of glomerular injury. This suggests that IgA deposition alone is not injurious.

Human studies

There is an extensive literature (for reviews see D'Amico, 1987; Woodroffe, 1988; Feehally, 1988; Emancipator & Lamm, 1989) describing a wide range of immunological phenomena in IgA nephropathy.

Glomerular deposits

Characterisation of the mesangial IgA deposits reveals that these are predominantly of IgA1 subclass (Feehally, 1988). This does not serve to localise the source of the IgA (mucosal on the one hand, or serum, and probably bone-marrow derived (Conley & Delacroix, 1987), on the other) as although 90% of serum IgA is IgA1, approximately 40% of mucosally derived IgA is also of this subclass. Of more significance is the probable polymeric nature of the glomerular IgA, as shown by elution studies (Monteiro *et al.*, 1985), the presence of J chain (Donini *et al.*, 1983) and the ability to bind secretory component (Bene, Faure & Duheille, 1982). The J chain is required for polymerisation of IgA monomers, and secretory component specifically recognises polymeric IgA and is involved in its transport across mucosal epithelia (Brandtzaeg, 1981). As serum IgA is largely monomeric, these observations suggest that the glomerular IgA is mucosally derived. There appears to be a higher than expected ratio of lambda to kappa light chains in the mesangial IgA (Lai *et al.*, 1986*a*), which is also more anionic than serum IgA (Monteiro *et al.*, 1985). Studies on the binding properties of eluted IgA are considered below in the section on possible antigens.

The co-deposition of C3 with IgA in the majority of cases, together with the presence of the membrane-attack complex (Rauterberg *et al.*, 1987) and usual absence of C1 and C4 in association with IgA (Tomino *et al.*, 1982*b*), suggests activation of complement via the alternative pathway, which aggregated IgA is known to do (Götze & Müller-Eberhard, 1971). The contribution of complement, and the IgG that is often found in the deposits as well, to glomerular injury is uncertain. There is a poor correlation between the amount of mesangial IgA deposition and severity of glomerulonephritis (Vangelista *et al.*, 1984), suggesting that other factors must be important in pathogenesis, but haematuria may occur in the absence of C3 and IgG (A report of the Southwest Pediatric Nephrology Study Group, 1982).

Serology

None of the serological abnormalities found in IgA nephropathy is specific for the condition, and as a result they are not of diagnostic use. Raised concentrations of total serum IgA are found in 20%–50% of patients (Clarkson, Woodroffe & Aarons, 1988). There is also an increased antigen-specific IgA response to a variety of antigens in response to oral or systemic immunisation (Woodroffe, 1988; Feehally, 1988). In over half the cases there is sharing of idiotypes on serum IgA between patients (Gonzalez-Cabrero *et al.*, 1987); this does not imply that there is necessarily any shared antigen recognition. Anti-endothelial antibodies, predominantly of the IgA class, are present in some patients and correlate with proteinuria, suggesting a possible role in pathogenesis (Yap *et al.*, 1988).

As the IgA deposited in the mesangium is polymeric (see above), studies of this minority fraction (approximately 10% of total serum IgA) may be particularly relevant (for review see Feehally, 1988). Such studies have given variable results, which may partly be explained by the presence of increased concentrations of polymeric IgA only during clinical relapses.

In addition to polymeric IgA, a variety of other forms of high molecular weight complexes that include IgA have been found. These include IgA–IC (for review see Feehally, 1988), in which the IgA is presumably bound to an antigen which in most cases is unknown (but see below), and mixed complexes that also include IgG (Czerkinsky *et al.*, 1986). Some reports find that the presence of IgA–IC correlates with disease activity, whereas others do not (Jones *et al.*, 1990). The mixed complexes may partly be due to the presence of IgA rheumatoid factors (Czerkinsky *et al.*, 1986); in any event, such complexes may be of particular significance, as the IgG component allows the fixation of complement, which IgA does poorly, if at all, whilst the IgA component inhibits the normal binding of IgG complexes to erythrocyte CR1 receptors (Waldo & Cochran, 1989*b*). These complexes may therefore not be efficiently cleared and are available for mesangial deposition, where the ability to fix complement may lead to injury. There is, however, no apparent association between IgA rheumatoid factors and glomerular IgG (Woodroffe, 1988).

Possible antigens

These can be considered under the broad headings of exogenous and endogenous. Exogenous antigens that might be involved include dietary, bacterial and viral antigens. Raised titres of IgA antibodies to many of these are found in patients with IgA nephropathy (see section on serology) but this of course does not necessarily imply a role in pathogenesis. Of particular interest are IgA antibodies to gliadin. Such antibodies are found in approximately 50% of adult patients with IgA nephropathy, as compared to less than 10% of cases of other forms of glomerular disease (Rostoker *et al.*, 1989); the findings in children, however, have been contradictory (Rodriguez-Soriano *et al.*, 1988). Attempts to identify antigens of potentially greater pathogenetic significance have involved examination of IgA–IC and antigens deposited in the glomerulus. Ovalbumin (Feehally *et al.*, 1987) and bovine serum albumin (Yap *et al.*, 1987), have been detected in IgA-IC, and other work has found deposition of food antigens in some cases (Russell *et al.*, 1986; Sato *et al.*, 1988).

Viral antigens include HBsAg, which may be found in the glomeruli of a significant proportion of HBsAg carriers with IgA nephropathy. The importance of this is uncertain. In some populations the incidence of hepatitis carriage is not significantly increased amongst patients with IgA nephropathy (Iida *et al.*, 1990), suggesting that the mesangial deposition of HBsAg represents non-specific trapping. In other areas, there does appear to be a substantial increase in the frequency of HBsAg carriage in patients (Lai *et al.*, 1988), which is consistent with a role in pathogenesis. Of even more obscure significance are the few reports of adenovirus and herpes simplex antigen deposition (Nagy *et al.*, 1984; Tomino *et al.*, 1987). A claim that cytomegalovirus (CMV) antigen deposition was present in 100% of cases (Gregory, Hammond & Brewer, 1988) could not be substantiated (Waldo *et al.*, 1989*a*) and was probably due to non-specificity of the antisera used for CMV antigen detection.

Turning to endogenous antigens, an IgM autoantibody to a nucleoprotein has been reported (Nomoto *et al.*, 1986), but the significance of this is unclear. The only endogenous antigen identified in IgA-IC is IgG, bound by IgA rheumatoid factor (Gonzalez-Cabrero *et al.*, 1987). IgA antibodies eluted from affected kidneys will rebind to mesangial areas of their source biopsy and a proportion of other patient's biopsies, but not to normal kidney (Tomino *et al.*, 1982*a*); similar observations have been found with IgA produced *in vitro* from Epstein Barr virus-transformed B cells from patients (Tomino *et al.*, 1990). The target of the eluted antibodies could either be an intrinsic glomerular antigen or an exogenous antigen deposited within the mesangium and acting as a planted antigen. Circulating IgA antibodies reactive with components of basement membrane collagen have been found in IgA nephropathy (Cederholm *et al.*, 1986), but such reactivity is mediated indirectly via fibronectin (Cederholm *et al.*, 1988) and in any event is presumably distinct from the anti-mesangial reactivity found in the elution studies. Polyspecific IgA autoantibodies appear to be a feature of IgA nephropathy, which suggests that the finding of the above apparently monospecific autoantibodies must be interpreted with caution (Matsiota *et al.*, 1990). One group has reported the presence of IgG antibodies with specificity for certain glomerular antigenic determinants in the sera of a proportion of patients (Ballardie *et al.*, 1988). An increase in such IgG autoantibodies did appear to be correlated with episodes of clinical relapse in some cases.

Cellular immunology

Studies in this area are particularly difficult to interpret as the results are often contradictory. No doubt, technical differences contribute to this, as well as heterogeneity of the patient population with respect to such factors as disease subtype and clinical state (relapse or remission).

An increase in IgA-bearing B lymphocytes in peripheral blood has been reported by some groups (Nomoto, Sakai & Arimori, 1979) but not by others (Fiorini *et al.*, 1982); this particular discrepancy may be explicable by non-specific Fc-mediated interactions, in that F(ab′)2 fragments of anti-IgA antibodies were used in the study that did not find an increase. Of perhaps greater relevance are studies of lymphocytes from mucosal sites; IgA-producing cells are not increased in the small bowel mucosa of patients with IgA nephropathy (Westberg *et al.*, 1983) but do appear to be present in greater numbers in the tonsils (Egido *et al.*, 1984*a*). In functional terms, an increase in *in vitro* IgA production, either spontaneous or following mitogen stimulation, has been found in some cases (Egido *et al.*, 1983; Hale *et al.*, 1986) but not in others (Linné & Wasserman, 1985; Rothschild & Chatenoud, 1984). Some of these differences may be due to the presence of abnormalities only during clinical relapse (Feehally *et al.*, 1986), although others have found no consistent relationship between clinical state and *in vitro* IgA synthesis (Hale *et al.*, 1986).

Attempts to define immunoregulatory abnormalities underlying the above functional changes have also produced inconsistent results (Wyatt *et al.*, 1988). An increased $CD4^+/CD8^+$ T cell ratio has often been noted (e.g. Egido *et al.*, 1983), but this may well not be specific for IgA nephropathy (Chatenoud & Bach, 1981). The fact that such an increased ratio has not been found in some studies (Linné & Wasserman, 1985) may in part be due to the presence of an increased $CD4^+/CD8^+$ ratio only during relapses (Feehally *et al.*, 1986). More specifically, an increase in IgA-specific help has been reported in some cases (Rothschild & Chatenoud, 1984) but not all (Hale *et al.*, 1986). Similarly a defect in IgA-specific suppression (Sakai, Nomoto & Arimori, 1979*a*) has not been found universally (Cosio *et al.*, 1982). $CD4^+$ T cells bearing receptors for IgA and capable of enhancing the class switch from IgM to IgA production by B cells are reportedly increased in the blood of patients and their relatives (Sakai *et al.*, 1989).

Cytokines

There is considerable interest in the possible role that cytokines might play in stimulating mesangial proliferation. In particular, IL–6 appears to act as an autocrine growth factor for mesangial cells (Horii *et al.*, 1989). The same study demonstrated that 50% of patients with mesangial proliferative glomerulonephritis (34/38 had IgA nephropathy) has detectable IL–6 in the urine, whereas very little was found in other glomerular diseases. There was also some relationship between the amount of urinary IL–6 and the stage of the disease.

Immune clearance mechanisms

The possible interference by IgA with normal IC clearance via erythrocyte CR1 receptors has been mentioned above. In addition, clearance of IgA–IC does not involve the erythrocyte system, and appears to be prolonged in some patients with IgA nephropathy (Roccatello et al., 1989), although this is not a universal finding (Rifai et al., 1989). Sera from patients also appears defective in its ability to solubilise glomerular immune deposits (Tomino et al., 1983). Impaired clearance via Fc or C3b receptor mechanisms has also been reported (Roccatello et al., 1985), but whether this is a primary abnormality or simply due to saturation of these pathways by an excess of IC is unclear; in view of the close correlation between IgA–IC and clearance half-life, the latter possibility is most likely.

Transplantation

There is a recurrence of IgA deposits in approximately 50% of patients transplanted for IgA disease (Clarkson, Woodroffe & Aarons, 1988). The clinical disease is relatively benign, with few episodes of macroscopic haematuria and a very low rate of progression to renal insufficiency (Berger, Noël & Nabarra, 1984). Of particular interest is the observation that kidneys with mesangial IgA deposits inadvertently used as transplants always seem to undergo resolution of these deposits (for review see Feehally, 1988).

Clinical subsets

A small minority of patients with IgA nephropathy develop features of an acute nephritic syndrome, usually in association with episodes of macroscopic haematuria; a proportion progress to acute azotemia (Clarkson et al., 1977). An acute crescentic glomerulonephritis is the usual histological finding, and, indeed, crescents may be found in the majority of cases during episodes of macroscopic haematuria even in the absence of renal impairment (Bennett & Kincaid-Smith, 1983). In addition to the deleterious effects of the crescentic process on renal function (see Chapter 8) there may also be an element of tubular damage secondary to the gross glomerular leakage of erythrocytes (Kincaid-Smith et al., 1983a); on occasion the mildness of the glomerular changes suggests that this tubular lesion is principally responsible for the renal impairment. These episodes of acute renal impairment usually resolve spontaneously (Kincaid-Smith et al., 1983a; Clarkson, Woodroffe & Aarons, 1988).

Another subset comprises patients with heavy proteinuria, often of nephrotic proportions. In some cases this appears to be a reflection of advanced glomerular disease (Katz, Walker & Landy, 1983), particularly with involvement of capillary walls and changes in sialic acid composition (Tomino *et al.*, 1986). In other cases, particularly in children, the nephrotic syndrome is accompanied by minimal mesangial lesions on light microscopy together with mesangial IgA deposition (Mustonen, Pasternack & Rantala, 1983). These features, together with the response to treatment with corticosteroids (see below), raise the possibility that such cases represent instances of minimal change nephropathy (see Chapter 7) occurring in individuals that coincidentally happen to have mesangial deposits of IgA (which in this case are of minimal pathological significance), or the non-specific trapping of IgA immune complexes secondary to increased glomerular permeability. Other authors, however, favour the hypothesis that this is a distinct variant of IgA nephropathy itself (Lai *et al.*, 1986c). The observation that successful treatment of such cases with steroids is associated with clearing of the mesangial IgA deposits (Cheng, Chan & Chan, 1989), which would be very unusual in IgA nephropathy, favours the former possibility.

Systemic features

In contrast to HSP (see below) there is controversy as to whether any other organ apart from the kidney is affected in IgA nephropathy. Although deposition of IgA in both muscle (Tomino *et al.*, 1981) and dermal vessels (Hené *et al.*, 1986) has been claimed, review of all published studies up to 1985 showed that the presence of IgA in dermal vessels was only marginally increased (76/138 cases in IgA nephropathy versus 169/510 in other renal disease; Hasbargen & Copley, 1985). Furthermore, cutaneous deposits of IgA may be found in a significant proportion of normal controls (Thompson *et al.*, 1980), suggesting that, in many cases, this is a non-specific observation.

Henoch-Schönlein purpura

In general, less information is available on HSP as, at least in the common childhood form, it is usually a relatively benign and self-limiting disease, preventing the accumulation of large numbers of chronic cases. However, most of the phenomenology described above in the context of IgA nephropathy has also been noted in HSP (reviewed in Feehally, 1988). Such observations support the suggestion that HSP is IgA nephropathy with the addition of a systemic vasculitis (Waldo, 1988). This is also consistent with the development of mesangial IgA deposits typical of IgA nephropathy in the transplants of patients whose original disease was HSP (Weiss *et al.*, 1978), and with the simultaneous occurrence in monozygotic twins of HSP in one twin and IgA nephropathy in the other in response to an upper respiratory tract infection (Meadow & Scott, 1985).

Points of difference between HSP and IgA nephropathy include the regular observation of deposits of IgA in dermal capillaries, and occasionally in the gut, in HSP (Stevenson *et al.*, 1982), which, as detailed above, are a controversial finding in IgA nephropathy. This presumably is a consequence of the systemic nature of HSP. Similarly, the finding of increased glomerular monocytes and T cells in HSP but not IgA nephropathy (Nolasco *et al.*, 1987) may simply be a reflection of the greater severity of the former condition. Anti-neutrophil cytoplasm antibodies (ANCA) of IgA class have been described in HSP (Van der Wall Bake *et al.*, 1987), but are also found in IgA nephropathy (Erb *et al.*, 1990); ANCA are discussed further in Chapter 8. There is little available information on the immunogenetics of HSP (see above). Considering the discrepancies in immunogenetic studies on IgA nephropathy, and the much smaller numbers involved in the studies on HSP, the immunogenetic data probably do not contribute significantly either way to the case for a unified pathogenesis underlying HSP and IgA nephropathy.

Secondary IgA nephropathy

It is likely that some of the disease associations reported with IgA nephropathy (Table 5.1) are coincidental; this is a common condition, and some associations are therefore bound to occur by chance alone. However, the incidence of IgA nephropathy in certain conditions is sufficiently high that a causal relationship is suggested. Thus mesangial IgA deposition is found in many forms of liver disease, especially in association with alcoholic cirrhosis (Newell, 1987), although this particular link has been questioned (Bene *et al.*, 1988). The latter condition is also distinguished from other liver disease by the deposition of IgA along hepatic sinusoids (Kater *et al.*, 1979). Although biliary obstruction in man does not lead to an increase in serum concentration of polymeric IgA (in contradistinction to the rat), total and polymeric IgA are raised in both alcoholic cirrhosis and other forms of liver disease (Kutteh *et al.*, 1982). Circulating IC are also increased (Coppo *et al.*, 1985) and there is impaired Fc mediated clearance of altered erythrocytes (Roccatello *et al.*, 1985). The particular association of IgA deposition with alcoholic liver disease may be connected with the ability of alcohol to increase intestinal permeability to macromolecules (Worthington, Meserole & Syrotuck, 1978).

The link between IgA nephropathy, on the one hand, and coeliac disease and dermatitis herpetiformis on the other (Katz, Dyck & Bear, 1979; Heironimus & Perry, 1986) is interesting in view of the occurrence of anti-gliadin antibodies in IgA nephropathy (see above). Increases in serum IgA and IC are also found in these two conditions (Asquith & Haeney, 1979). It seems clear that subclinical coeliac disease is very rare, if it occurs at all, in

IgA nephropathy, as reticulin and endomysial antibodies, which are more specific for coeliac disease than anti-gliadin antibodies, are absent (Kumar *et al.*, 1988). There do, however, appear to be some small bowel abnormalities in IgA nephropathy (Fornasieri *et al.*, 1987), and exclusion of gluten from the diet does reduce circulating IC (see below).

Raised concentrations of serum IgA are found in ankylosing spondylitis (Cowling, Ebringer & Ebringer, 1980), and increased amounts of immune complexes, in some cases IgA–IC, are present in a high proportion of patients with a variety of seronegative spondyloarthropathies (Rosenbaum *et al.*, 1981; Hall, Gerber & Lawley, 1984). These observations may be relevant to the association between IgA nephropathy and such arthropathies (Bruneau *et al.*, 1986), which are also, of course, linked to various enteric infections.

Therapeutic aspects

Treatment for IgA nephropathy has, in general, proved rather disappointing, no doubt due, in part, to our deficiencies concerning an understanding of the pathogenesis. However, this has not prevented the use of a variety of therapies aimed at possible disease mechanisms.

The close temporal association between infections and episodes of macroscopic haematuria in IgA nephropathy has led to attempts to reduce exposure to bacterial antigens. Both tonsillectomy and abscess drainage, combined with non-steroidal anti-inflammatory agents (Lagrue *et al.*, 1981), and prolonged treatment with doxycycline (Kincaid-Smith & Nicholls, 1983b) may indeed reduce the amount of haematuria, but it is unclear whether this has any effect on the long-term outlook. A similar attempt to limit exposure to exogenous antigens by the use of a gluten-free diet appears to modify some immunological abnormalities but to have no effect on the progression of renal impairment (Coppo *et al.*, 1990). A possible allergic component to the pathogenesis has led to a trial of sodium cromoglycate, which may reduce proteinuria in some cases (Sato *et al.*, 1990).

In an attempt to influence the IgA component of presumed pathogenic IgA–IC, two trials have examined the use of phenytoin, which significantly reduces serum IgA concentration (Clarkson *et al.*, 1980; Egido *et al.*, 1984b). Neither showed any useful effect on either histological or clinical measures of disease. A more direct attempt to remove IgA–IC, and other possible circulating mediators of disease, has led to the use of plasma exchange, usually in association with steroids and cytotoxic agents. There is anecdotal evidence for the efficacy of this approach, which has been recommended particularly for exacerbations of IgA nephropathy associated with significant renal deterioration, and in HSP (D'Amico, 1987). However, given that renal function may deteriorate abruptly when plasma exchange is stopped (Nicholls *et al.*, 1985), and that spontaneous remissions of these acute episodes are not uncommon, controlled data is required. Plasma exchange may also temporarily slow the rate of decline of chronically progressive IgA nephropathy, which in some cases may delay the initiation of dialysis (Nicholls *et al.*, 1990).

Immunosuppressive drugs have also been used alone. There seems little doubt that corticosteroids are effective at reducing proteinuria in the subset of patients with minimal glomerular lesions and mesangial IgA deposition (Mustonen, Pasternack & Rantala, 1983; Lai *et al.*, 1986*b*). As discussed above, such cases may be examples of minimal change nephropathy, which is well known to be steroid responsive (see Chapter 7). There is less evidence that steroids have any significant effect on IgA disease proper (Lai *et al.*, 1986*b*), although some encouraging results have been reported (Kobayashi *et al.*, 1986). The one controlled trial of cyclosporin demonstrated a significant reduction in proteinuria in the treated group, but at the expense of a significant fall in creatinine clearance (Lai *et al.*, 1987). However, renal function improved in most patients when the cyclosporin was stopped, whereas the reduction in proteinuria persisted for at least three months. A controlled trial of the combination of cyclophosphamide, warfarin and dipyridamole failed to show any effect on the progression of renal impairment, although proteinuria was reduced (Walker *et al.*, 1990).

Lastly, and probably not specific to IgA nephropathy, it may be possible to influence the mediators that may be responsible for progressive glomerular sclerosis. A suggestion that eicosapentaenoic acid was effective at preventing deterioration in renal function (Hamazaki, Tateno & Shishido, 1984) has not been confirmed (Bennett, Walker & Kincaid-Smith, 1989; Cheng, Chan & Chan, 1990). There are suggestions that angiotensin-converting enzyme inhibitors may have a role (Woodroffe, 1988).

Concluding remarks

Despite being probably the commonest form of glomerulonephritis, and the subject of extensive experimental investigation, there are still major unresolved issues concerning the pathogenesis of IgA nephropathy. These include the factors responsible for the unifying feature of the condition, namely mesangial IgA deposition, whether such IgA deposition is itself injurious and by what mechanisms injury is produced, and the relationship between the various forms of IgA nephropathy, both primary and secondary.

Patients with IgA nephropathy clearly have a milieu that favours mesangial deposition of IgA; this is demonstrated particularly well by, on the one hand, the recurrence of disease in kidneys transplanted into patients and, on the other, by the resolution of deposits when transplanted into non-IgA nephropathy recipients. The factors that could be contributing to this milieu include IgA autoantibodies reacting with glomerular components, increased permeability of mucosal surfaces favouring increased exposure to exogenous antigens (Davin, Forget & Mahieu, 1988), abnormalities of the IgA response to such mucosal antigens, and deficiencies in the clearance of the resultant immune complexes. There is some evidence for the presence of IgA autoantibodies (Cederholm *et al.*, 1986), but the clinical observation of infection-triggered relapses is perhaps more in favour of a significant role for exogenous antigens, presumably in the form of IgA–IC, whether formed *in situ* or deposited directly. There may well, of course, be a degree of heterogeneity; it has been suggested that the subset of patients with infection-related macroscopic haematuria are responding to intermittent exposure to an exogenous antigen, whereas the subgroup without such episodes are responding to more chronic exposure to an antigen, such as a food antigen or autoantigen (D'Amico, 1987).

The significance of the multitude of abnormalities of the IgA response described in IgA nephropathy is difficult to assess. The familial nature of some of these abnormalities, particularly their presence in unaffected relatives, is reasonably good evidence that they are not simply the result of the disease state. On the other hand, the lowering of serum IgA concentration by phenytoin has no significant effect on renal pathology, which suggests that this is a secondary phenomenon. Similarly, delayed clearance of immune complexes, although attractive as a pathogenetic mechanism, could simply be secondary to saturation of normal clearance routes by excess complexes (but see below on relationship between primary and secondary IgA nephropathy).

It is uncertain whether deposition of IgA by itself is sufficient (as opposed to necessary) to cause glomerular injury. There are clearly documented cases of mesangial IgA deposition in man occurring in the absence of glomerulonephritis (Waldherr *et al.*, 1989). On the other hand, haematuria may occur when the sole abnormality is IgA deposition (no complement components or IgG). The significance of this is difficult to interpret, as injury may be caused by short-lived deposits which are missed by the renal biopsy which only detects the persisting IgA. Together with the clear evidence from animal models that additional factors are required, it seems on balance that IgA deposition *per se* is probably not pathogenic. If the suggestion that a failure of oral tolerance is involved is correct (Gesualdo, Lamm & Emancipator, 1990), then IgA deposition may occur normally in response to challenge with oral antigens; it is only when such failure leads to the additional deposition of IgG and IgM that injury results.

There are a variety of processes that could cause glomerular injury, but whether any particular mechanism is involved, and the relative contribution of each, is unknown. Although IgA fixes complement poorly via the classical pathway, if at all, aggregated IgA can fix complement via the alternative pathway. The description of IgG autoantibodies (Ballardie *et al.*, 1988) is particularly interesting in view of the apparent correlation with episodes of clinical relapse; confirmation and extension of this observation is needed. It has been suggested that IgA deposition within the mesangium may overwhelm normal mesangial clearance mechanisms, allowing glomerular damage from a variety of secondary causes (D'Amico, 1987). Components of the cellular immune system are perhaps unlikely to play a significant role, at least as effector cells in the mediation of glomerular damage, simply because they are not present within the glomerulus. Finally, it has been speculated that alterations in glomerular haemodynamics may be as least as important as immunopathological mechanisms, particularly in the causation of the sclerosing process mainly responsible for deterioration in renal function (Woodroffe, 1988).

There is reasonably strong evidence that IgA nephropathy and HSP share a common pathogenesis, at least with respect to the renal findings. The factors responsible for the systemic vasculitis are obscure; the greater incidence of HSP in childhood points to a role for developmental and/or environmental influences rather than immunogenetic differences. This is reinforced by the example referenced above of the occurrence of HSP in one monozygotic twin and IgA nephropathy in the other.

Some of the secondary forms of IgA nephropathy may well be providing clues as to the aetiology of the primary disorder. In particular there is good evidence that the liver plays a major role in the normal disposal of immune complexes. The IgA deposition that occurs in association with liver disease may therefore be highlighting the causal importance of disturbances of normal clearance mechanisms in primary IgA nephropathy.

References

A report of the Southwest Pediatric Nephrology Study Group (1982). A multicenter study of IgA nephropathy in children. *Kidney International*, 22, 643–52.

Asquith, P. & Haeney, M. R. (1979). Coeliac disease. In *Immunology of the Gastrointestinal Tract*, ed. P. Asquith, pp. 66–94. London: Churchill Livingstone.

Ault, B. H., Stapleton, F. B., Rivas, M. L. et al. (1990). Association of Henoch–Schönlein purpura glomerulonephritis with C4B deficiency. *Journal of Pediatrics*, 117, 753–5.

Ballardie, F. W., Brenchley, P. E. C., Williams, S. & O'Donoghue, D. J. (1988). Autoimmunity in IgA nephropathy. *Lancet*, ii, 588–92.

Bene, M-C., Faure, G. & Duheille, J. (1982). IgA nephropathy: characterization of the polymeric nature of mesangial deposits by *in vitro* binding of free secretory component. *Clinical and Experimental Immunology*, 47, 527–34.

Bene, M. C., De Korwin, J. D., de Ligny, B. H., Aymard, B., Kessler, M. & Faure, G. C. (1988). IgA nephropathy and alcoholic liver cirrhosis. A prospective necropsy study. *American Journal of Clinical Pathology*, **89**, 769–73.

Bennett, W. M. & Kincaid-Smith, P. (1983). Macroscopic haematuria in mesangial IgA nephropathy: correlation with glomerular crescents and renal dysfunction. *Kidney International*, **23**, 393–400.

Bennett, W. M., Walker, R. G. & Kincaid-Smith, P. (1989). Treatment of IgA nephropathy with eicosapentaenoic acid (EPA): a two-year prospective trial. *Clinical Nephrology*, **31**, 128–31.

Berger, J. & Hinglais, N. (1968). Les dépôts intercapillaires d'IgA-IgG. *Journal of Urology and Nephrology*, **74**, 694–5.

Berger, J., Noël, L. H. & Nabarra, B. (1984). Recurrence of mesangial IgA nephropathy after renal transplantation. *Contributions in Nephrology*, **40**, 195–7.

Berthoux, F-C., Alamartine, E., Pommier, G. & Lepetit, J-C. (1988). HLA and IgA nephritis revisited 10 years later: HLA-B35 antigen as a prognostic factor. *New England Journal of Medicine*, **319**, 1609–10.

Berthoux, F. C., Gagne, A., Sabatier, J. C. *et al.* (1978). HLA-Bw35 and mesangial IgA glomerulonephritis. *New England Journal of Medicine*, **298**, 1034–5.

Beukhoff, J. R., Ockhuizen, T., Halie, L. M. *et al.* (1984). Subentities within adult primary IgA-nephropathy. *Clinical Nephrology*, **22**, 195–9.

Bignon, J. D., Houssin, A., Soulillou, J. P., Denis, J., Guimbretiere, J. & Guenel, J. (1980). HLA antigens and Berger's disease. *Tissue Antigens*, **16**, 108–11.

Brandtzaeg, P. (1981). Transport models for secretory IgA and secretory IgM. *Clinical and Experimental Immunology*, **44**, 221–32.

Brettle, R., Peters, D. K. & Batchelor, J. R. (1978). Mesangial IgA glomerulonephritis and HLA antigens. *New England Journal of Medicine*, **299**, 200.

Bruneau, C., Villiaumey, J., Avouac, B. *et al.* (1986). Seronegative spondyloarthropathies and IgA glomerulonephritis: a report of four cases and a review of the literature. *Seminars in Arthritis and Rheumatism*, **15**, 179–84.

Burns, A., Li, P., So, A., Feehally, J. & Rees, A. J. (1991). The DQw7 allele of the HLA-DQB1 locus is associated with susceptibility to mesangial IgA nephropathy in caucasoids. *Nephrology Dialysis and Transplantation* (in press).

Cederholm, B., Wieslander, J., Bygren, P. & Heinegard, D. (1986). Patients with IgA nephropathy have circulating anti-basement membrane antibodies reacting with structures common to collagen I, II and IV. *Proceedings of the National Academy of Sciences, USA*, **83**, 6151–5.

Cederholm, B., Wieslander, J., Bygren, P. & Heinegard, D. (1988). Circulating complexes containing IgA and fibronectin in patients with primary IgA nephropathy. *Proceedings of the National Academy of Sciences, USA*, **85**, 4865–8.

Chan, S. H., Ku, G. & Sinniah, R. (1981). HLA and Chinese IgA mesangial glomerulonephritis. *Tissue Antigens*, **17**, 351–2.

Chatenoud, L. & Bach, M-A. (1981). Abnormalities of T-cell subsets in glomerulonephritis and systemic lupus erythematosus. *Kidney International*, **20**, 267–74.

Cheng, I. K., Chan, P. C. & Chan, M. K. (1990). The effect of fish-oil dietary supplement on the progression of mesangial IgA glomerulonephritis. *Nephrology Dialysis and Transplantation*, **5**, 241–6.

Cheng, I. K. P., Chan, K-W. & Chan, M-K. (1989). Mesangial IgA nephropathy with steroid-responsive nephrotic syndrome: disappearance of mesangial IgA deposits following steroid-induced remission. *American Journal of Kidney Disease*, **14**, 361–4.

Clarkson, A. R., Seymour, A. E., Thompson, A. J., Haynes, W. D. G., Chan, Y-L. & Jackson, B. (1977). IgA nephropathy: a syndrome of uniform morphology, diverse clinical features and uncertain prognosis. *Clinical Nephrology*, **8**, 459–7.

Clarkson, A. R., Seymour, A. E., Woodroffe, A. J., McKenzie, P. E., Chan, Y-L. & Wootton, A. M. (1980). Controlled trial of phenytoin therapy in IgA nephropathy. *Clinical Nephrology*, 13, 215–18.

Clarkson, A. R., Woodroffe, A. J. & Aarons, I. (1988). IgA nephropathy and Henoch-Schönlein purpura. In *Diseases of the Kidney*, 4th edn, ed. R. W. Schrier & C. W. Gottschalk, pp. 2061–89. Boston/Toronto: Little, Brown and Company.

Conley, M. E. & Delacroix, D. L. (1987). Intravascular and mucosal immunoglobulin A: two separate, but related systems of immune defence? *Annals of Internal Medicine*, 106, 892–9.

Coppo, R., Aricò, S., Piccoli, G. *et al.* (1985). Presence and origin of IgA$_1$- and IgA$_2$-containing circulating immune complexes in chronic alcoholic liver diseases with and without glomerulonephritis. *Clinical Immunology and Immunopathology*, 35, 1–8.

Coppo, R., Roccatello, D., Amore, A. *et al.* (1990). Effects of a gluten-free diet in primary IgA nephropathy. *Clinical Nephrology*, 33, 72–86.

Cosio, F. G., Lam, S., Folami, A. O., Conley, M. E. & Michael, A. F. (1982). Immune regulation of immunoglobulin production in IgA nephropathy. *Clinical Immunology and Immunopathology*, 23, 430–6.

Counahan, R., Winterborn, M. H., White, R. H. R. *et al.* (1977). Prognosis of Henoch–Schönlein nephritis in children. *British Medical Journal*, ii, 11–14.

Cowling, P., Ebringer, R. & Ebringer, A. (1980). Association of inflammation with raised serum IgA in ankylosing spondylitis. *Annals of the Rheumatic Diseases*, 39, 545–9.

Czerkinsky, C., Koopman, W. J., Jackson, S. *et al.* (1986). Circulating immune complexes and immunoglobulin A rheumatoid factor in patients with mesangial immunoglobulin A nephropathies. *Journal of Clinical Investigation*, 77, 1931–8.

D'Amico, G. (1987). The commonest glomerulonephritis in the world: IgA nephropathy. *Quarterly Journal of Medicine*, 64, 709–27.

Davin, J. C., Forget, P. & Mahieu, P. R. (1988). Increased intestinal permeability to (51 Cr) EDTA is correlated with IgA immune complex-plasma levels in children with IgA-associated nephropathies. *Acta Paediatrica Scandinavica*, 77, 118–24.

Delacroix, D. L., Hodgson, H. J. F., McPherson, A., Dive, C. & Vaerman, J. P. (1982). Selective transport of polymeric Immunoglobulin A in bile. Quantitative relationships of monomeric and polymeric immunoglobulin A, immunoglobulin M, and other proteins in serum, bile and saliva. *Journal of Clinical Investigation*, 70, 230–41.

Demaine, A. G., Rambausek, M., Knight, J. F., Williams, D. G. & Ritz, E. (1988). Relation of mesangial IgA glomerulonephritis to polymorphisms of immunoglobulin heavy chain switch region. *Journal of Clinical Investigation*, 81, 611–14.

Donini, U., Casanova, C., Zini, N. & Zucchelli, P. (1983). The presence of J chain in mesangial immune deposits of IgA nephropathy. *Proceedings of the European Dialysis and Transplantation Association*, 19, 655–62.

Egido, J., Blasco, R., Sancho, J. & Lozano, L. (1983). T-cell dysfunction in IgA nephropathy: specific abnormalities in the regulation of IgA synthesis. *Clinical Immunology and Immunopathology*, 26, 201–12.

Egido, J., Blasco, R., Lozano, L., Sancho, J. & Garcia-Hoyo, R. (1984a). Immunological abnormalities in the tonsils of patients with IgA nephropathy: inversion in the ratio of IgA:IgG bearing lymphocytes and increased polymeric IgA synthesis. *Clinical and Experimental Immunology*, 57, 101–6.

Egido, J., Rivera, F., Sancho, J., Barat, A. & Hernando, L. (1984b). Phenytoin in IgA nephropathy: a long-term controlled trial. *Nephron*, 38, 30–9.

Egido, J., Julian, B. A. & Wyatt, R. J. (1987). Genetic factors in primary IgA nephropathy. *Nephrology Dialysis and Transplantation*, 2, 134–42.

Emancipator, S. N. (1988). Experimental models of IgA nephropathy. *American Journal of Kidney Disease*, 12, 415–19.

Emancipator, S. N., Gallo, G. R. & Lamm, M. E. (1983). Experimental IgA nephropathy induced by oral immunization. *Journal of Experimental Medicine*, **157**, 572–82.

Emancipator, S. N. & Lamm, M. E. (1989). IgA nephropathy: pathogenesis of the most common form of glomerulonephritis. *Laboratory Investigation*, **60**, 168–83.

Erb, A., Andrassay, K., Koderisch, J., Waldherr, E. & Ritz, E. (1990). Neutrophil cytoplasm IgA antibodies (ANCA-IgA) in patients with IgA nephritis (IgAN) Henoch–Schönlein purpura (HSP) and other forms of glomerulonephritis (GN). *Kidney International*, **37**, 1167.(Abstract).

Fauchet, R., Le Pogamp, P., Genetet, B. *et al.* (1980). HLA-DR4 antigen and IgA nephropathy. *Tissue Antigens*, **16**, 405–10.

Feehally, J., Dyer, P. A., Davidson, J. A., Harris, R. & Mallick, N. P. (1984). Immunogenetics of IgA nephropathy: experience in a UK centre. *Disease Markers*, **2**, 493–500.

Feehally, J., Beattie, J., Brenchley, P. E. C., Coupes, B. M., Mallick, N. P. & Postlethwaite, R. J. (1986). Sequential study of the IgA system in relapsing IgA nephropathy. *Kidney International*, **30**, 924–31.

Feehally, J., Beattie, T. J., Brenchley, P. E. C., Coupes, B. M., Mallick, N. P. & Postlethwaite, R. J. (1987). Response of circulating immune complexes to food challenge in relapsing IgA nephropathy. *Pediatric Nephrology*, **1**, 581–6.

Feehally, J. (1988). Immune mechanisms in glomerular IgA deposition. *Nephrology Dialysis and Transplantation*, **3**, 361–78.

Fiorini, G., Fornasieri, A., Sinico, R. *et al.* (1982). Lymphocyte populations in the peripheral blood from patients with IgA nephropathy. *Nephron*, **31**, 354–7.

Fornasieri, A., Sinico, R. A., Maldifassi, P., Bernasconi, P., Vegni, M. & D'Amico, G. (1987). IgA-antigliadin antibodies in IgA mesangial nephropathy (Berger's disease). *British Medical Journal*, **295**, 78–9.

Gesualdo, L., Lamm, M. E. & Emancipator, S. N. (1990). Defective oral tolerance promotes nephritogenesis in experimental IgA nephropathy induced by oral immunization. *Journal of Immunology*, **145**, 3684–91.

Gonzalez-Cabrero, J., Egido, J., Sancho, J. & Moldenhauer, F. (1987). Presence of shared idiotypes in serum and immune complexes in patients with IgA nephropathy. *Clinical and Experimental Immunology*, **68**, 694–702.

Gormly, A. A., Seymour, A. E., Clarkson, A. R. & Woodroffe, A. J. (1981). IgA glomerular deposits in experimental cirrhosis. *American Journal of Pathology*, **104**, 50–4.

Gregory, M. C., Hammond, M. E. & Brewer, E. D. (1988). Renal deposition of cytomegalovirus antigen in immunoglobulin-A nephropathy. *Lancet*, **i**, 11–14.

Götze, O. & Müller-Eberhard, H. J. (1971). The C3-activator system: an alternate pathway of complement activation. *Journal of Experimental Medicine*, **134**, 90S–108S.

Hale, G. M., McIntosh, S. L., Hiki, Y., Clarkson, A. R. & Woodroffe, A. J. (1986). Evidence for IgA-specific B cell hyperactivity in patients with IgA nephropathy. *Kidney International*, **29**, 718–24.

Hall, R. P., Gerber, L. H. & Lawley, T. J. (1984). IgA containing immune complexes in psoriatic arthritis. *Clinical and Experimental Rheumatology*, **2**, 221–5.

Hamazaki, T., Tateno, S. & Shishido, H. (1984). Eicosapentaenoic acid and IgA nephropathy. *Lancet*, **i**, 1017–18.

Hasbargen, J. A. & Copley, J. B. (1985). Utility of skin biopsy in the diagnosis of IgA nephropathy. *American Journal of Kidney Disease*, **6**, 100–2.

Heironimus, J. D. & Perry, E. L. (1986). Dermatitis herpetiformis and glomerulonephritis. Case report and review of the literature. *American Journal of Medicine*, **80**, 508–10.

Hené, R. J., Velthuis, P., van de Wiel, A., Klepper, D., Mees, E. J. D. & Kater, L. (1986). The relevance of IgA deposits in vessel walls of clinically normal skin. *Archives of Internal Medicine*, **146**, 745–9.

Hiki, Y., Kobayashi, Y., Tateno, S., Sada, M. & Kashiwagi, N. (1982). Strong association of DR4 with benign IgA nephropathy. *Nephron*, **32**, 222–6.

Hiki, Y., Kobayashi, Y., Ookubo, M. & Kashiwagi, N. (1990). The role of HLA-DR4 in the long-term prognosis of IgA nephropathy. *Nephron*, **54**, 264–5.

Horii, Y., Muraguchi, A., Iwano, M. *et al.* (1989). Involvement of IL-6 in mesangial proliferative glomerulonephritis. *Journal of Immunology*, **143**, 3949–55.

Iida, H., Izumino, K., Asaka, M., Fujita, M., Takata, M. & Sasayama, S. (1990). IgA nephropathy and hepatitis B virus. IgA nephropathy unrelated to hepatitis B surface antigenemia. *Nephron*, **54**, 18–20.

Imai, H., Nakamoto, Y., Asakura, K., Miki, K., Yasuda, T. & Miura, A. B. (1985). Spontaneous glomerular IgA deposition in ddy mice: an animal model of IgA nephritis. *Kidney International*, **27**, 756–61.

Isaacs, K. L. & Miller, F. (1982). Role of antigen size and charge in immune complex glomerulonephritis. I. Active induction of disease with dextran and its derivatives. *Laboratory Investigation*, **47**, 198–205.

Isaacs, K. L. & Miller, F. (1983). Antigen size and charge in immune complex glomerulonephritis. II. Passive induction of immune deposits with dextran–anti-dextran immune complexes. *American Journal of Pathology*, **111**, 298–306.

Jones, C. L., Powell, H. R., Kincaid-Smith, P. & Roberton, D. M. (1990). Polymeric IgA and immune complex concentrations in IgA-related renal disease. *Kidney International*, **38**, 323–31.

Julian, B. A., Woodford, S. Y., Baehler, R. W., McMorrow, R. G. & Wyatt, R. J. (1988). Familial clustering and immunogenetic aspects of IgA nephropathy. *American Journal of Kidney Disease*, **12**, 366–70.

Kasahara, M., Hamada, K., Okuyama, T. *et al.* (1982). Role of HLA in IgA nephropathy. *Clinical Immunology and Immunopathology*, **25**, 189–95.

Kashiwabara, H., Shishido, H., Tomura, S., Tuchida, H. & Miyajima, T. (1982). Strong association between IgA nephropathy and HLA-DR4 antigen. *Kidney International*, **22**, 377–82.

Kater, L., Jöbsis, C., Baart de la Faille-Kuyper, E. H., Vogten, A. J. M. & Grijm, R. (1979). Alcoholic hepatic disease. Specificity of IgA deposits in the liver. *American Journal of Clinical Pathology*, **71**, 51–7.

Katz, A., Dyck, R. F. & Bear, R. A. (1979). Coeliac disease with immune complex glomerulonephritis. *Clinical Nephrology*, **11**, 39–44.

Katz, A., Walker, J. F. & Landy, P. J. (1983). IgA nephritis with nephrotic range proteinuria. *Clinical Nephrology*, **20**, 67–71.

Kincaid-Smith, P., Bennett, W. M., Dowling, J. P. & Ryan, G. B. (1983a). Acute renal failure and tubular necrosis associated with haematuria due to glomerulonephritis. *Clinical Nephrology*, **19**, 206–10.

Kincaid-Smith, P. & Nicholls, K. (1983b). Mesangial IgA nephropathy. *American Journal of Kidney Disease*, **3**, 90–102.

Kobayashi, Y., Fuji, K., Hiki, Y. & Tateno, S. (1986). Steroid therapy in IgA nephropathy: a prospective pilot study in moderate proteinuric cases. *Quarterly Journal of Medicine*, **61**, 935–43.

Kohara, M., Naito, S., Arakawa, K. *et al.* (1985). The strong association of HLA-DR4 with spherical mesangial dense deposits in IgA nephropathy. *Journal of Clinical and Laboratory Immunology*, **18**, 157–60.

Komori, K., Nose, Y., Inouye, H., Tsuji, K., Nomoto, Y. & Sakai, H. (1979). Study on HLA system in IgA nephropathy. *Tissue Antigens*, **14**, 32–6.

Kumar, V., Sieniawska, M., Beutner, E. H. & Chorzelski, T. P. (1988). Are immunological markers of gluten-sensitive enteropathy detectable in IgA nephropathy. *Lancet*, **ii**, 1307.

Kutteh, W. H., Prince, S. J., Phillips, J. O., Spenney, J. G. & Mestecky, J. (1982). Properties of immunoglobulin A in serum of individuals with liver diseases and in hepatic bile. *Gastroenterology*, **82**, 184–93.

Lagrue, G., Sadreux, T., Laurent, J. & Hirbec, G. (1981). Is there a treatment of mesangial IgA glomerulonephritis? *Clinical Nephrology*, **16**, 161.

Lai, K. N., Chan, K. W., Mac-Moune, F. *et al.* (1986a). The immunochemical characterization of the light chains in the mesangial IgA deposits in IgA nephropathy. *American Journal of Clinical Pathology*, **85**, 548–51.

Lai, K. N., Lai, F. M., Ho, C. P. & Chan, K. W. (1986b). Corticosteroid therapy in IgA nephropathy with nephrotic syndrome: a long-term controlled trial. *Clinical Nephrology*, **26**, 174–80.

Lai, K. N., Mac-Moune, F., Chan, K. W., Ping, C., Leung, A. C. T. & Vallance-Owen, J. (1986c). An overlapping syndrome of IgA nephropathy and lipoid nephrosis. *American Journal of Clinical Pathology*, **86**, 716–23.

Lai, K. N., Lai, F. M-M., Li, P. K. T. & Vallance-Owen, J. (1987). Cyclosporin treatment of IgA nephropathy: a short term controlled trial. *British Medical Journal*, **295**, 1165–8.

Lai, K. N., Lai, F. M., Tam, J. S. & Vallance-Owen, J. (1988). Strong association between IgA nephropathy and hepatitis B surface antigenemia in endemic areas. *Clinical Nephrology*, **29**, 229–34.

Le Petit, J. C., Van Loghem, E., De lange, G., Berthoux, F. C., Chapuis-Cellier, C. & Serre, J. L. (1981). Gm, Am, Pi and Km markers in mesangial glomerulonephritis. *Journal of Immunogenetics*, **8**, 415–18.

Lemaître-Coelho, I., Jackson, G. D. F. & Vaerman, J-P. (1978). High levels of secretory IgA and free secretory component in the serum of rats with bile duct obstruction. *Journal of Experimental Medicine*, **147**, 934–9.

Lhotta, K., Konig, P., Hintner, H., Spielberger, M. & Dittrich, P. (1990). Renal disease in a patient with hereditary complete deficiency of the fourth component of complement. *Nephron*, **56**, 206–11.

Linné, T. & Wasserman, J. (1985). Lymphocyte subpopulations and immunoglobulin production in IgA nephropathy. *Clinical Nephrology*, **23**, 109–11.

MacDonald, I. M., Dumble, L. J. & Kincaid-Smith, P. (1976). HLA and glomerulonephritis. In *HLA and Disease*, pp. 203. Paris: INSERM.

Markham, R. V., Sutherland, J. C. & Mardiney, M. R. (1973). The ubiquitous occurrence of immune complex localization in the renal glomeruli of normal mice. *Laboratory Investigation*, **29**, 111–20.

Matsiota, P., Dosquet, P., Louzir, H., Druet, E., Druet, P. & Avrameas, S. (1990). IgA polyspecific autoantibodies in IgA nephropathy. *Clinical and Experimental Immunology*, **79**, 361–6.

Mclean, P. H., Wyatt, R. J. & Julian, B. A. (1984). Complement phenotypes in glomerulonephritis: increased frequency of homozygous null C4 phenotypes in IgA nephropathy and Henoch–Schönlein purpura. *Kidney International*, **26**, 855–60.

Meadow, S. R. & Scott, D. G. (1985). Berger disease: Henoch-Schönlein syndrome without the rash. *Journal of Pediatrics*, **106**, 27–32.

Melvin, T., Burke, B., Michael, A. F. & Kim, Y. (1983). Experimental IgA nephropathy in bile-duct ligated rats. *Clinical Immunology and Immunopathology*, **27**, 369–77.

Monteiro, R. C., Halbwachs-Mecarelli, L., Roque-Barreira, M. C., Noel, L-H., Berger, L. & Lesavre, P. (1985). Charge and size of mesangial IgA in IgA nephropathy. *Kidney International*, **28**, 666–71.

Moore, R., Medcraft, J., Sinico, R. *et al.* (1990a). Association of HLA-DQ gene polymorphism in European IgA nephropathy [IgAN]. *Nephrology Dialysis and Transplantation*, **5**, 681–2.(Abstract).

Moore, R., Medcraft, J., Sinico, R. *et al.* (1990*b*). HLA-DP region gene polymorphism in primary IgA nephropathy [IgAN]. *Nephrology Dialysis and Transplantation*, 5, 681.(Abstract).

Moore, R., Sinico, R., Medcraft, J., D'Amico, G. & Hitman, G. (1990*c*). Functional significance of HLA-DQ gene polymorphism in IgA nephropathy [IgAN]. *Nephrology Dialysis and Transplantation*, 5, 682.(Abstract).

Moore, R. H., Hitman, G. A., Sinico, R. A. *et al.* (1990*a*). Immunoglobulin heavy chain switch gene polymorphisms in glomerulonephritis. *Kidney International*, 38, 332–6.

Moore, R. H., Hitman, G. A., Lucas, E. Y. *et al.* (1990*b*). HLA DQ region gene polymorphism associated with primary IgA nephropathy. *Kidney International*, 37, 991–5.

Mustonen, J., Pasternack, A., Helin, H. *et al.* (1981). Circulating immune complexes, the concentration of serum IgA and the distribution of HLA antigens in IgA nephropathy. *Nephron*, 29, 170–5.

Mustonen, J., Pasternack, A. & Rantala, I. (1983). The nephrotic syndrome in IgA glomerulonephritis: response to corticosteroid therapy. *Clinical Nephrology*, 20, 172–6.

Nagy, J., Hámori, A., Ambrus, M. & Hernádi, E. (1979). More on IgA glomerulonephritis and HLA antigens. *New England Journal of Medicine*, 300, 92.

Nagy, J., Vj, M., Szücs, G., Trinn, C. & Burger, T. (1984). Herpes antigens and antibodies in kidney biopsies and sera of IgA glomerulonephritic patients. *Clinical Nephrology*, 21, 259–62.

Newell, G. C. (1987). Cirrhotic glomerulonephritis: incidence, morphology, clinical features, and pathogenesis. *American Journal of Kidney Disease*, 9, 183–90.

Nicholls, K., Walker, R. G., Kincaid-Smith, P. & Dowling, J. (1985). 'Malignant' IgA nephropathy. *American Journal of Kidney Disease*, 5, 42–6.

Nicholls, K., Becker, G., Walker, R., Wright, C. & Kincaid-Smith, P. (1990). Plasma exchange in progressive IgA nephropathy. *Journal of Clinical Apheresis*, 5, 128–32.

Nishimukai, H., Nakanishi, I., Takeuchi, Y. *et al.* (1989). Complement C6 and C7 polymorphisms in Japanese patients with chronic glomerulonephritis. *Human Hereditary*, 39, 150–5.

Nolasco, F. E. B., Cameron, J. S., Hartley, B., Coelho, A., Hildreth, G. & Reuben, R. (1987). Intraglomerular T cells and monocytes in nephritis: study with monoclonal antibodies. *Kidney International*, 31, 1160–6.

Nomoto, Y., Sakai, H. & Arimori, S. (1979). Increase of IgA-bearing lymphocytes in peripheral blood from patients with IgA nephropathy. *American Journal of Clinical Pathology*, 71, 158–60.

Nomoto, Y., Suga, T., Miura, M., Nomoto, H., Tomino, Y. & Sakai, H. (1986). Characterization of an acidic nuclear protein recognized by autoantibodies in sera from patients with IgA nephropathy. *Clinical and Experimental Immunology*, 65, 513–19.

Noël, L. H., Descamps, B., Jungers, P. *et al.* (1978). HLA antigen in three types of glomerulonephritis. *Clinical Immunology and Immunopathology*, 10, 19–23.

Nyulassy, S., Buc, M., Sasinka, M. *et al.* (1977). The HLA system in glomerulonephritis. *Clinical Immunology and Immunopathology*, 7, 319–23.

Oldstone, M. B. A. & Dixon, F. J. (1972). Disease accompanying *in utero* viral infection. The role of maternal antibody in tissue injury after transplacental infection with lymphocytic choriomeningitis virus. *Journal of Experimental Medicine*, 135, 827–38.

Ostergaard, J. R., Storm, K. & Lamm, L. U. (1990). Lack of association between HLA and Schönlein–Henoch purpura. *Tissue Antigens*, 35, 234–5.

Portis, J. L. & Coe, J. E. (1979). Deposition of IgA in renal glomeruli of mink affected with Aleutian disease. *American Journal of Pathology*, 96, 227–36.

Rambausek, M., van den Wall Bake, A. W., Schumacher-Ach, R. *et al.* (1987). Genetic polymorphism of C3 and Bf in IgA nephropathy. *Nephrology Dialysis and Transplantation*, 2, 208–11.

Rauterberg, E. W., Lieberknecht, H-M., Wingen, A-M. & Ritz, E. (1987). Complement membrane attack (MAC) in idiopathic IgA-glomerulonephritis. *Kidney International*, **31**, 820–9.

Richman, A. V., Mahoney, J. J. & Fuller, T. J. (1979). Higher prevalence of HLA-B12 in patients with IgA nephropathy. *Annals of Internal Medicine*, **90**, 201.

Rifai, A., Small, P. A., Teague, P. O. & Ayoub, E. M. (1979). Experimental IgA nephropathy. *Journal of Experimental Medicine*, **150**, 1161–73.

Rifai, A. & Mannik, M. (1983). Clearance kinetics and fate of mouse IgA immune complexes prepared with monomeric or dimeric IgA. *Journal of Immunology*, **130**, 1826–32.

Rifai, A. & Millard, K. (1985). Glomerular deposition of immune complexes prepared with monomeric or polymeric IgA. *Clinical and Experimental Immunology*, **60**, 363–8.

Rifai, A. (1987). Experimental models for IgA-associated nephritis. *Kidney International*, **31**, 1–7.

Rifai, A., Schena, F. P., Montinaro, V. *et al.* (1989). Clearance kinetics and fate of macromolecular IgA in patients with IgA nephropathy. *Laboratory Investigation*, **61**, 381–8.

Roccatello, D., Coppo, R., Piccoli, G. *et al.* (1985). Circulating Fc-receptor blocking factors in IgA nephropathies. *Clinical Nephrology*, **23**, 159–68.

Roccatello, D., Picciotto, G., Coppo, R. *et al.* (1989). Clearance of polymeric IgA aggregates in humans. *American Journal of Kidney Disease*, **14**, 354–60.

Rodriguez-Soriano, J., Arrieta, A., Vallo, A., Sebastian, M. J., Vitoria, J. C. & Masdevall, M. D. (1988). IgA antigliadin antibodies in children with IgA mesangial glomerulonephritis. *Lancet*, **i**, 1109–10.

Rosenbaum, J. T., Theofilopoulos, A. N., McDevitt, H. O., Pereira, A. B., Carson, D. & Calin, A. (1981). Presence of circulating immune complexes in Reiter's syndrome and ankylosing spondylitis. *Clinical Immunology and Immunopathology*, **18**, 291–7.

Rostoker, G., Delprato, S., Petit-Phar, M. *et al.* (1989). IgA antigliadin antibodies as a possible marker for IgA mesangial glomerulonephritis in adults with primary glomerulonephritis. *New England Journal of Medicine*, **320**, 1283–4.

Rothschild, E. & Chatenoud, L. (1984). T cell subset modulation of immunoglobulin production in IgA nephropathy and membranous glomerulonephritis. *Kidney International*, **25**, 557–64.

Russell, M. W., Mestecky, J., Julian, B. A. & Galla, J. H. (1986). IgA-associated renal diseases: antibodies to environmental antigens in sera and deposition of immunoglobulins and antigens in glomeruli. *Journal of Clinical Immunology*, **6**, 74–86.

Sakai, H., Nomoto, Y. & Arimori, S. (1979a). Decrease of IgA-specific suppressor T cell activity in patients with IgA nephropathy. *Clinical and Experimental Immunology*, **38**, 243–8.

Sakai, H., Nomoto, Y., Arimori, S., Komori, K., Inouye, H. & Tsuji, C. (1979b). Increase of IgA-bearing peripheral blood lymphocytes in families of patients with IgA nephropathy. *American Journal of Clinical Pathology*, **72**, 452–6.

Sakai, H., Miyazaki, M., Endoh, M. & Nomoto, Y. (1989). Increase of IgA-specific switch T cells in patients with IgA nephropathy. *Clinical and Experimental Immunology*, **78**, 378–82.

Sato, M., Ideura, T. & Koshikawa, S. (1986). Experimental IgA nephropathy in mice. *Laboratory Investigation*, **54**, 377–84.

Sato, M., Kojima, H., Takayama, K. & Koshikawa, S. (1988). Glomerular deposition of food antigens in IgA nephropathy. *Clinical and Experimental Immunology*, **73**, 295–9.

Sato, M., Takayama, K., Kojima, H. & Koshikawa, S. (1990). Sodium chromoglycate therapy in IgA nephropathy: a preliminary short-term trial. *American Journal of Kidney Disease*, **15**, 141–6.

Savi, M., Neri, T. M., Silvestri, M. G., Allegri, L. & Mignone, L. (1979). HLA antigens and IgA mesangial glomerulonephritis. *Clinical Nephrology*, **12**, 45–6.

Schifferli, J. A., Steiger, G., Paccaud, J-P., Sjöholm, A. G. & Hauptmann, G. (1986). Difference in the biological properties of the two forms of the fourth component of human complement (C4). *Clinical and Experimental Immunology*, **63**, 473–7.

Smith, S. M., Yu, G. S. & Tsukamoto, H. (1990). IgA nephropathy in alcohol abuse. An animal model. *Laboratory Investigation*, **62**, 179–84.

Stevenson, J. A., Leong, L. A., Cohen, A. H. & Border, W. A. (1982). Henoch-Schönlein purpura. Simultaneous demonstration of IgA deposits in involved skin, intestine and kidney. *Archives of Pathology and Laboratory Medicine*, **106**, 192–5.

Takeuchi, E., Doi, T., Shimada, T., Muso, E., Maruyama, N. & Yoshida, H. (1989). Retroviral gp70 antigen in spontaneous mesangial glomerulonephritis of ddY mice. *Kidney International*, **35**, 638–46.

Thompson, A. J., Chan, Y-L., Woodroffe, A. J., Clarkson, A. R. & Seymour, A. E. (1980). Vascular IgA deposits in clinically normal skin of patients with renal disease. *Pathology*, **12**, 407–13.

Tomino, Y., Nomoto, Y., Endoh, M. & Sakai, H. (1981). Deposition of IgA-dominant immune-complexes in muscular vessels from patients with IgA nephropathy. *Acta Pathologica Japonica*, **31**, 361–5.

Tomino, Y., Endoh, M., Nomoto, Y. & Sakai, H. (1982a). Specificity of eluted antibody from renal tissues of patients with IgA nephropathy. *American Journal of Kidney Disease*, **1**, 276–80.

Tomino, Y., Endoh, M., Nomoto, Y. & Sakai, H. (1982b). Double immunofluorescence studies of immunoglobulins, complement components and their control proteins in patients with IgA nephropathy. *Acta Pathologica Japonica*, **32**, 251–6.

Tomino, Y., Sakai, H., Suga, T. et al. (1983). Impaired solubilization of glomerular immune deposits by sera from patients with IgA nephropathy. *American Journal of Kidney Disease*, **3**, 48–53.

Tomino, Y., Sakai, H., Miura, M. et al. (1986). Effect of immunoglobulin depositions of glomerular sialic acids in patients with IgA nephropathy. *American Journal of Nephrology*, **6**, 187–92.

Tomino, Y., Yagame, M., Omata, F., Nomoto, Y. & Sakai, H. (1987). A case of IgA nephropathy with adeno- and herpes simplex viruses. *Nephron*, **47**, 258–61.

Tomino, Y., Koide, H., Yagame, M., Sakai, H. & Tanaka, S. (1990). Preliminary study on specificity of IgA released from lymphocytes by EB virus transformation in patients with IgA nephropathy. *American Journal of the Medical Sciences*, **299**, 374–8.

Van der Wall Bake, A. W. L., Lobatto, S., Jonges, L., Daha, M. R. & Van Es, L. A. (1987). IgA antibodies directed against cytoplasmic antigens of polymorphonuclear leucocytes in patients with Henoch-Schonlein purpura. *Advances in Experimental and Medical Biology*, **216B**, 1593–8.

Vangelista, A., Frascà, G. M., Mondini, S. & Bonomini, V. (1984). Idiopathic IgA mesangial nephropathy: immunohistological features. *Contributions in Nephrology*, **40**, 167–73.

Waldherr, R., Rambausek, M., Duncker, W. D. & Ritz, E. (1989). Frequency of mesangial IgA deposits in a non-selected autopsy series. *Nephrology Dialysis and Transplantation*, **4**, 943–6.

Waldo, F. B. (1988). Is Henoch–Schönlein purpura the systemic form of IgA nephropathy? *American Journal of Kidney Disease*, **12**, 373–7.

Waldo, F. B., Britt, W. J., Tomana, M., Julian, B. A. & Mestecky, J. (1989a). Non-specific mesangial staining with antibodies to cytomegalovirus in immunoglobulin-A nephropathy. *Lancet*, **i**, 129–31.

Waldo, F. B. & Cochran, A. M. (1989b). Mixed IgA-IgG aggregates as a model of immune complexes in IgA nephropathy. *Journal of Immunology*, **142**, 3841–6.

Walker, R. G., Yu, S. H., Owen, J. E. & Kincaid-Smith, P. (1990). The treatment of mesangial IgA nephropathy with cyclophosphamide, dipyridamole and warfarin: a two-year prospective trial. *Clinical Nephrology*, **34**, 103–7.

Weiss, J. H., Bhathena, D. B., Curtis, J. J., Lucas, B. A. & Luke, R. G. (1978). A possible relationship between Henoch–Schönlein syndrome and IgA nephropathy (Berger's disease). *Nephron*, **22**, 582–91.

Welch, R. W., Beischel, L. S. & Choi, E. M. (1989). Molecular genetics of C4B deficiency in IgA nephropathy. *Human Immunology*, **26**, 353–63.

Welch, T. R. & Berry, A. (1987). C3 alleles in diseases associated with C3 activation. *Disease Markers*, **5**, 81–7.

Westberg, N. G., Baklien, K., Schmekel, B., Gillberg, R. & Brandtzaeg, P. (1983). Quantitation of immunoglobulin-producing cells in small intestinal mucosa of patients with IgA nephropathy. *Clinical Immunology and Immunopathology*, **26**, 442–5.

Woodroffe, A. J., Clarkson, A. R., Seymour, A. E. & Lomax-Smith, J. D. (1982). Mesangial IgA nephritis. *Springer Seminars in Immunopathology*, **5**, 321–32.

Woodroffe, A. J. (1988). IgA nephropathy: toward an understanding of its pathogenesis. In *Immunopathology of Renal Disease. Contemporary Issues in Nephrology. 18*, ed. C. B. Wilson, B. M. Brenner & J. H. Stein, pp. 197–211. New York, Edinburgh, London, Melbourne: Churchill Livingstone.

Worthington, B. D., Meserole, L. & Syrotuck, J. A. (1978). Effect of daily ethanol on intestinal permeability to macromolecules. *American Journal of Digestive Diseases*, **23**, 23–32.

Wyatt, R. J., Julian, B. A., Galla, J. H. & McLean, R. H. (1984). Increased frequency of C3 fast alleles in IgA nephropathy. *Disease Markers*, **2**, 419–28.

Wyatt, R. J., Valenski, W. R., Stapleton, F. B. *et al.* (1988). Immunoregulatory studies in patients with IgA nephropathy. *Journal of Clinical and Laboratory Immunology*, **25**, 109–14.

Wyatt, R. J., Rivas, M. L., Schena, F. P., Bin, J. & Julian, B. A. (1990). Regional variation in C4 phenotype in patients with IgA nephropathy. *Journal of Pediatrics*, **116**, S72–7.

Yap, H. K., Sakai, R. S., Woo, K. T., Lim, C. H. & Jordan, S. C. (1987). Detection of bovine serum albumin in the circulating IgA immune complexes of patients with IgA nephropathy. *Clinical Immunology and Immunopathology*, **43**, 395–402.

Yap, H. K., Sakai, R. S., Bahn, L. *et al.* (1988). Anti-vascular endothelial cell antibodies in patients with IgA nephropathy: frequency and clinical significance. *Clinical Immunology and Immunopathology*, **49**, 450–62.

–6–
Mesangiocapillary glomerulonephritis

Mesangiocapillary glomerulonephritis (MCGN), also known as membrano-proliferative glomerulonephritis and, in the past, as hypocomplementaemic persistent glomerulonephritis, was first characterised in the 1960s (Habib *et al.*, 1961; Gotoff *et al.*, 1965; West *et al.*, 1965). The lesion may occur as a primary glomerulopathy or in the context of a number of systemic diseases (see Table 6.1); this chapter will be concerned mainly with the primary forms, which, as with the secondary causes, are heterogeneous. The inter-relationship of these forms is discussed at the end of this chapter.

The histological features, common to all the primary forms of MCGN, are mesangial expansion, due to an increase in both matrix and mesangial cells, and thickening of capillary loops due to peripheral extension of mesangial cells and matrix. This extension takes the form of an interposition between the endothelial cells and basement membrane and results in the deposition of fresh basement material at the interface between endothelial cell and

Table 6.1. *Secondary causes of mesangiocapillary glomerulonephritis*

Infection (particularly chronic)
    Bacterial (infective endocarditis, leprosy)
    Viral (hepatitis B)
    Protozoal (schistosomiasis)

Neoplasia
    Light chain disease
    Lymphoma, carcinoma

Systemic lupus erythematosus

Cryoglobulinaemia

Sickle cell anaemia

interposed matrix; this produces the characteristic double contouring or 'tram-tracking' of the capillary wall. In addition there may be a contribution to the proliferation from endothelial cells and polymorphs, and occasionally extracapillary proliferation in the form of crescents. Immunofluorescence and ultrastructural studies reveal differences between the primary forms. In type I MCGN, immunofluorescence demonstrates deposits, particularly of C3 but also of IgG and IgM, both in mesangial areas and in capillary loops in a subendothelial or endomembranous (within the internal lamina of the GBM) location. Ultrastructurally, electron dense deposits are found at the same sites. Type II MCGN is a distinctive entity, actually described before the recognition of MCGN as a separate, hypocomplementaemic form of nephritis (Berger & Galle, 1963). It is defined by intramembranous dense deposits on electron microscopy (dense deposit disease); such deposits are usually associated with the histological appearance of MCGN but occasionally a focal sclerosing pattern may be seen (Kashtan et al., 1990). By immunofluorescence, C3 is deposited in a linear pattern along the capillary loops and in a granular fashion in the mesangium; immunoglobulins are occasionally present (usually IgM). Dense deposits and C3 deposition may also be found in the basement membranes of Bowman's capsule, tubules, blood vessels, and, occasionally, in basement membranes in the spleen (Thorner & Baumal, 1982). In addition, various ocular abnormalities have also been noted in type II MCGN (Duvall-Young et al., 1989), and dense deposit material has been found in Bruch's membrane in the eye (Duvall-Young, MacDonald & McKechnie, 1989). A number of different lesions have been classified as 'type III' MCGN and it is not clear that this is a distinct category as opposed to representing morphological variants of type I MCGN. The lesions described include a superimposed pattern similar to stage I membranous nephropathy, with epimembranous deposits and protrusions of basement membrane material (Burkholder, Marchand & Krueger, 1970), and a variant in which the glomerular basement membrane has a disrupted and fenestrated appearance (Anders et al., 1977; Strife et al., 1977).

In clinical terms, primary MCGN has a more uniform picture. The disease tends to occur in children and young adults and presents as the nephrotic syndrome in 50%–75% of cases. Other presentations include an abnormal urine sediment or the clinical picture of a rapidly progressive glomerulonephritis; this latter may occur more frequently in type II MCGN (Habib et al., 1975). Type I is considerably more common than type II, with the latter accounting for 15%–30% of MCGN in most series (Glassock et al., 1986; Donadio, 1988). Overall, the disease is found in approximately 7% of childhood and 12% of adult cases of the nephrotic syndrome (Glassock et al., 1986). A characteristic finding is hypocomplementaemia, which occurs to a variable extent in all types of MCGN (discussed further below). The disease usually progresses to renal failure at a variable rate, with the prognosis perhaps being worse in type II MCGN (Cameron et al., 1983).

Immunogenetics

The MHC

There are reports of an increased frequency of B7 in type II MCGN (Noël et al., 1978) and of A2 (p < 0.02) and Bw44 (p < 0.002) in unspecified (but probably type I) MCGN (Rashid et al., 1983); none of these was significant after correction for multiple comparisons. A study of 35 patients with type I or type III MCGN found significant increases in the frequencies of B8 and DR3, and a non-significant increase in the frequency of the C4A*Q0 null allele of C4 (Welch et al., 1986). All of these increased frequencies could be entirely accounted for by the increased frequency in patients of a particular extended MHC haplotype (B8,DR3,SC01,GLO2, where SC01 represents Bf*S,C2*C,C4A*Q0,C4B*1 and GLO2 represents glyoxalase I 2). Presence of this haplotype was associated with a relative risk of 14.79 (p = 0.0006), and occurred with an equally increased frequency in both type I and type III MCGN. Interestingly the frequency of a very similar haplotype, differing only in glyoxalase allotype (B8,DR3,SC01,GLO1), was not increased, suggesting that B8, DR3 and/or C4A*Q0 alleles are unlikely to be primarily involved in this linkage. Genetic C2 deficiency may also predispose to type I MCGN (Holland, de Bracco & Christian, 1972; Kim et al., 1977).

As with membranous nephropathy (see Chapter 3), the reported association between MCGN and C4B*2.9 (Wank et al., 1984) may be an artefact due to the acquisition of this complement variant in uraemia (Welch & Beischel, 1985). The nature of the alloantigen found on B cells in 75% of patients with type I MCGN (versus 17% in controls; relative risk 16.6, p < 0.0005) is unclear (Friend et al., 1977). The typing sera from multiparous women (mothers of the patients studied) was absorbed to remove anti-class I MHC specificities, but undefined anti-class II reactivity could well be responsible.

Nephritic factor is associated particularly with type II MCGN (see below), and although there does not seem to be any direct information on class II alleles the finding of DR7 in 8 out of 11 patients with nephritic factor (Rees, 1984) is probably of most relevance to this type.

Other loci

The histological pattern of type I (and type III) MCGN is seen in a variety of genetically determined complement abnormalities. These include deficiencies of components of the classical pathway (see above), C3 (Berger *et al.*, 1983), terminal complement components (C6,C7,C8; Coleman *et al.*, 1983), C1 esterase inhibitor deficiency (Hory & Haultier, 1989), and an inherited abnormality of the alternative pathway C3 convertase (Marder *et al.*, 1983). Type II MCGN is not found in these conditions, but there is a suggestion that the C3F allelic variant of C3 occurs more frequently in cases of type II MCGN as compared to both controls and type I MCGN (McLean & Winkelstein, 1984). There is no significant difference between controls and type I MCGN cases with respect to C3 allele frequencies (McLean & Winkelstein, 1984; Welch & Berry, 1987). Both type II MCGN and partial lipodystrophy (see below) have been found in association with a hypomorphic variant of C3F (McLean & Winkelstein, 1984).

The genetic basis for some of the familial cases of MCGN (for review see Berry *et al.*, 1981) is uncertain; others of these familial cases are due to inherited complement deficiencies. An increase in IgM-bearing B cells has been found in the peripheral blood of patients with type I and II MCGN and also of their relatives (Sakai *et al.*, 1979); the significance of this is obscure.

Immunopathology

Animal studies

A lesion resembling type I MCGN is part of the spectrum of disease that can be induced by experimental immune complex nephritis; this experimental model is considered further in Chapter 1. More specifically, some Finnish Landrace lambs develop a disease very similar to type I MCGN as part of a more generalised immune complex-type disease (Angus *et al.*, 1980). The affected lambs are deficient in C3; although C3 is found deposited in the glomeruli, C3 deficiency may be the primary genetic lesion rather than being secondary to complement activation. Dogs may also develop a glomerulonephritis with an MCGN pattern (Center *et al.*, 1987), on occasion in association with specific infections (Grauer *et al.*, 1988; Ludders *et al.*, 1988). Mice suffering from haemolytic anaemia due to a hereditary defect in spectrin also have an associated MCGN (Maggio-Price *et al.*, 1988). This is of particular interest, given the occurrence of MCGN in human sickle cell disease (see below).

There are no animal models of type II MCGN.

Human studies

Most interest in the immunopathology of human MCGN has centred on the complement system. Serum concentrations of C3 and CH50 are lowered in up to 50% of cases of type I (and probably type III) MCGN at diagnosis, and in nearly all cases of type II MCGN (Donadio, 1988). This reduction in complement is prolonged, in contrast to poststreptococcal glomerulonephritis, and was one of the features that first defined MCGN as a separate entity. Concentrations of earlier components of the classical (C1q, C4) and alternative (factor B, properdin) pathways may be low in type I MCGN (Ooi, Vallota & West, 1976; Michael *et al.*, 1973), but C1q and C4 are usually normal in type II MCGN (Ooi, Vallota & West, 1976; Donadio *et al.*, 1979). C5 catabolism is not increased in type II MCGN despite active C3 consumption (Sissons *et al.*, 1977), probably reflecting the fact that, in order to function as a C5 convertase, the alternative pathway C3 convertase must be attached to a cell surface and have additional molecules of C3b. In contrast, terminal complement components (C5-C9) are reduced in types I and III (Clardy *et al.*, 1989). The reduction in C5 correlates with the reduction in C3; late terminal components are activated to a greater extent in type III MCGN as compared to type I despite approximately equal C5 activation (Clardy *et al.*, 1989). The main contribution to these reductions in complement components is probably increased catabolism. However, exogenous labelled C3 is not catabolised at an increased rate (Peters *et al.*, 1972); this may be explained by either reduced synthesis or lack of access of exogenous C3 to the pool in which catabolism is occurring. A large proportion of this basic complement phenomenology can now be explained in terms of circulating factors that activate the complement system in a number of ways.

Nephritic factor, partial lipodystrophy and type II MCGN

A factor capable of activating C3 (C3NeF, NeF) was first found in the serum of a patient with MCGN (Spitzer *et al.*, 1969). Subsequent work has shown a strong association between NeF and type II MCGN (present in over 60%) and a weaker association with type I (present in 10%–20%) (Glassock *et al.*, 1986). There is also an association between NeF and patients with partial lipodystrophy, who in turn may also suffer from MCGN, usually type II (Sissons *et al.*, 1976; Eisenger, Shortland & Moorhead, 1972; Peters *et al.*, 1973). All combinations have been noted: patients with NeF, MCGN and partial lipodystrophy; NeF and partial lipodystrophy without renal involvement; and even NeF in apparent isolation (Karstrop, 1976; Tedesco *et al.*, 1985), or in association with chronic urticaria in the absence of lipodystrophy or renal disease (Borradori *et al.*, 1989). MCGN, lipodystrophy and NeF have also been described as coexisting within members of a single family spanning two generations (Power, Ng & Simpson, 1990). It is interesting that partial lipodystrophy, or variants, have been associated with other abnormalities of the complement system (Frank, Gelfand & Atkinson, 1976; Sissons *et al.*, 1976) .

Classical NeF is an IgG autoantibody (Thompson, 1972; Davis *et al.*, 1977) which binds to and stabilises the alternative pathway C3 convertase C3bBb (Daha, Fearon & Austen, 1976). It thus permanently activates the alternative pathway and its presence is usually associated with profound C3 depletion, although occasionally very low concentrations of NeF are compatible with a normal C3 concentration (Ohi *et al.*, 1990). The binding site for NeF on C3bBb is unknown, but is likely to be the same for most if not all NeFs. The evidence for this is the similar functional characteristics, and the sharing of a common idiotype. Evidence for this last point comes from a study that used monoclonal NeFs, produced by Epstein Barr virus transformation of B cells from patients with NeF, to purify antibodies with antiidiotypic activity specific for NeF (Tsokos *et al.*, 1989). Such antiidiotypic antibodies crossreacted with all monoclonal and polyclonal NeFs tested. Interestingly, antiidiotypic antibodies can be detected in normal individuals as well as patients with Nef, although in the latter case a much higher percentage of the antiidiotypes resembled the C3bBb ligand of NeF (internal image antiidiotypes; Spitzer, Stitzel & Tsokos, 1990*b*). In fact, it is also possible to demonstrate NeF production from normal individuals by mitogen stimulation of peripheral blood lymphocytes (Spitzer, Stitzel & Tsokos, 1990*a*). The fact that the affinity of this NeF from normal individuals appeared to be approximately the same as that from patients raises the possibility that NeF might have a physiological role.

The connection between NeF and MCGN on the one hand, and partial lipodystrophy on the other, remains speculative. The two main classes of explanation for the association with renal disease (Pusey, Venning & Peters, 1988) are first, that the complement deficiency produced by NeF leads to inability to handle immune complexes and therefore the diseases typical of inherited complement deficiencies (see Chapter 4 on lupus nephritis); and second, it is possible that complement activation *per se* is nephrotoxic. Attempts to reproduce MCGN in animals by continual activation of the complement system have been unsuccessful (Verroust, Wilson & Dixon, 1974; Simpson *et al.*, 1978), but these are not perfect models of the action of NeF. The possible connections with nephritis are discussed further in the final section of this chapter.

There have been a number of developments with respect to possible connections between the complement system and adipose tissue. It has been known for some time that fat cells produce a serine protease called adipsin (Cook *et al.*, 1985). There is indirect evidence that adipsin is involved in adipose tissue metabolism in that increased adipsin mRNA is associated with catabolic states and decreased mRNA with some (but not all) experimental models of obesity (Flier *et al.*, 1987). It has recently become clear that not only does adipsin share identical functional characteristics with the alternative complement pathway component factor D, but that there is a high degree of sequence homology between the two and, in fact, adipsin will serve as well as factor D in the C3 dependent cleavage of factor B (Rosen *et al.*, 1989). It is most probable that factor D and adipsin are one and the same. This fascinating observation must have some bearing on the link between NeF and partial lipodystrophy, although the mechanism is unknown at present; one speculative possibility is considered at the end of the chapter.

Nephritic factors in types I and III MCGN

These conditions are more heterogeneous than type II MCGN, and in turn a variety of complement activating mechanisms seem to be involved. Circulating immune complexes are found in some cases (Davis, Marder & West, 1981) and these can activate complement via the classical pathway. Other ill-defined C3 activating factors, which are clearly not NeF, have also been described (Bartlow, Roberts & Lewis, 1979). More recently, a factor which causes C3 activation after prolonged *in vitro* incubation (Mollnes *et al.*, 1986), in contrast to NeF which leads to rapid C3 lysis, has been detected in nearly every hypocomplementaemic serum from cases of type I and III MCGN (Clardy *et al.*, 1989). This factor also appears to be an IgG and has been termed $NeF_{I/III}$, in contrast to the classical NeF_{II} (Clardy *et al.*, 1989). $NeF_{I/III}$ differs from NeF_{II} not only in the speed with which it activates C3, but also in being dependent on properdin, and in being able to activate the terminal components of complement. The fact that there is a good correlation between *in vitro* C3 activation by $NeF_{I/III}$ and *in vivo* C3 concentration suggests that this factor is of pathophysiological relevance, and not simply an *in vitro* artefact. Further analysis suggests that hypocomplementaemia in type II MCGN is mainly due to NeF_{II}, in type III MCGN to $NeF_{I/III}$, and in type I MCGN is uniquely multifactorial, with contributions from both types of NeF as well as activation via the classical pathway due to immune complexes (Varade, Forristal & West, 1990). Type I MCGN is also associated, in a higher percentage of cases than types II and III, with autoantibodies to a neoantigen on C1q (Strife *et al.*, 1990), and with the presence of a C4 nephritic factor that stabilises the classical pathway C3 convertase C4b2a (Seino *et al.*, 1990).

In addition to abnormalities of complement components, a variety of other areas has been more briefly investigated:

Cellular immune system

A decreased ratio of $CD4^+$ to $CD8^+$ T cells together with a decrease in non-specific $CD8^+$-mediated suppression has been found in one study (Brando *et al.*, 1983), whereas there were no disturbances in T cell subsets in two others (Chatenoud & Bach, 1981; Fornasieri *et al.*, 1983); the type of MCGN was not given in these studies but was likely to have been type I.

Platelets

There has been some interest in the role of platelets, both in glomerular disease in general (Cameron, 1984), and in MCGN in particular. Platelet antigens have been found in the glomeruli in MCGN (Miller, Dresner & Michael, 1980; Duffus *et al.*, 1982), and a shortened platelet survival time demonstrated *in vivo* (George *et al.*, 1974). None of these findings is unique to MCGN, and the failure of therapeutic manoeuvres aimed at platelets to influence the course of the disease (Donadio & Offord, 1989; discussed further below) casts some doubt on their relevance to pathogenesis.

Nature of dense deposit material in type II MCGN

This remains unknown. Biochemical analysis reveals rather few differences from normal basement membrane, with only a decrease in cystine and an increase in sialic acid (Galle & Mahieu, 1975). This led to the suggestion that the material was a reflection of a systemic abnormality which causes *in situ* alteration of normal basement membrane components. Certainly the material does not stain for immunoglobulin or complement components, but neither does it react with an antiserum raised to glomerular basement membrane (Kim *et al.*, 1979). Although it does react with thioflavin T (Churg, Duffy & Bernstein, 1979), suggesting some similarity with amyloid, this is a relatively non-specific reagent. There is some evidence that the material has a lipid component (Muda, Barsotti & Marinozzi, 1988).

Recurrence of MCGN in renal allografts

This is particularly characteristic of type II MCGN, and intramembranous dense deposits are found in the allograft of a very high proportion of patients transplanted for this disease (88% in one review, Cameron, 1982). Of note is the fact that recurrence of dense deposits despite normal complement concentrations is well described (Leibowitch *et al.*, 1979). It is, however, much less common for recurrent type II MCGN to cause renal failure, with an estimated graft loss due to recurrent disease of approximately 10% (Cameron, 1982). Type I MCGN probably recurs in approximately 25%–30% of grafts (Donadio, 1988) and again produces allograft failure in about 10% of cases (Cameron, 1982).

Secondary forms of MCGN (see Table 6.1)

Many of these are dealt with in greater depth elsewhere in this volume. In general these diseases are often associated with immune complex formation, hypocomplementaemia, and a type I MCGN pattern. In many cases, other patterns of glomerulopathy are more commonly seen, as, for instance, in systemic lupus erythematosus, where an MCGN pattern is a rather unusual variant of type IV lupus nephritis (see Chapter 4). Similarly, chronic hepatitis B infection is more usually associated with a membranous nephropathy (Chapter 3), or possibly IgA nephropathy (Chapter 5), but MCGN has also been described (Nagy et al., 1979; Venkataseshan et al., 1990), although as usual it is difficult to exclude non-specific trapping of hepatitis antigens in diseased glomeruli. The renal lesion found in haematological malignancies, especially Hodgkin's disease, tends to be a minimal change nephropathy, and that in carcinomas a membranous nephropathy, but there are a few reports of MCGN in both groups of neoplasms (Morel-Maroger Striker & Striker, 1985). The occurrence of an MCGN pattern (of varying severity) in a high proportion of patients with sickle cell anaemia (Pardo et al., 1975) is intriguing in view of a similar observation in a mouse model of haemolytic anaemia (see above). This suggests that chronic haemolysis per se in some way predisposes to MCGN.

Therapeutic aspects

The studies considered in this section have all dealt with primary MCGN; the secondary forms are more appropriately treated by attention to the primary disease. Another general point is that, because of the relative rarity of type II MCGN, most of the evaluable data concerns type I (and in some cases type III) MCGN.

An initial uncontrolled report claimed that triple therapy with cyclophosphamide, dipyridamole and warfarin gave considerably improved renal survival as compared to a retrospectively analysed untreated group (Kincaid-Smith, 1972). However, the renal mortality in this untreated group was unusually high, and two subsequent controlled studies of this form of treatment have failed to demonstrate significant benefit (Tiller et al., 1981; Cattran et al., 1985), and indeed have shown significant and serious side effects of the treatment (Tiller et al., 1981). Only cases of type I MCGN were entered into one of these studies (Tiller et al., 1981), and, although the other trial contained 12 cases of type II MCGN, this was was insufficient to allow any firm conclusions as to the value or otherwise of treatment in this disease.

One group has reported a number of uncontrolled studies of the use of corticosteroids in children with all primary types of MCGN, although types I and III predominated (McEnery, McAdams & West, 1985). In general, improvements in renal survival and glomerular histology were claimed with only minimal side effects. A controlled trial of corticosteroids in type I MCGN found a non-significant trend towards improved maintenance of renal function in the treatment versus control group (International study of kidney disease in children, 1982); however, if severe steroid side effects were taken into account then there was no treatment advantage.

The final form of therapy that has been studied in a controlled fashion is the use of anti-platelet agents. One trial combined dipyridamole with warfarin and showed better preservation of renal function with a between-patient comparison of treatment versus control (Zimmerman et al., 1983). However, there was no difference on a within-patient comparison (patients crossed over from one group to another) and there were significant haemorrhagic complications. A trial of dipyridamole and aspirin showed an initial short-term advantage of treatment in terms of preservation of renal function (Donadio et al., 1984) but long-term follow-up has shown no significant differences in renal survival (Donadio & Offord, 1989).

Plasma exchange has been used as an uncontrolled treatment of MCGN (McGinley et al., 1985). Some of the patients with type I MCGN (but neither of the two with type II MCGN) experienced a stabilisation of their deteriorating renal function whilst regular plasma exchange was continued. A single case report describes the use of plasma exchange in the treatment of recurrent type II MCGN in a renal allograft (Oberkircher et al., 1988). A number of long-term uncontrolled studies of the use of non-steroidal antiinflammatory drugs (NSAIDs), or various combinations of NSAIDs, immunosuppressants and/or anti-platelet drugs, have been published (for review see Donadio & Offord, 1989). This review points out that, although improved renal survival versus historical controls is claimed for these various treatments, this form of analysis is biased by comparing survival from date of clinical onset of disease. The survival curves in the treated groups are then almost certain to show an improvement (shift to the right), as patients must at least have survived to the initiation of treatment whereas those in the control groups are under no such constraint. The conclusion was that no form of treatment, including the subjects of the controlled studies mentioned above, has been shown to be of value in MCGN. This conclusion has also been reached by other reviewers (Schena & Cameron, 1988).

Concluding remarks

Although undoubtedly heterogeneous, it seems likely that types I and III MCGN are immune complex diseases. Their occurrence in hereditary complement deficiencies, the immunofluorescent and ultrastructural features, and the occurrence of a similar pattern in experimental models of immune complex disease and in diseases with a known immune complex pathogenesis all support this. What is less clear is the relationship of the hypocomplementaemia to the renal lesion. No doubt the relative deficiency of complement components found in idiopathic MCGN leads to the same abnormality of handling of immune complexes as is found in the hereditary complement deficiencies; the pathophysiological consequences of this are discussed further in the chapter on lupus nephritis. Why extra-renal lesions are not found in MCGN is unclear, as is the reason for the prolonged deficiency of complement which is often found. It may be that some underlying abnormality of immune complex handling is responsible both for the hypocomplementaemia and the particular pattern of renal injury, but it is also possible that the prolonged complement activation may be nephrotoxic in itself; this possibility is discussed further below. The contribution of the slow acting nephritic factors identified in types I and III MCGN is unclear at present, but their presence strengthens the analogy between these types and type II MCGN (see below); further work is required to evaluate the importance of these interesting factors.

Type I and type III MCGN are probably closely related variants. There is overlap in the histological features and many of the complement abnormalities are common to the two forms, in distinction to the more unique findings in type II MCGN. Whether the subtle differences in activation of terminal complement components found between types I and II can account for (or are caused by) the differing glomerular lesions is unknown.

By contrast, type II MCGN is an homogeneous, and considerably more enigmatic disease, with major unanswered questions concerning the relationship between the complement abnormalities on the one hand, and lipodystrophy and the renal lesion on the other. With respect to the first of these, the identification of adipsin as factor D is most intriguing. The physiological relevance, if any, of the changes in adipsin mRNA associated with different metabolic states is unclear, but it remains possible that adipsin may have some role in adipose tissue metabolism distinct from its role as factor D. However, it is perhaps more likely that partial lipodystrophy, in which there is loss of fat cells, is connected with the cytotoxic capacities of the complement system. One suggestion (due to D.K.Peters) follows from the observation that the alternative pathway is constantly turning over at a low rate due to C3b-dependent positive feedback; this turnover can be rapidly amplified in the presence of activators that interfere with the normal control by inhibitory proteins (Fearon & Austen, 1977). Such control is likely to be particularly critical in the vicinity of adipocytes, which are actively secreting factor D, a key enzyme in this amplification process. If NeF is present, then the C3bBb alternative pathway convertase is protected from inhibition, and rapid complement activation can occur next to the fat cell. This could lead to fat cell damage and lipodystrophy. It is perhaps relevant that partial lipodystrophy often follows measles (Lachmann & Peters, 1982), a condition in which the capillaries will allow easy access of circulating NeF to the extravascular fluid bathing the fat cells.

One problem with the above hypothesis is that NeF does not seem to cause activation of the terminal components of complement from C5 to C9 (Clardy *et al.*, 1989), but it is possible that opsonisation by attachment of C3b to the cell, and the generation of biologically active fragments such as C3a, Bb and Ba, are sufficiently injurious. Other factors that require an explanation are the rather selective distribution of adipocyte loss in partial lipodystrophy, and the fact that, although a nephritic factor appears to be present in MCGN types I and III (Clardy *et al.*, 1989), these conditions are only very rarely associated with partial lipodystrophy (Chartier, Buzzanga & Paquin, 1987).

Despite these developments concerning connections between the complement system and fat tissue, the link between NeF and type II MCGN remains obscure. It seems unlikely that an immune complex aetiology secondary to the complement deficiency induced by NeF is responsible: dense deposit disease is, in general, not associated with hereditary complement deficiencies, and the unique ultrastructural features are quite unlike those seen in other immune complex diseases, either clinical or experimental. The attempts to test the other main explanation for the association (nephrotoxicity of complement activation by NeF *per se*) are somewhat inconclusive. First, the result of complement activation differs from that produced by NeF. In the model of chronic administration of cobra venom factor (which behaves as a C3b resistant to the natural inhibitors H and I) the native C3bBb produced is not complexed with NeF, and treatment was only continued for three months (Simpson *et al.*, 1978). Similarly, the chronic activation of the alternative pathway by daily injections of inulin or zymosan (Verroust, Wilson & Dixon, 1974) will produce a normal C3bBb molecule. The potential importance of these differences is shown by the fact that other abnormalities of the alternative pathway C3 convertase in man that result in chronic activation are not associated with the development of dense deposits (Marder *et al.*, 1983). Secondly, there are differences in the complement receptors present in the glomeruli of the animals used in these experiments (mice and rabbits respectively) and man: a C3b receptor is present on visceral epithelial cells in man but not in other species (Moran & Peters, 1979). It therefore remains possible that complement activation by NeF, perhaps due to particular properties of the C3bBb–NeF complex, or a particular affinity for C3 by human glomerular receptors, is directly nephrotoxic. Progress in determining the nature of the dense deposit material would be most helpful in suggesting possible mechanisms for such toxicity.

Finally, it has been suggested that the alteration in basement membrane in type II MCGN, which is not confined to the kidney and usually recurs in transplanted kidneys even in the absence of complement abnormalities, may be the primary lesion, with activation of the alternative pathway and the development of NeF a secondary event or epiphenomenon (Levy, Gubler & Habib, 1979). It is difficult to exclude this, although it is perhaps less likely than a direct causal link between NeF and the dense deposits, with their occurrence in the face of apparently normal complement concentrations perhaps due to amounts of NeF insufficient to deplete C3. In any event the recurrence in allografts demonstrates that a circulating factor of some sort is presumably involved.

References

Anders, D., Agricola, B., Sippel, M. & Thoenes, W. (1977). Basement membrane changes in membranoproliferative glomerulonephritis. II. Characterization of a third type by silver impregnation of ultra thin sections. *Virchows Archives [A]*, **376**, 1–19.

Angus, K. W., Gardiner, A. C., Mitchell, B. & Thomson, D. (1980). Mesangiocapillary glomerulonephritis in lambs: the ultrastructure and immunopathology of diffuse glomerulonephritis in newly born Finnish Landrace lambs. *Journal of Pathology*, **131**, 65–74.

Bartlow, B. G., Roberts, J. L. & Lewis, E. J. (1979). Nonimmunoglobulin C3 activating factor in membranoproliferative glomerulonephritis. *Kidney International*, **15**, 294–302.

Berger, J. & Galle, P. (1963). Dépôts denses au sein des basales du rein: étude en microscopies optique et élèctronique. *Presse Medicale*, **71**, 2351–4.

Berger, M., Balow, J. E., Wilson, C. B. & Frank, M. M. (1983). Circulating immune complexes and glomerulonephritis in a patient with congenital absence of the third component of complement. *New England Journal of Medicine*, **308**, 1009–12.

Berry, P. L., McEnery, P. T., McAdams, A. J. & West, C. D. (1981). Membranoproliferative glomerulonephritis in two sibships. *Clinical Nephrology*, **16**, 101–6.

Borradori, L., Rybojad, M., Morel, P., Puissant, A. & Weiss, L. (1989). Chronic urticaria and moderate leukocytoclastic vasculitis associated with C3 nephritic factor activity. *Archives of Dermatology*, **125**, 1589–90.

Brando, B., Busnach, G., Bertoli, S., Nova, M. L. & Minetti, L. (1983). T-suppressor cell abnormalities in type I membranoproliferative glomerulonephritis. *Proceedings of the European Dialysis and Transplantation Association*, **19**, 669–72.

Burkholder, P. M., Marchand, A. & Krueger, R. P. (1970). Mixed membranous and proliferative glomerulonephritis. A correlative light, immunofluorescence, and electron microscopic study. *Laboratory Investigation*, **23**, 459–79.

Cameron, J. S. (1982). Glomerulonephritis in renal transplants. *Transplantation*, **34**, 237–45.

Cameron, J. S., Turner, D. R., Heaton, J. et al. (1983). Idiopathic mesangiocapillary glomerulonephritis. Comparison of types I and II in children and adults and long-term prognosis. *American Journal of Medicine*, **74**, 175–92.

Cameron, J. S. (1984). Platelets in glomerular disease. *Annual Review of Medicine*, **35**, 175–80.

Cattran, D. C., Cardella, C. J., Roscoe, J. H. et al. (1985). Results of a controlled drug trial in membranoproliferative glomerulonephritis. *Kidney International*, **27**, 436–41.

Center, S. A., Smith, C. A., Wilkinson, E., Erb, H. N. & Lewis, R. M. (1987). Clinicopathologic, renal immunofluorescent, and light microscopic features of glomerulonephritis in the dog: 41 cases (1975–1985). *Journal of the American Veterinary Medical Association*, **190**, 81–90.

Chartier, S., Buzzanga, J. B. & Paquin, F. (1987). Partial lipodystrophy associated with a type 3 form of membranoproliferative glomerulonephritis. *Journal of the American Academy of Dermatology*, **16**, 201–5.

Chatenoud, L. & Bach, M-A. (1981). Abnormalities of T-cell subsets in glomerulonephritis and systemic lupus erythematosus. *Kidney International*, **20**, 267–74.

Churg, J., Duffy, J. L. & Bernstein, J. (1979). Identification of dense deposit disease. *Archives of Pathology & Laboratory Medicine*, **103**, 67–72.

Clardy, C., Forristal, J., Strife, C. F. & West, C. D. (1989). Serum terminal complement component levels in hypocomplementemic glomerulonephritides. *Clinical Immunology and Immunopathology*, **50**, 307–20.

Clardy, C. W., Forristal, J., Strife, C. F. & West, C. D. (1989). A properdin dependent nephritic factor slowly activating C3, C5, and C9 in membranoproliferative glomerulonephritis, types I and III. *Clinical Immunology and Immunopathology*, **50**, 333–47.

Coleman, T. H., Forristal, J., Kosaka, T. & West, C. D. (1983). Inherited complement component deficiencies and membranoproliferative glomerulonephritis. *Kidney International*, **24**, 681–90.

Cook, K. S., Groves, D. L., Min, H. Y. & Spiegelman, B. M. (1985). A developmentally regulated mRNA from 3T3 adipocytes encodes a novel serine protease homologue. *Proceedings of the National Academy of Sciences, USA*, **82**, 6480–4.

Daha, M. R., Fearon, D. T. & Austen, K. F. (1976). C3 nephritic factor (C3Nef): stabilization of fluid phase and cell-bound alternative pathway convertase. *Journal of Immunology*, **116**, 1–7.

Davis, A. E., Ziegler, J. B., Gelfand, E. W., Rosen, F. S. & Alper, C. A. (1977). Heterogeneity of nephritic factor and its identification as an immunoglobulin. *Proceedings of the National Academy of Sciences USA*, **74**, 3980–3.

Davis, C. A., Marder, H. & West, C. D. (1981). Circulating immune complexes in membranoproliferative glomerulonephritis. *Kidney International*, **20**, 728–32.

Donadio, J. V., Slack, T. K., Holley, K. E. & Ilstrup, D. M. (1979). Idiopathic membranoproliferative (mesangiocapillary) glomerulonephritis. A clinicopathological study. *Mayo Clinic Proceedings*, **54**, 141–50.

Donadio, J. V., Anderson, C. F., Mitchell, J. C. *et al.* (1984). Membranoproliferative glomerulonephritis. A prospective clinical trial of platelet-inhibitor therapy. *New England Journal of Medicine*, **310**, 1421–6.

Donadio, J. V. (1988). Membranoproliferative glomerulonephritis. In *Diseases of the Kidney*, 4th edn, ed. R. W. Schrier & C. W. Gottschalk, pp. 2035–60. Boston/Toronto: Little, Brown and Company.

Donadio, J. V. & Offord, K. P. (1989). Reassessment of treatment results in membranoproliferative glomerulonephritis, with emphasis on life-table analysis. *American Journal of Kidney Disease*, **14**, 445–51.

Duffus, P., Parbtani, A., Frampton, G. & Cameron, J. S. (1982). Intraglomerular localization of platelet related antigens, platelet factor 4 and β-thromboglobulin in glomerulonephritis. *Clinical Nephrology*, **17**, 288–97.

Duvall-Young, J., MacDonald, M. K. & McKechnie, N. M. (1989). Fundus changes in (type II) mesangiocapillary glomerulonephritis simulating drusen: a histopathological report. *British Journal of Ophthalmology*, **73**, 297–302.

Duvall-Young, J., Short, C. D., Raines, M. F., Gokal, R. & Lawler, W. (1989). Fundus changes in mesangiocapillary glomerulonephritis type II: clinical and fluorescein angiographic findings. *British Journal of Ophthalmology*, **73**, 900–6.

Eisenger, A. J., Shortland, J. R. & Moorhead, P. J. (1972). Renal disease in partial lipodystrophy. *Quarterly Journal of Medicine*, **41**, 343–54.

Fearon, D. T. & Austen, K. F. (1977). Activation of the alternative complement pathway due to resistance of zymosan-bound amplification convertase to endogenous regulatory mechanisms. *Proceedings of the National Academy of Sciences, USA*, **74**, 1683–7.

Flier, J. S., Cook, K. S., Usher, P. & Spiegelman, B. M. (1987). Severely impaired adipsin expression in genetic and acquired obesity. *Science*, **237**, 405–8.

Fornasieri, A., Sinico, R., Fiorini, G. *et al.* (1983). T-lymphocyte subsets in primary and secondary glomerulonephritis. *Proceedings of the European Dialysis and Transplantation Association*, **19**, 635–41.

Frank, M. M., Gelfand, J. A. & Atkinson, J. P. (1976). Hereditary angioedema: the clinical syndrome and its management. *Annals of Internal Medicine*, **84**, 580–93.

Friend, P. S., Yunis, E. J., Noreen, H. J. & Michael, A. F. (1977). B-cell alloantigen associated with chronic mesangiocapillary glomerulonephritis. *Lancet*, **i**, 562–4.

Galle, P. & Mahieu, P. (1975). Electron dense alteration of kidney basement membranes. A renal lesion specific of a systemic disease. *American Journal of Medicine*, **58**, 749–64.

George, C. R. P., Slichter, S. J., Quadracci, L. J., Striker, G. E. & Harker, L. A. (1974). A kinetic evaluation of hemostasis in renal disease. *New England Journal of Medicine*, **291**, 1111–15.

Glassock, R. J., Adler, S. G., Ward, H. J. & Cohen, A. H. (1986). Primary glomerular diseases. In *The Kidney*, 3rd edn, ed. B. M. Brenner & F. C. Rector, pp. 929–1013. Philadelphia: W.B.Saunders Company.

Gotoff, S. P., Fellers, F. X., Vawter, G. F., Janeway, C. A. & Rosen, F. S. (1965). The beta$_{1c}$ globulin in childhood nephrotic syndrome. Laboratory diagnosis of progressive glomerulonephritis. *New England Journal of Medicine*, **273**, 524–9.

Grauer, G. F., Burgess, E. C., Cooley, A. J. & Hagee, J. H. (1988). Renal lesions associated with Borrelia burgdorferi infection in a dog. *Journal of the American Veterinary Medical Association*, **193**, 237–9.

Habib, R., Michielsen, P., de Montera, E., Hinglais, N., Galle, P. & Hamburger, J. (1961). In *Ciba Foundation Symposium on Renal Biopsy*, ed. G. E. W. Wolstenholme & M. P. Cameron, pp. 70. London: Ciba Foundation.

Habib, R., Gubler, M-C., Loirat, C., Maïz, H. B. & Levy, M. (1975). Dense deposit disease: a variant of membranoproliferative glomerulonephritis. *Kidney International*, **7**, 204–15.

Holland, N. H., de Bracco, M. M. E. & Christian, C. L. (1972). Pathways of complement activation in glomerulonephritis. *Kidney International*, **1**, 106–14.

Hory, B. & Haultier, J. J. (1989). Glomerulonephritis and hereditary angioedema: report of 2 cases. *Clinical Nephrology*, **31**, 259–63.

International study of kidney disease in children (1982). Alternate day steroid therapy in membranoproliferative glomerulonephritis: a randomised controlled clinical trial. *Kidney International*, **21**, 150.(Abstract).

Karstrop, A. (1976). C3 activator and hypocomplementaemia in a 'healthy' woman. *British Medical Journal*, **I**, 501–2.

Kashtan, C. E., Burke, B., Burch, G., Gustav Fisker, S. & Kim, Y. (1990). Dense intramembranous deposit disease: a clinical comparison of histological subtypes. *Clinical Nephrology*, **33**, 1–6.

Kim, Y., Friend, P. S., Dresner, I. G., Yunis, E. J. & Michael, A. F. (1977). Inherited deficiency of the second component of complement (C2) with membranoproliferative glomerulonephritis. *American Journal of Medicine*, **62**, 765–71.

Kim, Y., Vernier, R. L., Fish, A. J. & Michael, A. F. (1979). Immunofluorescence studies of dense deposit disease. The presence of railroad tracks and mesangial rings. *Laboratory Investigation*, **40**, 474–80.

Kincaid-Smith, P. (1972). The treatment of chronic mesangiocapillary (membranoproliferative) glomerulonephritis with impaired renal function. *Medical Journal of Australia*, **2**, 587–92.

Lachmann, P. J. & Peters, D. K. (1982). Complement. In *Clinical Aspects of Immunology*, 4th edn, ed. P. J. Lachmann & D. K. Peters, pp. 18–49. Oxford: Blackwell Scientific Publications.

Leibowitch, J., Halbwachs, L., Wattel, S., Gaillard, M-H. & Droz, D. (1979). Recurrence of dense deposits in transplanted kidney: II. Serum complement and nephritic factor profiles. *Kidney International*, 15, 396–403.

Levy, M., Gubler, M-C. & Habib, R. (1979). New concepts on membranoproliferative glomerulonephritis. In *Progress in glomerulonephritis*, ed. P. Kincaid-Smith, A. J. F. d'Apice & R. C. Atkins, pp. 177–205. New York: John Wiley and Sons.

Ludders, J. W., Grauer, G. F., Dubielzig, R. R., Ribble, G. A. & Wilson, J. W. (1988). Renal microcirculatory and correlated histologic changes associated with dirofilariasis in dogs. *American Journal of Veterinary Research*, 49, 826–30.

Maggio-Price, L., Russell, R., Wolf, N. S., Alpers, C. E. & Engel, D. (1988). Clinicopathologic features of young and old sph^ha/sph^ha mice. *American Journal of Pathology*, 132, 461–73.

Marder, H. K., Coleman, T. H., Forristal, J., Beischel, L. & West, C. D. (1983). An inherited defect in the C3 convertase, C3b,Bb, associated with glomerulonephritis. *Kidney International*, 23, 749–58.

McEnery, P. T., McAdams, A. J. & West, C. D. (1985). The effect of prednisone in a high-dose, alternate-day regime on the natural history of idiopathic membranoproliferative glomerulonephritis. *Medicine*, 64, 401–24.

McGinley, E., Watkins, R., McLay, A. & Boulton-Jones, J. M. (1985). Plasma exchange in the treatment of mesangiocapillary glomerulonephritis. *Nephron*, 40, 385–90.

McLean, R. H. & Winkelstein, J. A. (1984). Genetically determined variation in the complement system: relationship to disease. *Journal of Pediatrics*, 105, 179–88.

Michael, A. F., McLean, R. H., Roy, L. P. et al. (1973). Immunologic aspects of the nephrotic syndrome. *Kidney International*, 3, 105–15.

Miller, K., Dresner, I. G. & Michael, A. F. (1980). Localization of platelet antigen in human kidney disease. *Kidney International*, 18, 472–9.

Mollnes, T. E., Ng, Y. C., Peters, D. K., Lea, T., Tschopp, J. & Harboe, M. (1986). Effect of nephritic factor on C3 and on the terminal pathway of complement *in vivo* and *in vitro*. *Clinical and Experimental Immunology*, 65, 73–9.

Moran, J. E. & Peters, D. K. (1979). Studies on the glomerular C3b receptor. In *Progress in Glomerulonephritis*, ed. P. Kincaid-Smith, A. J. F. d'Apice & R. C. Atkins, pp. 109–17. New York: John Wiley & Sons.

Morel-Maroger Striker, L. & Striker, G. E. (1985). Glomerular lesions in malignancies. *Contributions in Nephrology*, 48, 111–22.

Muda, A. O., Barsotti, P. & Marinozzi, V. (1988). Ultrastructural histochemical investigations of 'dense deposit disease'. Pathogenetic approach to a special type of mesangiocapillary glomerulonephritis. *Virchows Archives [A]*, 413, 529–37.

Nagy, J., Bajtai, G., Brasch, H. et al. (1979). The role of hepatitis B surface antigen in the pathogenesis of glomerulonephritis. *Clinical Nephrology*, 12, 109–16.

Noël, L. H., Descamps, B., Jungers, P. et al. (1978). HLA antigen in three types of glomerulonephritis. *Clinical Immunology and Immunopathology*, 10, 19–23.

Oberkircher, O. R., Enama, M., West, J. C., Campbell, P. & Moran, J. (1988). Regression of recurrent membranoproliferative glomerulonephritis type II in a transplanted kidney after plasmapheresis therapy. *Transplantation Proceedings*, 20, 1 suppl. 1, 418–23.

Ohi, H., Watanabe, S., Fujita, T., Seki, M. & Hatano, M. (1990). Detection of C3bBb-stabilizing activity (C3 nephritic factor) in the serum from patients with membranoproliferative glomerulonephritis. *Journal of Immunological Methods*, 131, 71–6.

Ooi, Y. M., Vallota, E. H. & West, C. D. (1976). Classical complement pathway activation in membranoproliferative glomerulonephritis. *Kidney International*, 9, 46–53.

Pardo, V., Strauss, J., Kramer, H., Ozawa, T. & McIntosh, R. M. (1975). Nephropathy associated with sickle cell anemia: an autologous immune complex nephritis. II. Clinicopathologic study of seven patients. *American Journal of Medicine*, **59**, 650–9.

Peters, D. K., Martin, A., Weinstein, A. *et al.* (1972). Complement studies in membranoproliferative glomerulonephritis. *Clinical and Experimental Immunology*, **11**, 311–20.

Peters, D. K., Williams, D. G., Charlesworth, J. A. *et al.* (1973). Mesangiocapillary nephritis, partial lipodystrophy, and hypocomplementaemia. *Lancet*, **ii**, 535–8.

Power, D. A., Ng, Y. C. & Simpson, J. G. (1990). Familial incidence of C3 nephritic factor, partial lipodystrophy and membranoproliferative glomerulonephritis. *Quarterly Journal of Medicine*, **75**, 387–98.

Pusey, C. D., Venning, M. C. & Peters, D. K. (1988). Immunopathology of glomerular and interstitial disease. In *Diseases of the Kidney*, 4th edn, ed. R. W. Schrier & C. W. Gottschalk, pp. 1827–83. Boston/Toronto: Little, Brown and Company.

Rashid, H. U., Papiha, S. S., Agroyannis, B. *et al.* (1983). The association of HLA and other genetic markers with glomerulonephritis. *Human Genetics*, **63**, 38–44.

Rees, A. J. (1984). The HLA complex and susceptibility to glomerulonephritis. *Plasma Therapy*, **5**, 455–71.

Rosen, B. S., Cook, K. S., Yaglom, J. *et al.* (1989). Adipsin and complement factor D activity: an immune-related defect in obesity. *Science*, **244**, 1483–7.

Sakai, H., Nomoto, Y., Arimori, S., Itoh, H. & Hasegawa, O. (1979). Increase of IgM-bearing peripheral blood lymphocytes in patients with idiopathic membranoproliferative glomerulonephritis (MPGN) and their family members. *Clinical Nephrology*, **12**, 210–15.

Schena, F. P. & Cameron, J. S. (1988). Treatment of proteinuric idiopathic glomerulonephritides in adults: a retrospective survey. *American Journal of Medicine*, **85**, 315–26.

Seino, J., Kinoshita, Y., Sudo, K. *et al.* (1990). Quantitation of C4 nephritic factor by an enzyme-linked immunosorbent assay. *Journal of Immunological Methods*, **128**, 101–8.

Simpson, I. J., Moran, J., Evans, D. J. & Peters, D. K. (1978). Prolonged complement activation in mice. *Kidney International*, **13**, 467–71.

Sissons, J. G. P., West, R. J., Fallows, J. *et al.* (1976). The complement abnormalities of lipodystrophy. *New England Journal of Medicine*, **294**, 461–5.

Sissons, J. G. P., Leibowitch, J., Amos, N. & Peters, D. K. (1977). Metabolism of the fifth component of complement, and its relation to metabolism of the third component, in patients with complement activation. *Journal of Clinical Investigation*, **59**, 704–15.

Spitzer, R. E., Vallota, E. H., Forristal, J. *et al.* (1969). Serum C'3 lytic system in patients with glomerulonephritis. *Science*, **164**, 436–7.

Spitzer, R. E., Stitzel, A. E. & Tsokos, G. C. (1990a). Production of IgG and IgM autoantibody to the alternative pathway C3 convertase in normal individuals and patients with membranoproliferative glomerulonephritis. *Clinical Immunology and Immunopathology*, **57**, 10–18.

Spitzer, R. E., Stitzel, A. E. & Tsokos, G. C. (1990b). Human anti-idiotypic responses to autoantibody against the alternative pathway C3 convertase. *Clinical Immunology and Immunopathology*, **57**, 19–31.

Strife, C. F., McEnery, P. T., McAdams, A. J. & West, C. D. (1977). Membranoproliferative glomerulonephritis with disruption of the glomerular basement membrane. *Clinical Nephrology*, **7**, 65–72.

Strife, C. F., Prada, A. L., Clardy, C. W., Jackson, E. & Forristal, J. (1990). Autoantibody to complement neoantigens in membranoproliferative glomerulonephritis. *Journal of Pediatrics*, **116**, s98–s102.

Tedesco, F., Tovo, P. A., Tamaro, G., Basaglia, M., Perticarari, S. & Villa, M. A. (1985). Selective C3 deficiency due to C3 nephritic factor in an apparently healthy girl. *Ricerca in Clinica e in Laboratorio*, **15**, 323–9.

REFERENCES

131

Thompson, R. A. (1972). C3 inactivating factor in the serum of a patient with chronic hypocomplementaemic proliferative glomerulo-nephritis. *Immunology*, 22, 147–58.

Thorner, P. & Baumal, R. (1982). Extraglomerular dense deposits in dense deposit disease. *Archives of Pathology and Laboratory Medicine*, 106, 628–31.

Tiller, D. J., Clarkson, A. R., Mathew, T. *et. al.* (1981). A prospective randomized trial in the use of cyclophopshamide, dipyridamole and warfarin in membranous and mesangiocapillary glomerulonephritis. In *Eighth International Congress of Nephrology: Advances in Basic and Clinical Nephrology*, ed. W. Zurukzoglu, M. Papadimitriou, M. Sion *et. al.*, pp. 345–51. Basel: Karger.

Tsokos, G. C., Stitzel, A. E., Patel, A. D., Hiramatsu, M., Balow, J. E. & Spitzer, R. E. (1989). Human polyclonal and monoclonal IgG and IgM complement 3 nephritic factors: evidence for idiotypic commonality. *Clinical Immunology and Immunopathology*, 53, 113–22.

Varade, W. S., Forristal, J. & West, C. D. (1990). Patterns of complement activation in idiopathic membranoproliferative glomerulonephritis, types I, II, III. *American Journal of Kidney Disease*, 16, 196–206.

Venkataseshan, V. S., Lieberman, K., Kim, D. U. *et al.* (1990). Hepatitis-B-associated glomerulonephritis: pathology, pathogenesis, and clinical course. *Medicine*, 69, 200–16.

Verroust, P. J., Wilson, C. B. & Dixon, F. J. (1974). Lack of nephritogenicity of systemic activation of the alternate complement pathway. *Kidney International*, 6, 157–69.

Wank, R., Schendel, D. J., O'Neil, G. J., Riethmüller, G., Held, E. & Feucht, H. E. (1984). Rare variant of complement C4 is seen in high frequency in patients with primary glomerulo-nephritis. *Lancet*, i, 872–4.

Welch, T. R. & Beischel, L. (1985). C4 uremic variant: an acquired C4 allotype. *Immunogenetics*, 22, 553–62.

Welch, T. R., Beischel, L., Balakrishnan, K., Quinlan, M. & West, C. D. (1986). Major-histocompatibility-complex extended haplotypes in membranoproliferative glomerulonephritis. *New England Journal of Medicine*, 314, 1476–81.

Welch, T. R. & Berry, A. (1987). C3 alleles in diseases associated with C3 activation. *Disease Markers*, 5, 81–7.

West, C. D., McAdams, A. J., McConville, J. M., Davis, N. C. & Holland, N. H. (1965). Hypocomplementemic and normocomplementemic persistant (chronic) glomerulonephritis; clinical and pathologic characteristics. *Journal of Pediatrics*, 67, 1089–112.

Zimmerman, S. W., Moorthy, A. V., Dreher, W. H., Friedman, A. & Varanasi, U. (1983). Prospective trial of warfarin and dipyridamole in patients with membranoproliferative glomerulonephritis. *American Journal of Medicine*, 75, 920–7.

−7−
Minimal change nephropathy and focal segmental glomerulosclerosis

It is not clear that these two conditions should necessarily be considered together. To begin with, although minimal change nephropathy forms a relatively homogeneous clinicopathological entity, there is almost certainly considerable heterogeneity amongst cases of focal segmental glomerulosclerosis. Furthermore, the evidence that an immunological disturbance underlies the pathogenesis is considerably stronger for minimal change nephropathy (but even here such evidence is indirect). However, there is, at least superficially, some overlap between the two conditions, and it is commonly supposed that at least one subset of cases of focal segmental glomerulosclerosis represents an evolutionary phase of minimal change nephropathy. These issues have been extensively debated (see, for instance, Cameron, 1979) and are considered further at the end of the chapter, but for convenience the two conditions will be discussed together. Also included in this chapter are certain conditions, such as IgM nephropathy and mesangial proliferative nephropathy, that may represent variants of minimal change nephropathy or focal segmental glomerulosclerosis; their possible interrelationships are also discussed further below.

Minimal change nephropathy is an important disease, being responsible for over three-quarters of cases of the nephrotic syndrome in children (International study of kidney disease in children, 1978), and for up to 30% in adults (Sharpstone, Ogg & Cameron, 1969). Clinically, the picture is uniform, with the presentation nearly always being with the nephrotic syndrome; hypertension is occasionally found, particularly in adults. The condition is usually idiopathic, but is sometimes related to malignancy (particularly Hodgkin's disease) or to an immunological disturbance such as allergy or immunisation. Histologically, the absence of significant glomerular changes by light microscopy led to the designation 'minimal change' (Churg, Habib & White, 1970). The presence of lipid droplets in proximal

Table 7.1. *Conditions associated with focal sclerosing lesions*

Following focal proliferative nephritis
Reflux nephropathy
Hyperfiltration in remnant kidney
Drugs (heroin and analgesic abuse)
HIV infection
Alport's syndrome
Sickle cell disease
Renal transplantation (in allograft)
Malignancy
Obesity
Diabetes mellitus

tubules led to the old name of lipoid nephrosis. By electron microscopy there is fusion of the podocyte foot processes, a relatively non-specific consequence of proteinuria (Roy, Vernier & Michael, 1972). Immunofluorescence is characteristically negative for immunoglobulins or complement components. Occasional variants are found in which there is very mild mesangial proliferation, and sometimes deposition of IgM in the mesangium; these are discussed further in the section on immunopathology. The long-term prognosis, at least of the steroid responsive majority (see section on therapeutic aspects), is excellent (Lewis *et al.*, 1989).

The entity of focal segmental glomerulosclerosis (also known as focal glomerulosclerosis, focal and segmental hyalinosis, and by a number of similar synonyms) was first described as a previously unrecognised finding in minimal change nephropathy (Rich, 1957), but similar pathological changes are found in a diverse range of conditions (see Table 7.1; this is not an exhaustive listing). The idiopathic condition accounts for 10%–20% of cases of the nephrotic syndrome in both children and adults (Glassock *et al.*, 1986), but asymptomatic proteinuria, hypertension and renal impairment (which can be rapidly progressive: Brown *et al.*, 1978) are considerably more common than in uncomplicated minimal change nephropathy. The lesion probably affects the juxtamedullary glomeruli first, and consists of segmental sclerosis affecting only some glomeruli (focal). There is increased mesangial matrix with collapse of capillary loops and deposition of subendothelial hyaline material. In advanced cases, there may be global sclerosis of most glomeruli. Findings on electron microscopy reflect these changes and may also show fine granular paramesangial and subendothelial deposits (Silva & Hogg, 1989). The characteristic immunofluorescence appearance is of granular IgM and C3, usually in association with the areas of sclerosis. The occasional description of linear IgG staining is of uncertain significance, but is not associated with anti-glomerular basement membrane antibodies

(Matalon *et al.*, 1974). A good response to treatment is much less frequent than in minimal change nephropathy, and the long-term prognosis considerably worse, although there is considerable heterogeneity (Cameron, 1988).

Immunogenetics

Much of the immunogenetic data is based on the clinical entity of steroid-responsive nephrotic syndrome in children, and, unless otherwise stated, this is the subject of the studies reviewed below. Although histopathological confirmation is often not available, the vast majority of this group will consist of minimal change nephropathy.

The MHC

The first study of MHC alleles in steroid-responsive nephrotic syndrome demonstrated an association with B12, with a relative risk of 6.3 (Thomson *et al.*, 1976). There was also a link between B12 and atopy (which was significantly more common in patients than controls), and the presence of atopy and B12 gave a relative risk of 13. However, a follow-up study from the same unit, whilst confirming the B12 link with the nephrotic syndrome, could not confirm the B12 association with atopy, although the incidence of atopy was again increased (Trompeter *et al.*, 1980). The follow-up study did, however, confirm the initial finding of a link between B12 and tendency to relapse after cyclophosphamide. Other MHC class I associations noted include B8 and B18 in an Irish population (with no association with B12; O'Regan *et al.*, 1980) and B8 and B13 in a German population (Noss, Bachman & Olbing, 1981).

The initial report of an MHC class II association was from Australia, and in this series the diagnosis of minimal change nephropathy was confirmed on biopsy (Alfiler *et al.*, 1980). The finding of a significant link with DR7 (relative risk 5.9) has since been confirmed in a number of other populations, including German (Lenhard *et al.*, 1980*b*), French (de Mouzon-Cambon *et al.*, 1981), and Spanish (Nuñez-Roldan *et al.*, 1982); the latter study also found a significant decrease in the frequency of DR2 in patients (10%) versus controls (30%). A recent study on 40 Caucasoid children using DR, DQ and DP typing by RFLP methods showed a significant increase in DR7 ($p = 2 \times 10^{-5}$, aetiological fraction 0.6) and DQw2 (specifically, the DQB1 β chain gene of the DQw2; $p = 2 \times 10^{-4}$, aetiological fraction 0.7), and a weak association with an uncommon DP allele, DP-CP63 (Clark *et al.*, 1990). DQw2 and DR7 are in linkage disequilibrium, and the contributions of these two alleles to susceptibility as a primary influence as opposed to being secondary to this disequilibrium is unclear. The authors of this report felt that DQw2 was unlikely to be the sole primary association, as the frequency of DR3, which is also in linkage disequilibrium with DQw2, was not increased. However, an increased frequency of DR3 in combination with DR7 has been noted (Cambon-Thomsen *et al.*, 1986; Ruder *et al.*, 1990, although in the former study this may have been principally in patients with FSGS; see below), and a study of extended HLA haplotypes in American caucasians found significant increases in the frequencies of the [A1,B8,DR3,DRw52,SC01] and [B44,DR7,DRw53,FC31] haplotypes (Lagueruela *et al.*, 1990). This latter study did not find any significant association with any individual allele (after correction for multiple comparisons) except for DQw2, which was present in 5 out of 11 incidences of the B8,DR3 extended haplotype, and in all 10 incidences of the B44,DR7 extended haplotype. The authors suggest that the increased incidence of these extended haplotypes could explain the findings of increased frequencies of B8, DR3, DR7 (see above), Bf*F (McLean *et al.*, 1983) and C4A*Q0 (McLean *et al.*, 1987), although they themselves could find no association with alleles of any of the MHC-encoded complement components (Lagueruela *et al.*, 1990).

The linkage disequilibrium manifested by the presence of these extended MHC haplotypes may also contribute to the increased frequency of the rare DP allele mentioned above, which appeared to segregate with DR7 (Clark *et al.*, 1990); although there is a recombination hot spot between DQ and DR, on the one hand, and DP on the other (Bodmer & Bodmer, 1984), weak linkage between DR and DP alleles has been described (Shaw, Duquesnoy & Smith, 1981).

It is possible that the associations reviewed above are peculiar to *childhood* minimal change nephropathy. One study could find no evidence of a DR7 link in adult patients, although this link was present in patients with disease onset before 15 years of age (Laurent *et al.*, 1983). As is usual, there are population differences, and, in the Japanese, in whom DR7 is relatively rare, there appear to be associations with DRw8 and DQw3 (Kobayashi *et al.*, 1985); in particular, the frequencies of all but one of the DR alleles associated with DQw3 (DR4,5,w8,w9) were increased, suggesting that DQw3 was a major susceptibility marker. This latter study was also performed on adult subjects. There is also an increase in DRw53 in Japanese patients with minimal change nephropathy (Naito, Kohara & Arakawa, 1987).

Much less immunogenetic information is available on focal segmental glomerulosclerosis, perhaps reflecting the relative difficulty of defining an homogeneous group of patients in this condition. A few studies have found no particularly striking associations (Lenhard *et al.*, 1980*a*; Noël *et al.*, 1978; Komori *et al.*, 1983). A group of steroid resistant nephrotic patients (which would probably contain a significant proportion of cases of focal segmental glomerulosclerosis) had an increased incidence of DR3, and, in particular, patients who were DR3/DR7 heterozygotes appeared to be at increased risk of an early onset of disease and the development of focal sclerosis (Cambon-Thomsen et al., 1986). Another study of a similar steroid-resistant population found a significant increase in the combination of B8, DR3 and DR7 (Ruder et al., 1990). Certain subtypes of DR3 and DR7 have also been found at higher frequency in the steroid-resistant population (Mytilineos et al., 1990), and there is a single report of an increased incidence of DR4, most striking in adult onset cases (Glicklich et al., 1988). Familial focal segmental glomerulosclerosis has been noted, and it is intriguing that the reported cases appear to share the DRw8 allele in the majority of instances, even though this is rare in the background population (Tejani et al., 1983; McCurdy, Butera & Wilson, 1987).

IgM nephropathy, a possible variant within this group of diseases (see below) may also occur in a familial pattern (Scolari et al., 1990); it is of interest that an extended MHC haplotype recurred in nine out of ten affected members.

Other loci

There is little information on other genetic loci in these conditions. Significant associations between minimal change nephropathy and polymorphisms of complement components C6 and C7 have been reported (Nishimukai et al., 1989). It is unclear whether the increased familial incidence of minimal change nephropathy (White, 1973) is due to the MHC associations reviewed above or to other loci.

Immunopathology

Animal studies

There is very little information from animal models that is at all likely to be relevant to the immunopathogenesis of the human diseases. Although lesions very similar to minimal change nephropathy may be induced by, for instance, the injection of adriamycin or the aminonucleoside of puromycin into rats (Bertani et al., 1982; Diamond & Karnovsky, 1986), this is most unlikely to bear much relationship to the aetiology of the human condition. Similarly, there is a wide range of models of glomerulosclerosis, again particularly in the rat (for review see Remuzzi & Bertani, 1990), whose relevance to human focal segmental glomerulosclerosis probably lies mainly in the demonstration of the diversity of stimuli that can give rise to a single non-specific histopathological entity. Some of these models are, however, relevant to the debate concerning the relationship between minimal change nephropathy and focal segmental glomerulosclerosis in that they demonstrate a clear evolutionary relationship between the two experimental analogues (Okuda et al., 1986; Fogo et al., 1988); this aspect is considered further at the end of the chapter.

Human studies

As with the immunogenetic studies considered above, many of the studies in man have concentrated on the entity of steroid responsive nephrotic syndrome in children; as before this will be assumed to be composed mainly of cases of minimal change nephropathy.

A wide range of immunological abnormalities have been described in minimal change nephropathy and, to a lesser extent, in focal segmental glomerulosclerosis. In many cases, it is possible that these abnormalities are the result simply of the nephrotic state, rather than having a more fundamental connection with pathogenesis. Certain topics, notably the role of abnormalities of glomerular charge in the aetiology of proteinuria (for discussion see Schnaper & Robson, 1988), are somewhat outside the scope of this chapter, although it is clearly possible that such mechanisms are the pathways by which any putative immunological aetiological factors might act.

Abnormalities of the humoral immune system

Although IgM concentrations are raised in minimal change nephropathy, there is a significant decrease in IgG concentration (Giangiacomo et al., 1975); IgE concentrations are increased (see below). Despite a decrease in mitogen-induced IgG synthesis found in vitro (Heslan et al., 1982), spontaneous synthesis is, if anything, increased (Beale et al., 1983). A defect in specific antibody production, particularly in the steroid-resistant subgroup, may contribute to the increased susceptibility to pneumococcal infections (Spika et al., 1982). There are a number of reports of the detection of circulating immune complexes in both minimal change nephropathy and focal segmental glomerulosclerosis (Border, 1979; Cairns, London & Mallick, 1982). There may be some relationship between such complexes and proteinuria (Levinsky et al., 1978). It is possible that the presence of immune complexes may, in part, be due to impaired Fc receptor function, although such impairment does not correlate well with the concentration of complexes (Davin, Foidart & Mahieu, 1983).

Abnormalities of the cellular immune system

A slight decrease in T cell and increase in B cell numbers has been noted during relapse (Sasdelli *et al.*, 1980), but, in general, no marked or consistent abnormalities in T or B cell subset distribution have been described (Feehally *et al.*, 1984). The *in vitro* proliferative response to mitogens may be depressed (Minchin, Turner & Bower, 1980; Chapman *et al.*, 1982), and this has been attributed in part to suppressive serum factors (Beale *et al.*, 1980; see next section). The possible *in vivo* correlates of this depressed reactivity include decreased xenogeneic activity of lymphocytes from patients with minimal change nephropathy injected into rats (Matsumoto, 1982), and decreased reactivity on skin testing to a variety of recall antigens (Fodor *et al.*, 1982). Increased suppressor cell function might explain some of these observations and this has indeed been noted, at least as measured by concanavalin A-induced suppression (Osakabe & Matsumoto, 1981; Wu & Moorthy, 1982). As mentioned at the start of this section, there is evidence that many of these phenomena are simply secondary to the nephrotic state (Taube, Brown & Williams, 1984).

In terms of increased responses, direct lymphocytoxicity to renal tubular cells has been noted (Eyres, Mallick & Taylor, 1976), but could be the result of renal damage, and subsequent sensitisation to neoantigens, rather than the cause of such damage. Decreased suppressor cell activity, which might predispose to increased responsiveness, has been found by some and attributed to a prolonged effect of cyclophosphamide (Taube, Brown & Williams, 1981). However, a more comprehensive study of a group of children in remission from minimal change nephropathy could find no evidence of a defect in suppression attributable to either the disease or cyclophosphamide treatment (Feehally *et al.*, 1984).

Inhibitory and suppressive factors

A variety of serum factors have been described (for review see Schnaper & Robson, 1988), ranging from inhibitors of mitogen-induced proliferation (Beale *et al.*, 1980; Chapman *et al.*, 1982) to actual lymphocytotoxins (Ooi, Orlina & Masaitis, 1974). In many cases these findings are not specific for minimal change nephropathy (Taube *et al.*, 1981), and may even be found in normal serum (Thomson & Kraft, 1987). An initial characterisation of some such factors has been performed (Barna *et al.*, 1983); such characterisation is probably most advanced in the case of soluble immune response suppressor (SIRS). SIRS is found in the urine and serum of certain nephrotic patients and can inhibit in a non-specific fashion both *in vivo* and *in vitro* immune responses (Schnaper, Pierce & Aune, 1984; Schnaper & Aune, 1985). There is a striking correlation between steroid responsiveness of proteinuria and steroid-induced inhibition of SIRS (Schnaper, Aune & Roby, 1987). Sera from nephrotic patients activate $CD8^+$ lymphocytes to produce SIRS and there is preliminary characterisation of this SIRS-inducing activity with the suggestion that it is produced by $CD4^+$ lymphocytes (Schnaper, 1990). Although SIRS could clearly be involved in the aetiology of the variety of depressed immune responses mentioned above, the connection with proteinuria, if any, is obscure, particularly as chronic administration of SIRS to mice apparently does not result in proteinuria (unpublished observations referred to in Schnaper, 1990).

Miscellaneous immunological abnormalities

Lymphocytes may produce a factor that increases the permeability of vessel walls to macromolecules (Lagrue et al., 1975). This has been confirmed by more recent work (Boulton Jones & Simpson, 1980; Tomizawa et al., 1985), but the presence of this factor does not seem to be specific for minimal change nephropathy, and in particular there is no direct relationship between the presence of the factor and increased glomerular permeability (Bakker et al., 1982). Concentrations of complement components are usually normal, although decreased concentrations of factor D (Ballow et al., 1982) and factor B (McLean et al., 1977; Anderson et al., 1979), and increased levels of immunoconglutinin have been noted (Ngu, Barratt & Soothill, 1970). Neutrophil function may be depressed (Anderson et al., 1979).

Relationship of minimal change nephropathy to allergy

There is a high incidence of allergic manifestations in minimal change nephropathy (Lagrue & Laurent, 1982; Lin et al., 1990), and on occasion a particular allergy appears to be directly implicated in the aetiology (Sandberg et al., 1977; Lagrue et al., 1985). The suggestion has been made that minimal change nephropathy may, in fact, be an allergic disease (Lagrue & Laurent, 1982), and in apparent support of this is the observation that serum IgE concentrations are frequently raised both in children (Groshong et al., 1973) and adults (Lagrue et al., 1984) with minimal change nephropathy. However, it is possible that this elevation in IgE, which may persist during remission, is not associated with the aetiology of minimal change nephropathy but is simply another manifestation of a more fundamental immunological disturbance.

Possibly related to this connection with atopy are the associations seen with drugs, notably non-steroidal antiinflammatory agents (Warren et al., 1989, and see Chapter 9), and events such as reactions to insect bites and stings (Swanson & Leveque, 1990) and contact dermatitis (Rytand, 1948).

Relationship of minimal change nephropathy to malignancy

The classical malignancy found in association with minimal change nephropathy is Hodgkin's disease, although a number of other neoplastic associations have also been recorded, notably lymphomas (Morel-Maroger Striker & Striker, 1985). The close relationship is particularly well illustrated by cases in which chemotherapy, or local radiotherapy, of Hodgkin's disease leads to remission of the minimal change nephropathy, and recurrence of lymphoma is accompanied by relapse of the renal lesion.

The link with Hodgkin's disease was one of the factors considered by Shalhoub in formulating his original hypothesis that minimal change nephropathy represented the renal manifestation of a disorder of T cell function (Shalhoub, 1974). The fact that the nature of the malignant cell in Hodgkin's disease remains uncertain, and may well, in at least some cases, be a B and not a T cell (Weiss *et al.*, 1986), does not detract from the inference that a circulating factor produced by (neoplastic) cells of the immune system can cause minimal change nephropathy. Some initial attempts to explore possible mechanisms have shown that serum from patients with Hodgkin's disease will suppress *in vitro* lymphocyte responses, and that this suppression is partially reversed after treatment of the Hodgkin's disease (Crowley, Ree & Esparza, 1982).

Possible variants of minimal change nephropathy and focal segmental glomerulosclerosis

The original description of deposits of IgM in the mesangium of cases with the clinical features of minimal change nephropathy led to the proposal that this was a distinct entity, termed mesangial IgM nephropathy (Cohen, Border & Glassock, 1978; Bhasin *et al.*, 1978). This distinction remains controversial, as does the influence on prognosis (Cohen & Border, 1982). It has been suggested that mesangial IgM deposition, particularly in association with mesangial hypercellularity (see below), has a worse prognosis than minimal change nephropathy without these features (Cohen, Border & Glassock, 1978; Bhasin *et al.*, 1978; Cohen & Border, 1982). On the other hand, there is evidence that such cases, particularly when mesangial IgM deposition is the sole abnormality, behave identically to minimal change nephropathy, both in terms of response to treatment and prognosis (Vilches *et al.*, 1982), and that the presence of IgM is neither constant within an individual on repeat biopsy nor associated with any particular subgroup (Ji-Yun *et al.*, 1984; Habib *et al.*, 1988). It is possible that IgM deposition may represent non-specific trapping secondary to disturbed mesangial function rather than a separate disease. However, the familial occurrence of this entity (see above) lends some support to the concept that it is a distinct disease.

A significant proportion of children with otherwise typical minimal change nephropathy will manifest some degree of mesangial hypercellularity or expansion (27/521 and 16/521 respectively in one large series: International study of kidney disease in children, 1981b); these changes may be even commoner in certain racial groups (Chen, Wang & Zou, 1989). Although on occasion the hypercellularity is sufficiently pronounced that some authorities classify this as a distinct disease (mesangial proliferative glomerulonephritis, often with mesangial IgM deposits; Glassock et al., 1986), there are many clinical and pathological features that overlap with both minimal change nephropathy and focal segmental glomerulosclerosis. It has therefore been suggested that all these entities are part of the same spectrum of disease (Habib et al., 1984). In any event there seems to be general agreement that mesangial hypercellularity or expansion seen in the context of otherwise typical minimal change nephropathy carries a worse prognosis (Waldherr et al., 1978; Cameron, 1988). Although not as clear cut, there may be similar implications for focal segmental glomerulosclerosis (Schoeneman, Bennett & Greifer, 1978; Ito et al., 1984).

As mentioned at the start of this chapter, it is likely that focal segmental glomerulosclerosis is a heterogeneous entity. However, one subgroup that has been distinguished is so-called 'malignant' focal segmental glomerulosclerosis (Brown et al., 1978). These cases are characterised by rapid deterioration of renal function together with marked proteinuria which is resistant to any form of treatment, and which may require renal ablation even at end-stage renal failure (McCarron et al., 1976). Recurrence of focal segmental glomerulosclerosis in transplanted kidneys is well known and may occur in up to 40% of cases (Glassock et al., 1986), but this 'malignant' subgroup appears to be at particular risk (Axelsen et al., 1984; Cameron et al., 1989).

Therapeutic aspects

The response of these conditions to immunosuppressive treatment is of particular importance as one of the principal pieces of evidence for an underlying immunological disturbance.

On the rare occasion that a precipitating factor can be identified, then treatment of this may result in remission of minimal change nephropathy; this has been noted in allergy (Sandberg et al., 1977), malignancy (Crowley, Ree & Esparza, 1982), and drug-associated (Finkelstein et al., 1982) minimal change nephropathy. Because of the suggestion that an allergic disturbance may underlie a significant proportion of apparently idiopathic cases of minimal change nephropathy (see above), treatment with disodium cromoglycate has been tried, with occasional anecdotal success (Lagrue *et al.*, 1985).

The vast majority of patients with the idiopathic condition will respond to treatment with corticosteroids (International study of kidney disease in children, 1981*a*; Zech *et al.*, 1982), although subsequent relapses are frequent (Grupe, 1979). The presence of mesangial hypercellularity (International study of kidney disease in children, 1981*b*) and immune deposits (Allen *et al.*, 1982) may be associated with a lower response rate to steroids. With the possible exception of an increase in relapse rate in cases with increased mesangial cellullarity (Allen *et al.*, 1982), frequency of relapse does not appear to correlate with the histopathological findings (International study of kidney disease in children, 1982); however, the development of steroid resistance in an initially steroid responsive case (or steroid resistance *ab initio*) may reflect the presence of focal segmental glomerulosclerosis.

Cyclophosphamide is usually used in cases of frequently relapsing or steroid-dependent minimal change nephropathy, and is of undoubted benefit (International study of kidney disease in children, 1974). As for corticosteroids, its mode of action in this condition is unknown. It produces lymphopaenia, which particularly affects CD4$^+$ T cells (Feehally *et al.*, 1984); this change reverts to normal 6 to 12 months after treatment although the therapeutic benefit in terms of freedom from relapse may persist for much longer. Chlorambucil can be used as an alternative to cyclophosphamide, and may result in fewer relapses (Grupe, Makker & Ingelfinger, 1976; Elzouki & Jaiswal, 1990); as it is also an alkylating agent its mode of action may well be similar to that of cyclophosphamide.

Other immunomodulatory drugs that have been used in minimal change nephropathy include levamisole, with rather variable results (Niaudet *et al.*, 1984), and cyclosporin A (Meyrier, 1987; Ponticelli & Rivolta, 1990). This latter agent, although it does appear to be effective in some cases of steroid and cyclophosphamide resistant minimal change nephropathy, is unfortunately nephrotoxic, which limits its usefulness. It is also of note that spontaneous remissions may occur after measles infection (Yuceoglu, Berkovich & Chiu, 1969), which is known to be immunosuppressive (Joffe & Rabson, 1978).

In contrast to minimal change nephropathy, focal segmental glomerulosclerosis is much more resistant to therapy. A response to corticosteroids is occasionally seen, particularly in children (in about 30%; Arbus *et al.*, 1982). Cyclophosphamide does not appear to confer any additional benefit over and above that obtained with steroids alone (International study of kidney disease in children, 1983). Other treatments that have been tried include anti-platelet agents in addition to immunosuppression (Futrakul, Poshyachinda & Mitrakul, 1978) and meclofenamate, a non-steroidal antiinflammatory drug which is capable of reducing proteinuria (Velosa *et al.*, 1985). The existence, suggested by some of the data reviewed in the previous section, of a circulating factor that induces proteinuria, is further supported by a report of reduction of proteinuria induced by plasma exchange and immunoadsorption of plasma to protein A (Dantal *et al.*, 1990).

Because of the poor prognosis and generally disappointing results of traditional immunosuppressive treatment in focal segmental glomerulosclerosis, there is considerable interest in the use of cyclosporin A and, possibly, allied compounds. As with minimal change nephropathy, cyclosporin can induce remissions in cases of focal segmental glomerulosclerosis resistant to treatment with steroids and cytotoxic drugs (Meyrier, 1987; Meyrier & Simon, 1988; Ponticelli & Rivolta, 1990). The new immunosuppressant FK 506 probably has a related mode of action to cyclosporin in that, although the cytoplasmic binding proteins are distinct, these both have the same enzymatic activity (Harding *et al.*, 1989). FK 506 is considerably more potent than cyclosporin and of greater importance is its apparent lack of nephrotoxicity (Starzl *et al.*, 1989). A report of complete remission induced by FK 506 in a case of steroid and cyclophosphamide resistant focal segmental glomerulosclerosis is therefore of great interest (McCauley *et al.*, 1990), and further evaluation of this agent is clearly required.

Concluding remarks

Two of the most interesting issues relevant to this disease are the extent to which immunological abnormalities contribute to pathogenesis, and the relationship between minimal change nephropathy and focal segmental glomerulosclerosis.

The circumstantial evidence that led to the initial proposals that minimal change nephropathy is the result of disordered immune function (Shalhoub, 1974; Mallick, 1977) has, if anything, strengthened with time. This evidence can be summarised as follows: 1) the immunogenetic associations; 2) the association with allergy and the precipitation of disease by allergic and other immunological stimuli; 3) the association with neoplasms of the lymphoid system, notably Hodgkin's disease; 4) the many abnormalities of humoral and cellular immunity and the various inhibitory factors that have been described (with the caveat that an uncertain proportion of these may simply be secondary to the nephrotic state); 5) the response to immunosuppression, whether therapeutic, or induced by measles. The evidence with respect to focal segmental glomerulosclerosis is more sparse, and the difficulty compounded by the probable heterogeneous aetiology of this pattern of glomerular injury. However, some cases undoubtedly respond to immunosuppressive treatment, and the evidence outlined above could apply to a certain extent to the subset of focal segmental glomerulosclerosis that may be related to minimal change nephropathy (see below).

Unfortunately, despite the almost overwhelming body of indirect evidence, direct evidence in support of the immunological abnormality hypothesis is lacking. One of the difficulties in pursuing the question further is the lack of an animal model which is at all likely to be closely related to human minimal change nephropathy. However, it may be possible to make some progress by the identification of circulating factors in human disease that can induce proteinuria in animals. Evidence for the existence of such factors is provided by the remission of the renal lesion with treatment of associated Hodgkin's disease, the recurrence of both minimal change nephropathy (Mauer et al., 1979) and focal segmental glomerulosclerosis in renal allografts, and the remission seen in one case of focal segmental glomerulosclerosis following protein A absorption of plasma (Dantal et al., 1990). There is some preliminary evidence that infusion of serum from certain patients with focal segmental glomerulosclerosis into rats will induce proteinuria (Zimmerman & Mann, 1984), and that culture supernatants of peripheral blood mononuclear cells from patients with minimal change nephropathy will do the same (Yoshizawa et al., 1989; Maruyama et al., 1989). Further characterisation of the factor(s) responsible for this may allow the cell of origin to be identified (hypothesised to be a component of the immune system), and thus provide a direct connection between proteinuria and immunological abnormalities.

With respect to the relationship between minimal change nephropathy and focal segmental glomerulosclerosis, it seems clear that a variety of processes can culminate in the final common pathway of focal segmental glomerulosclerosis. The principal debate has focused on whether minimal change nephropathy per se is such a process, whether a particular subset of cases of minimal change nephropathy is predisposed to the development of glomerulosclerosis, or whether the two diseases are distinct entities, with sampling errors on the biopsy accounting for the confusion. To deal with the last point first, if sampling errors are responsible, then apparent transitions both ways (from apparent minimal change nephropathy to focal segmental glomerulosclerosis and vice versa) would be expected. In fact, it is extremely rare for a re-biopsy of a case of focal segmental glomerulosclerosis to show minimal change nephropathy, if this occurs at all. For example, one study found focal segmental sclerosis on the second biopsy of ten individuals with an initial diagnosis of minimal change nephropathy; a third biopsy from six of these showed focal segmental sclerosis in all (Fogo et al., 1990). The main question, therefore, appears to be whether all patients with minimal change nephropathy are at risk of progression to focal segmental glomerulosclerosis, or only a particular subset. It seems reasonably clear that many patients with minimal change nephropathy have a very benign course. Prolonged follow-up studies of steroid-sensitive biopsy-proven minimal change nephropathy have shown no evidence of progression to renal failure (Lewis *et al.*, 1989), and, in fact, there are very few documented cases of the development of renal failure in patients whose proteinuria is abolished by steroids (six cases in the literature, for review see Cameron, 1988).

We are therefore left with the perhaps unsurprising conclusion that a particular subset of patients with minimal change nephropathy is at particular risk of progression. Important remaining issues include the identification of features that will allow this subset to be defined, and an elucidation of the mechanisms involved: do these patients have a distinct disease *ab initio*, or is some more aggressive process superimposed on otherwise typical minimal change nephropathy, and if so, what is the stimulus for this? There has been some progress on the first of these points. As mentioned above, the presence of IgM is probably not associated with a worse prognosis, but mesangial hypercellularity is. However, this latter finding is relatively rare (2.5% of cases), and perhaps of more promise is the presence of glomerular hypertrophy (Fogo *et al.*, 1990). This study showed that 32 children with persisting benign minimal change nephropathy had a mean glomerular area that was the same as that of normal controls, whereas ten children who progressed from minimal change nephropathy to focal segmental glomerulosclerosis had a highly significant increase in their mean glomerular area on their initial biopsy. All children (there were only four) whose mean glomerular area was more than $1.75 \times$ control showed this progression. As the authors state, further improvement in the use of glomerular area as a discriminatory marker for a subgroup with a worse prognosis can be anticipated with the use of age-matched controls to allow for variation of glomerular size with growth.

The mechanisms that are responsible for the progression of minimal change nephropathy to focal segmental glomerulosclerosis, or the development of glomerulosclerosis in general, remain unknown. Several have been proposed, including hyperfiltration (Brenner, Meyer & Hostetter, 1982), lipid abnormalities (Moorhead *et al.*, 1982; Keane, Kasiske & O'Donnell, 1988; Diamond & Karnovsky, 1988), glomerular hypertrophy (Yoshida, Fogo & Ichikawa, 1989), and altered glomerular permeability to macromolecules (Remuzzi & Bertani, 1990). It is beyond the scope of this volume to discuss these further; future progress will depend upon a more detailed understanding of the pathogenesis of these disorders than is presently available.

References

Alfiler, C. A., Roy, L. P., Doran, T., Sheldon, A. & Bashier, H. (1980). HLA-DRw7 and steroid-responsive nephrotic syndrome of childhood. *Clinical Nephrology*, 14, 71–4.

Allen, W. R., Travis, L. B., Cavallo, T., Brouhard, B. H. & Cunningham, R. J. (1982). Immune deposits and mesangial hypercellularity in minimal change nephrotic syndrome: clinical relevance. *Journal of Pediatrics*, 100, 188–91.

Anderson, D. C., York, T. L., Rose, G. & Smith, C. W. (1979). Assessment of serum factor B, serum opsonins, granulocyte chemotaxis, and infection in nephrotic syndrome of children. *Journal of Infectious Disease*, 140, 1–11.

Arbus, G. S., Poucell, S., Bacheyie, G. S. & Baumal, R. (1982). Focal segmental glomerulosclerosis with idiopathic nephrotic syndrome. *Journal of Pediatrics*, 101, 40–5.

Axelsen, R. A., Seymour, A. E., Mathew, T. H., Fisher, G., Canny, A. & Pascoe, V. (1984). Recurrent focal glomerulosclerosis in renal transplants. *Clinical Nephrology*, 21, 110–14.

Bakker, W. W., Beukhof, J. R., van Luijk, W. H. J. & Van der Hem, G. K. (1982). Vascular permeability increasing factor (VPF) in IgA nephropathy. *Clinical Nephrology*, 18, 165–7.

Ballow, M., Kennedy, T. L., Gaudio, K. M., Siegel, N. J. & McLean, R. H. (1982). Serum hemolytic factor D values in children with steroid-responsive idiopathic nephrotic syndrome. *Journal of Pediatrics*, 100, 192–6.

Barna, B. P., Makker, S., Kallen, R. *et al.* (1983). A lymphocytotoxic factors(s) in plasma of patients with minimal change nephrotic syndrome: partial characterization. *Clinical Immunology and Immunopathology*, 27, 272–82.

Beale, M. G., Hoffsten, P. E., Robson, A. M. & MacDermott, R. P. (1980). Inhibitory factors of lymphocyte transformation in sera from patients with minimal change nephrotic syndrome. *Clinical Nephrology*, 13, 271–6.

Beale, M. G., Nash, G. S., Bertovich, M. J. & MacDermott, R. P. (1983). Immunoglobulin synthesis by peripheral blood mononuclear cells in minimal change nephrotic syndrome. *Kidney International*, 23, 380–6.

Bertani, T., Poggi, A., Pozzoni, R. *et al.* (1982). Adriamycin-induced nephrotic syndrome in rats. Sequence of pathologic events. *Laboratory Investigation*, 46, 16–23.

Bhasin, H. K., Abuelo, J. G., Nayak, R. & Esparza, A. R. (1978). Mesangial proliferative glomerulonephritis. *Laboratory Investigation*, 39, 21–9.

Bodmer, J. & Bodmer, W. (1984). Histocompatibility 1984. *Immunology Today*, 5, 251–4.

Border, W. A. (1979). Immune complex detection in glomerular diseases. *Nephron*, 24, 105–13.

Boulton Jones, J. M. & Simpson, S. (1980). Immunological studies of minimal-change nephropathy. *British Medical Journal*, 280, 291–2.

Brenner, B. M., Meyer, T. W. & Hostetter, T. H. (1982). Dietary protein intake and the progressive nature of kidney disease: the role of hemodynamically mediated glomerular injury in the pathogenesis of progressive glomerular sclerosis in aging, renal ablation, and intrinsic renal disease. *New England Journal of Medicine*, 307, 652–9.

Brown, C. B., Cameron, J. S., Turner, D. R. *et al.* (1978). Focal segmental glomerulosclerosis with rapid decline in renal function ('malignant FSGS'). *Clinical Nephrology*, 10, 51–61.

Cairns, S. A., London, R. A. & Mallick, N. P. (1982). Circulating immune complexes in idopathic glomerular disease. *Kidney International*, 21, 507–12.

Cambon-Thomsen, A., Bouissou, F., Abbal, M. *et al.* (1986). HLA et Bf dans le syndrome néphrotique idiopathique de l'enfant: differences entre les formes corticosensibles et corticorésistantes. *Pathologie Biologie*, 34, 725–30.

Cameron, J. S. (1979). The problem of focal segmental glomerulosclerosis. In *Progress in Glomerulonephritis*, ed. P. Kincaid-Smith, A. J. F. d'Apice & R. W. Atkins, pp. 209–28. New York: John Wiley & Sons Inc.

REFERENCES

Cameron, J. S. (1988). The long-term outcome of glomerular diseases. In *Diseases of the Kidney*, 4th edn, ed. R. W. Schrier & C. W. Gottschalk, pp. 2127–89. Boston/Toronto: Little, Brown and Company.

Cameron, J. S., Senguttuvan, P., Hartley, B. *et al.* (1989). Focal segmental glomerulosclerosis in fifty-nine renal allografts from a single centre; analysis of risk factors for recurrence. *Transplantation Proceedings*, **21**, 2117–18.

Chapman, S., Taube, D., Brown, Z. & Williams, D. G. (1982). Impaired lymphocyte transformation in minimal change nephropathy in remission. *Clinical Nephrology*, **18**, 34–8.

Chen, Y. P., Wang, H. Y. & Zou, W. Z. (1989). Non-IgA mesangial proliferative glomerulonephritis. Clinical and pathological analysis of 77 cases. *Chinese Medical Journal*, **102**, 510–5.

Churg, J., Habib, R. & White, R. H. R. (1970). Pathology of the nephrotic syndrome in children. A report for the International Study of Kidney Disease in Children. *Lancet*, **i**, 1299–302.

Clark, A. G. B., Vaughan, R. W., Stephens, H. A. F., Chantler, C., Williams, D. G. & Welsh, K. I. (1990). Genes encoding the β-chains of HLA-DR7 and HLA-DQw2 define major susceptibility determinants for idiopathic nephrotic syndrome. *Clinical Science*, **78**, 391–7.

Cohen, A. H., Border, W. A. & Glassock, R. J. (1978). Nephrotic syndrome with glomerular mesangial IgM deposits. *Laboratory Investigation*, **38**, 610–19.

Cohen, A. H. & Border, W. A. (1982). Mesangial proliferative glomerulonephritis. *Seminars in Nephrology*, **2**, 228–40.

Crowley, J. P., Ree, H. J. & Esparza, A. (1982). Monocyte-dependent serum suppression of lymphocyte blastogenesis in Hodgkin's disease: an association with nephrotic syndrome. *Journal of Clinical Immunology*, **2**, 270–5.

Dantal, J., Testa, A., Bigot, E. & Soulillou, J. P. (1990). Disappearance of proteinuria after immunoadsorption in a patient with focal glomerulosclerosis. *Lancet*, **336**, 190.

Davin, J. C., Foidart, J. B. & Mahieu, P. R. (1983). Fc-receptor function in minimal change nephrotic syndrome of childhood. *Clinical Nephrology*, **20**, 280–4.

de Mouzon-Cambon, A., Bouissou, F., Dutau, G. *et al.* (1981). HLA-DR7 in children with idiopathic nephrotic syndrome. *Tissue Antigens*, **17**, 518–24.

Diamond, J. R. & Karnovsky, M. J. (1986). Focal and segmental glomerulosclerosis following a single intravenous dose of puromycin aminonucleoside. *American Journal of Pathology*, **122**, 481–7.

Diamond, J. R. & Karnovsky, M. J. (1988). Focal and segmental glomerulosclerosis: analogies to atherosclerosis. *Kidney International*, **33**, 917–24.

Elzouki, A. Y. & Jaiswal, O. P. (1990). Evaluation of chlorambucil therapy in steroid-dependent cyclophosphamide-resistant children with nephrosis. *Pediatric Nephrology*, **4**, 459–62.

Eyres, K., Mallick, N. P. & Taylor, G. (1976). Evidence for cell-mediated immunity to renal antigens in minimal-change nephrotic syndrome. *Lancet*, **i**, 1158–9.

Feehally, J., Beattie, T. J., Brenchley, P. E. C. *et al.* (1984). Modulation of cellular immune function by cyclophosphamide in children with minimal-change nephropathy. *New England Journal of Medicine*, **310**, 415–20.

Finkelstein, A., Fraley, D. S., Stachura, I., Feldman, H. A., Gandy, D. R. & Bourke, E. (1982). Fenoprofen nephropathy: lipoid nephrosis and interstitial nephritis. A possible T-lymphocyte disorder. *American Journal of Medicine*, **72**, 81–7.

Fodor, P., Saitúa, M., Rodriguez, E., González, B. & Schlesinger, L. (1982). T-cell dysfunction in minimal-change nephrotic syndrome of childhood. *American Journal of Diseases of Children*, **136**, 713–17.

Fogo, A., Yoshida, Y., Glick, A. D., Homma, T. & Ichikawa, I. (1988). Serial micropuncture analysis of glomerular function in two rat models of glomerular sclerosis. *Journal of Clinical Investigation*, **82**, 322–30.

Fogo, A., Hawkins, E. P., Berry, P. L. *et al.* (1990). Glomerular hypertrophy in minimal change disease predicts subsequent progression to focal glomerular sclerosis. *Kidney International*, **38**, 115–23.

Futrakul, P., Poshyachinda, M. & Mitrakul, C. (1978). Focal sclerosing glomerulonephritis: a kinetic evaluation of hemostasis and the effect of anticoagulant therapy: a controlled study. *Clinical Nephrology*, **10**, 180–6.

Giangiacomo, J., Cleary, T. G., Cole, B. R., Hoffsten, P. & Robson, A. M. (1975). Serum immunoglobulins in the nephrotic syndrome. A possible cause of minimal-change nephrotic syndrome. *New England Journal of Medicine*, **293**, 8–12.

Glassock, R. J., Adler, S. G., Ward, H. J. & Cohen, A. H. (1986). Primary glomerular diseases. In *The Kidney*, 3rd edn, ed. B. M. Brenner & F. C. Rector, pp. 929–1013. Philadelphia: W.B.Saunders Company.

Glicklich, D., Haskell, L., Senitzer, D. & Weiss, R. A. (1988). Possible genetic predisposition to idiopathic focal segmental glomerulosclerosis. *American Journal of Kidney Disease*, **12**, 26–30.

Groshong, T., Mendelson, L., Mendoza, S., Bazaral, M., Hamburger, R. & Tune, B. (1973). Serum IgE in patients with minimal-change nephrotic syndrome. *Journal of Pediatrics*, **83**, 767–71.

Grupe, W. E., Makker, S. P. & Ingelfinger, J. R. (1976). Chlorambucil treatment of frequently relapsing nephrotic syndrome. *New England Journal of Medicine*, **295**, 746–9.

Grupe, W. E. (1979). Childhood nephrotic syndrome. Clinical associations and response to therapy. *Postgraduate Medicine*, **65/no.5**, 229–36.

Habib, R., Churg, J., Bernstein, J. *et al.* (1984). Minimal change disease, mesangial proliferative glomerulonephritis and focal sclerosis: individual entities or a spectrum of disease? In *Nephrology*, ed. R. R. Robinson, pp. 634. New York: Springer-Verlag.

Habib, R., Girardin, E., Gagnadoux, M. F., Hinglais, N., Levy, M. & Broyer, M. (1988). Immunopathological findings in idiopathic nephrosis: clinical significance of glomerular 'immune deposits'. *Pediatric Nephrology*, **2**, 402–8.

Harding, M. W., Galat, A., Uehling, D. E. & Schreiber, S. L. (1989). A receptor for the immunosuppressant FK506 is a *cis–trans* peptidyl–prolyl isomerase. *Nature*, London, **341**, 758–60.

Heslan, J. M., Lautie, J. P., Intrator, L., Blanc, C., Lagrue, G. & Sobel, A. T. (1982). Impaired IgG synthesis in patients with the nephrotic syndrome. *Clinical Nephrology*, **18**, 144–7.

International study of kidney disease in children (1974). Prospective, controlled trial of cyclophosphamide therapy in children with the nephrotic syndrome. *Lancet*, **ii**, 423–7.

International study of kidney disease in children (1978). Nephrotic syndrome in children: prediction of histopathology from clinical and laboratory characteristics at time of diagnosis. *Kidney International*, **13**, 159–65.

International study of kidney disease in children (1981*a*). The primary nephrotic syndrome in children. Identification of patients with minimal change nephrotic syndrome from initial response to prednisone. *Journal of Pediatrics*, **98**, 561–4.

International study of kidney disease in children (1981*b*). Primary nephrotic syndrome in children: clinical significance of histopathologic variants of minimal change and of diffuse mesangial hypercellularity. *Kidney International*, **20**, 765–71.

International study of kidney disease in children (1982). Early identification of frequent relapsers among children with minimal change nephrotic syndrome. *Journal of Pediatrics*, **101**, 514–18.

International study of kidney disease in children (1983). Cyclophosphamide therapy in focal segmental glomerular sclerosis: a controlled clinical trial. *European Journal of Paediatrics*, **140**, 149.(Abstract).

Ito, H., Yoshikawa, N., Aozai, F. *et al.* (1984). Twenty-seven children with focal segmental glomerulosclerosis: correlation between the segmental location of the glomerular lesions and prognosis. *Clinical Nephrology*, **22**, 9–14.

Ji-Yun, Y., Melvin, T., Sibley, R. & Michael, A. F. (1984). No evidence for a specific role of IgM in mesangial proliferation of idiopathic nephrotic syndrome. *Kidney International*, **25**, 100–6.

Joffe, M. I. & Rabson, A. R. (1978). Dissociation of lymphokine production and blastogenesis in children with measles infections. *Clinical Immunology and Immunopathology*, **10**, 335–43.

Keane, W. F., Kasiske, B. L. & O'Donnell, M. P. (1988). Hyperlipidemia and the progression of renal disease. *American Journal of Clinical Nutrition*, **47**, 157–60.

Kobayashi, Y., Chen, X-M., Hiki, Y., Fujii, K. & Kashiwagi, N. (1985). Association of HLA-DRw8 and DQw3 with minimal change nephrotic syndrome in Japanese adults. *Kidney International*, **28**, 193–7.

Komori, K., Nose, Y., Inouye, H. *et al.* (1983). Immunogenetical study in patients with chronic glomerulonephritis. *Tokai Journal of Experimental and Clinical Medicine*, **8**, 135–48.

Lagrue, G. & Laurent, J. (1982). Is lipoid nephrosis an 'allergic' disease? *Transplantation Proceedings*, **14**, 485–8.

Lagrue, G., Xheneumont, S., Branallec, A., Hirbec, G. & Weil, B. A. (1975). Vascular permeability factor elaborated from lymphocytes. I. Demonstration in patients with nephrotic syndrome. *Biomedicine*, **23**, 37–40.

Lagrue, G., Laurent, J., Hirbec, G. *et al.* (1984). Serum IgE in primary glomerular diseases. *Nephron*, **36**, 5–9.

Lagrue, G., Laurent, J., Belghiti, D. & Sainte-Laudy, J. (1985). Food sensitivity and idiopathic nephrotic syndrome. *Lancet*, **ii**, 777.

Lagueruela, C. C., Buettner, T. L., Cole, B. R., Kissane, J. M. & Robson, A. M. (1990). HLA extended haplotypes in steroid-sensitive nephrotic syndrome of childhood. *Kidney International*, **38**, 145–50.

Laurent, J., Ansquer, J. C., de Mouzon-Cambon, A., Bracq, C. & Lagrue, G. (1983). Adult onset lipoid nephrosis is not DR7 associated. *Tissue Antigens*, **22**, 229–30.

Lenhard, V., Muller-Wiefel, D. E., Dippell, J., Schroder, D., Seidl, S. & Scharer, K. (1980*a*). HLA in minimal change nephrotic syndrome (MC) and focal segmental glomerulosclerosis (FSS). *Pediatric Research*, **14**, 1003.(Abstract).

Lenhard, V., Dippell, J., Müller-Wiefel, D. E., Schröder, D., Siedl, S. & Schärer, K. (1980*b*). HLA antigens in children with idiopathic nephrotic syndrome. *Proceedings of the European Dialysis and Transplantation Association*, **17**, 673–7.

Levinsky, R. J., Malleson, P. N., Barratt, T. M. & Soothill, J. F. (1978). Circulating immune complexes in steroid-responsive nephrotic syndrome. *New England Journal of Medicine*, **298**, 126–9.

Lewis, M. A., Baildom, E. M., Davis, N., Houston, I. B. & Postlethwaite, R. J. (1989). Nephrotic syndrome: from toddlers to twenties. *Lancet*, **i**, 255–9.

Lin, C. Y., Lee, B. H., Lin, C. C. & Chen, W. P. (1990). A study of the relationship between childhood nephrotic syndrome and allergic disease. *Chest*, **97**, 1408–11.

Mallick, N. P. (1977). The pathogenesis of minimal change nephropathy. *Clinical Nephrology*, **7**, 87–95.

Maruyama, K., Tomizawa, S., Shimabukuro, N., Fukuda, T., Johshita, T. & Kuroume, T. (1989). Effect of supernatants derived from T lymphocyte culture in minimal change nephrotic syndrome on rat kidney capillaries. *Nephron*, **51**, 73–6.

Matalon, R., Katz, L., Gallo, G., Waldo, E., Cabaluna, C. & Eisinger, R. P. (1974). Glomerular sclerosis in adults with nephrotic syndrome. *Annals of Internal Medicine*, **80**, 488–95.

Matsumoto, K. (1982). Impaired local graft-versus-host reaction in lipod nephrosis. *Nephron*, 31, 281–2.

Mauer, S. M., Hellerstein, S., Cohn, R. A., Sibley, R. K. & Vernier, R. L. (1979). Recurrence of steroid-responsive nephrotic syndrome after renal transplantation. *Journal of Pediatrics*, 95, 261–4.

McCarron, D. A., Rubin, R. J., Barnes, B. A., Harrington, J. T. & Millan, V. G. (1976). Therapeutic bilateral renal infarction in end-stage renal disease. *New England Journal of Medicine*, 294, 652.

McCauley, J., Tzakis, A. G., Fung, J. J., Todo, S. & Starzl, T. E. (1990). FK506 in steroid-resistant focal sclerosing glomerulonephritis of childhood. *Lancet*, 335, 674.

McCurdy, F. A., Butera, P. J. & Wilson, R. (1987). The familial occurrence of focal segmental glomerular sclerosis. *American Journal of Kidney Disease*, 10, 467–9.

McLean, R. H., Forsgren, A., Björkstén, B., Kim, Y., Quie, P. G. & Michael, A. F. (1977). Decreased serum factor B concentration associated with decreased opsonization of *Escherichia coli* in the idiopathic nephrotic syndrome. *Pediatric Research*, 11, 910–16.

McLean, R. H., Kennedy, T. L., Ballow, M., Gaudio, K. M. & Siegel, N. J. (1983). Increased frequency of factor B fast variant ($BF*F$) in the idiopathic nephrotic syndrome of childhood. *Disease Markers*, 1, 25–32.

McLean, R. H., Bias, W. B., Tina, L., Ruley, J. & Bock, G. H. (1987). Variability of C4 gene number in the nephrotic syndrome. *American Society of Nephrology*, 18A.(Abstract).

Meyrier, A. (1987). Treatment with cyclosporin of patients with idiopathic nephrotic syndrome. *Springer Seminars in Immunopathology*, 9, 441–50.

Meyrier, A. & Simon, P. (1988). Treatment of corticoresistant idiopathic nephrotic syndrome in the adult: minimal change disease and focal segmental glomerulosclerosis. *Advances in Nephrology*, 17, 127–50.

Minchin, M. A., Turner, K. J. & Bower, G. D. (1980). Lymphocyte blastogenesis in nephrotic syndrome. *Clinical and Experimental Immunology*, 42, 241–6.

Moorhead, J. F., El Nakos, M., Chan, M. K. & Varghese, Z. (1982). Lipid nephrotoxicity in chronic progressive glomerular and tubulo-interstitial disease. *Lancet*, ii, 1309–10.

Morel-Maroger Striker, L. & Striker, G. E. (1985). Glomerular lesions in malignancies. *Contributions in Nephrology*, 48, 111–22.

Mytilineos, J., Konrad, M., Scherer, S. *et al.* (1990). RFLP DRβ typing in patients with idiopathic nephrotic syndrome. *Nephrology Dialysis and Transplantation*, 5, 656.(Abstract).

Naito, S., Kohara, M. & Arakawa, K. (1987). Association of Class II antigens of HLA with primary glomerulopathies. *Nephron*, 45, 111–14.

Ngu, J. L., Barratt, T. M. & Soothill, J. F. (1970). Immunoconglutinin and complement changes in steroid sensitive relapsing nephrotic syndrome of childhood. *Clinical and Experimental Immunology*, 6, 109–16.

Niaudet, P., Drachman, R., Gagnadoux, M. F. & Broyer, M. (1984). Treatment of idiopathic nephrotic syndrome with levamisole. *Acta Paediatrica Scandinavica*, 73, 637–41.

Nishimukai, H., Nakanishi, I., Takeuchi, Y. *et al.* (1989). Complement C6 and C7 polymorphisms in Japanese patients with chronic glomerulonephritis. *Human Hereditary*, 39, 150–5.

Noss, G., Bachman, H. J. & Olbing, H. (1981). Association of minimal change nephrotic syndrome (MCNS) with HLA-B8 and B13. *Clinical Nephrology*, 15, 172–4.

Noël, L. H., Descamps, B., Jungers, P. *et al.* (1978). HLA antigen in three types of glomerulonephritis. *Clinical Immunology and Immunopathology*, 10, 19–23.

Nuñez-Roldan, A., Villechenous, E., Fernandez-Andrade, C. & Martin-Govantes, J. (1982). Increased HLA-DR7 and decreased DR2 in steroid-responsive nephrotic syndrome. *New England Journal of Medicine*, 306, 366–7.

O'Regan, D., O'Callaghan, U., Dundon, S. & Reen, D. J. (1980). HLA antigens and steroid responsive nephrotic syndrome of childhood. *Tissue Antigens*, 16, 147–51.

Okuda, S., Oh, Y., Tsuruda, H., Onoyama, K., Fujimi, S. & Fujishima, M. (1986). Adriamycin-induced nephropathy as a model of chronic progressive glomerular disease. *Kidney International*, **29**, 502–10.

Ooi, B. S., Orlina, A. R. & Masaitis, L. (1974). Lymphocytotoxins in primary renal disease. *Lancet*, **ii**, 1348–50.

Osakabe, K. & Matsumoto, K. (1981). Concanavalin A-induced suppressor cell activity in lipoid nephrosis. *Scandinavian Journal of Immunology*, **14**, 161–6.

Ponticelli, C. & Rivolta, E. (1990). Ciclosporin in minimal-change glomerulopathy and in focal segmental glomerular sclerosis. *American Journal of Nephrology*, **10** Suppl. 1, 105–9.

Remuzzi, G. & Bertani, T. (1990). Is glomerulosclerosis a consequence of altered glomerular permeability to macromolecules? *Kidney International*, **38**, 384–94.

Rich, A. F. (1957). A hitherto undescribed vulnerability of the juxtamedullary glomeruli in lipoid nephrosis. *Bulletin of the Johns Hopkins Hospital*, **100**, 173–86.

Roy, L. P., Vernier, R. L. & Michael, A. F. (1972). Effect of protein-load proteinuria on glomerular polyanion. *Proceedings of the Society for Experimental Biology and Medicine*, **141**, 870–4.

Ruder, H., Scharer, K., Opelz, G. *et al.* (1990). Human leukocyte antigens in idiopathic nephrotic syndrome in children. *Pediatric Nephrology*, **4**, 478–81.

Rytand, D. A. (1948). Fatal anuria, the nephrotic syndrome and glomerular nephritis as sequels of the dermatitis of poison oak. *American Journal of Medicine*, **5**, 548–60.

Sandberg, D. H., McIntosh, R. M., Bernstein, C. W., Carr, R. & Strauss, J. (1977). Severe steroid-responsive nephrosis associated with hypersensitivity. *Lancet*, **i**, 388–91.

Sasdelli, M., Rovinetti, C., Cagnoli, L., Beltrandi, E., Barboni, F. & Zucchelli, P. (1980). Lymphocyte subpopulations in minimal-change nephropathy. *Nephron*, **25**, 72–6.

Schnaper, H. W. (1990). A regulatory system for soluble immune response suppressor production in steroid-responsive nephrotic syndrome. *Kidney International*, **38**, 151–9.

Schnaper, H. W. & Aune, T. M. (1985). Identification of the lymphokine soluble immune response suppressor in urine of nephrotic children. *Journal of Clinical Investigation*, **76**, 341–9.

Schnaper, H. W., Aune, T. M. & Roby, R. K. (1987). Steroid-sensitive mechanism of soluble immune response suppressor production in steroid-responsive nephrotic syndrome. *Journal of Clinical Investigation*, **79**, 257–64.

Schnaper, H. W., Pierce, C. W. & Aune, T. M. (1984). Identification and initial characterization of concanavalin A- and interferon-induced human suppressor factors: evidence for a human equivalent of murine soluble immune response suppressor (SIRS). *Journal of Immunology*, **132**, 2429–35.

Schnaper, H. W. & Robson, A. M. (1988). Nephrotic Syndrome: Minimal Change Disease, Focal Glomerulosclerosis, and Related Disorders. In *Diseases of the Kidney*, 4th edn, ed. R. W. Schrier & C. W. Gottschalk, pp. 1949–2004. Boston: Little, Brown & Company.

Schoeneman, M. J., Bennett, B. & Greifer, I. (1978). The natural history of focal segmental glomerulosclerosis with and without mesangial hypercellularity in children. *Clinical Nephrology*, **9**, 45–54.

Scolari, F., Scaini, P., Savoldi, S. *et al.* (1990). Familial IgM nephropathy: a morphologic and immunogenetic study of three pedigrees. *American Journal of Nephrology*, **10**, 261–8.

Shalhoub, R. J. (1974). Pathogenesis of lipoid nephrosis: a disorder of T cell function. *Lancet*, **ii**, 556–60.

Sharpstone, P., Ogg, C. S. & Cameron, J. S. (1969). Nephrotic syndrome due to primary renal disease in adults: I. Survey of incidence in South-East England. *British Medical Journal*, **2**, 533–5.

Shaw, S., Duquesnoy, R. J. & Smith, P. L. (1981). Population studies of the HLA-linked SB antigens. *Immunogenetics*, **14**, 153–62.

Silva, F. G. & Hogg, R. J. (1989). Minimal change nephrotic syndrome-focal sclerosis complex (including IgM nephropathy and diffuse mesangial hypercellularity). In *Renal Pathology with Clinical and Functional Correlations*, ed. C. C. Tisher & B. M. Brenner, pp. 265–339. Philadelphia: J.B.Lippincott Company.

Spika, J. S., Halsey, N. A., Fish, A. J. *et al.* (1982). Serum antibody response to pneumococcal vaccine in children with nephrotic syndrome. *Pediatrics*, **69**, 219–23.

Starzl, T. E., Todo, S., Fung, J., Demetris, A. J., Venkataramman, R. & Jain, A. (1989). FK506 for liver, kidney, and pancreas transplantation. *Lancet*, **ii**, 1000–4.

Swanson, G. P. & Leveque, J. A. (1990). Nephrotic syndrome associated with ant bite. *Texas Medicine*, **86**, 39–41.

Taube, D., Brown, Z. & Williams, D. G. (1981). Long-term impairment of suppressor-cell function by cyclophosphamide in minimal-change nephropathy and its association with therapeutic response. *Lancet*, **i**, 235–8.

Taube, D., Brown, Z. & Williams, D. G. (1984). Impaired lymphocyte and suppressor cell function in minimal change nephropathy, membranous nephropathy and focal glomerulosclerosis. *Clinical Nephrology*, **22**, 176–82.

Taube, D., Chapman, S., Brown, Z. & Williams, D. G. (1981). Depression of normal lymphocyte transformation by sera of patients with minimal change nephropathy and other forms of nephrotic syndrome. *Clinical Nephrology*, **15**, 286–90.

Tejani, A., Nicastri, A., Phadke, K. *et al.* (1983). Familial focal segmental glomerulosclerosis. *International Journal of Pediatric Nephrology*, **4**, 231–4.

Thomson, N. M. & Kraft, N. (1987). Normal human serum also contains the lymphotoxin found in minimal change nephropathy. *Kidney International*, **31**, 1186–93.

Thomson, P. D., Barratt, T. M., Stokes, C. R., Turner, M. W. & Soothill, J. F. (1976). HLA antigens and atopic features in steroid-responsive nephrotic syndrome of childhood. *Lancet*, **ii**, 765–8.

Tomizawa, S., Maruyama, K., Nagasawa, N., Suzuki, S. & Kuroume, T. (1985). Studies of vascular permeability factor derived from T lymphocytes and inhibiting effect of plasma on its production in minimal change nephrotic syndrome. *Nephron*, **41**, 157–60.

Trompeter, R. S., Barratt, T. M., Kay, R., Turner, M. W. & Soothill, J. F. (1980). HLA, atopy, and cyclophosphamide in steroid-responsive childhood nephrotic syndrome. *Kidney International*, **17**, 113–17.

Velosa, J. A., Torres, V. E., Donadio, J. V., Wagoner, R. D., Holley, K. E. & Offord, K. P. (1985). Treatment of severe nephrotic syndrome with meclofenamate: an uncontrolled pilot study. *Mayo Clinic Proceedings*, **60**, 586–92.

Vilches, A. R., Turner, D. R., Cameron, J. S., Ogg, C. S., Chantler, C. & Williams, D. G. (1982). Significance of mesangial IgM deposits in 'minimal change' nephrotic syndrome. *Laboratory Investigation*, **46**, 10–15.

Waldherr, R., Gubler, M-C., Levy, M. *et al.* (1978). The significance of pure diffuse mesangial proliferation in idiopathic nephrotic syndrome. *Clinical Nephrology*, **10**, 171–9.

Warren, G. V., Korbet, S. M., Schwartz, M. M. & Lewis, E. J. (1989). Minimal change glomerulopathy associated with nonsteroidal antiinflammatory drugs. *American Journal of Kidney Disease*, **13**, 127–30.

Weiss, L. M., Strickler, J. G., Hu, E., Warnke, R. A. & Sklar, J. (1986). Immunoglobulin gene rearrangements in Hodgkin's disease. *Human Pathology*, **17**, 1009–14.

White, R. H. R. (1973). The familial nephrotic syndrome. I. A European survey. *Clinical Nephrology*, **1**, 215–19.

Wu, M. J. & Moorthy, A. V. (1982). Suppressor cell function in patients with primary glomerular disease. *Clinical Immunology and Immunopathology*, **22**, 442–7.

Yoshida, Y., Fogo, A. & Ichikawa, I. (1989). Glomerular hemodynamic changes vs. hypertrophy in experimental glomerular sclerosis. *Kidney International*, **35**, 654–60.

Yoshizawa, N., Kusumi, Y., Matsumoto, K. *et al.* (1989). Studies of a glomerular permeability factor in patients with minimal-change nephrotic syndrome. *Nephron*, **51**, 370–6.

Yuceoglu, A. M., Berkovich, S. & Chiu, J. (1969). Effect of live measles virus vaccine on childhood nephrosis. *Journal of Pediatrics*, **74**, 291–3.

Zech, P., Colon, S., Pointet, P. H., Deteix, P., Labeeuw, M. & Leitienne, P. H. (1982). The nephrotic syndrome in adults aged over 60: etiology, evolution and treatment of 76 cases. *Clinical Nephrology*, **17**, 232–6.

Zimmerman, S. W. & Mann, S. (1984). Increased urinary protein excretion in the rat produced by serum from a patient with recurrent focal segmental glomerular sclerosis after renal transplantation. *Clinical Nephrology*, **22**, 32–8.

—8—
Systemic vasculitis and crescentic glomerulonephritis

Systemic vasculitis is characterised by necrotising inflammation of blood vessel walls; practically any organ system can be involved, leading to protean clinical manifestations. A variety of classifications has been applied to this group of diseases, with some differences in nomenclature between countries. One such classification, based on size of vessel and type of inflammation, is shown in Table 8.1. The difficulties are illustrated by the overlaps that exist within this scheme; polyarteritis, for instance, may well represent a spectrum, with classical polyarteritis nodosa and microscopic polyarteritis at either end, and with many cases in practice falling between these extremes. Classification criteria for a variety of vasculitides have also been established (Hunder *et al.*, 1990 and succeeding articles).

Renal involvement is most commonly and characteristically seen in the small vessel vasculitides, Wegener's granulomatosis and microscopic polyarteritis, which are the main focus of this chapter. The lesion is usually a focal proliferative glomerulonephritis, often with necrosis and/or crescent

Table 8.1. *Classification of vasculitis by size of vessel and type of inflammation*

Size of vessel	Type of inflammation	
	Granulomatous	Non-granulomatous
Large	Takayasu's arteritis Giant cell arteritis	
Intermediate	Churg–Strauss syndrome	Polyarteritis nodosa Kawasaki disease
Small	Wegener's granulomatosis	Microscopic polyarteritis Henoch–Schönlein purpura

formation; some subtle differences between the lesions seen with polyarteritis and Wegener's granulomatosis have been reported (Antonovych *et al.*, 1989). The occurrence of such a lesion in the absence of extra-renal disease is commonly termed idiopathic crescentic glomerulonephritis, although there are a number of synonyms (Atkins & Thomson, 1988). The histological similarities between the idiopathic condition and that occurring in the context of vasculitis, together with the subsequent appearance of vasculitis in a substantial proportion of the idiopathic cases (Woodworth *et al.*, 1987), suggests close similarities in pathogenesis. This is supported by the occurrence of anti-neutrophil cytoplasm antibodies (ANCA; see below) in a variable proportion of all three conditions. The increasing availability of ANCA as a diagnostic test is showing that this group of diseases is probably considerably more common than previously supposed: one survey found a combined incidence of Wegener's granulomatosis and microscopic polyarteritis of 1.5/million/year which quadrupled to 6.1/million/year following the introduction of an assay for ANCA (Andrews *et al.*, 1990). There may also have been an increase in incidence that predates the use of ANCA (Woodrow *et al.*, 1990).

Wegener's granulomatosis is a systemic vasculitis characterised by glomerulonephritis and granulomatous inflammation of the upper and lower airways. Not all components are necessarily present, and in particular limited forms are distinguished with disease restricted to the respiratory tract (Carrington & Liebow, 1966; Deremee *et al.*, 1976). The term microscopic polyarteritis (actually, microscopic form of periarteritis nodosa) was originally proposed to distinguish glomerulonephritis occurring in the context of systemic vasculitis from the predominantly ischaemic glomerular changes seen in classical macroscopic polyarteritis with aneurysm formation (Davson, Ball & Platt, 1948). Soon after, the term hypersensitivity angiitis was used to describe the small vessel vasculitis seen in association with drugs, sera and infections (Zeek, 1952). In many cases, however, there was no obvious precipitating factor, and the term came to be used synonymously with microscopic polyarteritis, particularly in the United States. More recently, hypersensitivity angiitis has tended to be equated with cutaneous (leukocytoclastic) vasculitis (Balow & Fauci, 1988). Microscopic polyarteritis is a term commonly used in the UK but not in other European countries, where it is often considered to be a subset of Wegener's granulomatosis (Rasmussen, Borregaard & Wiik, 1987). Many cases classified as crescentic nephritis in the context of a systemic vasculitis in Europe would be termed idiopathic crescentic glomerulonephritis in the United States (Couser, 1988).

Wegener's granulomatosis and microscopic polyarteritis, together with idiopathic crescentic glomerulonephritis, make up the bulk of cases of acute crescentic nephritis. This histological picture is also characteristic of the

Table 8.2. *Conditions that may be associated with crescentic nephritis*

Anti-glomerular basement membrane disease
ANCA-associated renal disease:
 Microscopic polyarteritis
 Wegener's granulomatosis
 'Idiopathic' or 'pauci-immune' crescentic glomerulonephritis
 Churg-Strauss syndrome
Diseases associated with damage to the glomerular basement membrane:
 IgA nephropathy and Henoch-Schönlein purpura
 Lupus nephritis
 Other 'connective tissue' diseases (rheumatoid arthritis, mixed connec-
  tive tissue diseases)
 Membranous nephropathy
 Mesangiocapillary glomerulonephritis
 Cryoglobulinaemia
 Infection related (poststreptococcal, nephritis associated with infective
  endocarditis, infected ventriculo-atrial shunts and visceral abscess)
 Other possible vasculitides (ANCA status uncertain):
  Behçets syndrome, relapsing polychondritis,
  Takayasu's disease
 Accelerated hypertension; systemic sclerosis
Truly idiopathic crescentic glomerulonephritis

---

rarer anti-glomerular basement membrane disease, and may occur in a variety of other primary renal conditions or systemic diseases (see Table 8.2). Many of these other conditions will have characteristic findings when the glomeruli are examined by immunofluorescence and electron microscopy; such studies are usually negative in the context of Wegener's granulomatosis or microscopic polyarteritis (Balow & Fauci, 1988). Cases of idiopathic crescentic glomerulonephritis may or may not have associated immune deposits (Atkins & Thomson, 1988), with the latter sometimes referred to as 'pauci-immune', but the availability of ANCA is resulting in a re-evaluation and re-classification of this group (see final section of this chapter).

Immunogenetics

The MHC

Rather little is known concerning the immunogenetics of this group of diseases. The situation will change rapidly now that efficient means of typing at class II subloci are available, and also because it is possible to define more homogeneous groups of patients on the basis of autoantibody production (see below).

The first reported study found a link between Wegener's granulomatosis and B8 (present in 38.7% of patients versus 18.9% of controls; $p < 0.01$, but probably not corrected for multiple comparisons; Katz et al., 1979). A later study found a very similar increase in B8 but this was not significant after correction (Elkon et al., 1983). There was, however, a significant association between Wegener's granulomatosis and DR2 ($p_{corr} < 0.008$). There were no other significant associations between Wegener's granulomatosis and the other MHC antigens that were examined, nor between polyarteritis nodosa and Churg-Strauss vasculitis and any antigen. Most recently, an increase in DQw7 has been found in both Wegener's granulomatosis and microscopic polyarteritis (Spencer et al., 1991); this increase was accompanied by all the linked DR alleles DR4, DR5 and DR6. There was a suggestion that DQw7, DR4 individuals were more likely to become ANCA negative; 50% of patients with a persistently positive ANCA were DR2$^+$.

A study of the immunogenetics of idiopathic crescentic glomerulonephritis also found an increased incidence of DR2 in patients versus controls (relative risk 3.54, $p < 0.01$; Müller et al., 1984). The incidence of MT3 (relative risk 3.33, $p < 0.025$) and the complement allotype BfF (relative risk 4.85, $p < 0.001$) were also increased; it is unclear whether any of these p values are corrected or not. The population studied was said to have 'immune complex mediated' crescentic glomerulonephritis. All had glomerular deposits of IgG and/or IgM, and conditions such as anti-glomerular basement membrane disease and lupus were excluded. This is the type of study that needs to be repeated now that ANCA is available to aid in the classification.

Other loci

At present, there is no information on this point.

Immunopathology

Animal studies

Unfortunately, there are no good animal models of the main entity considered in this chapter, namely crescentic glomerulonephritis with scanty immune deposits, with or without systemic vasculitis. Although there are many animal models that encompass both vasculitis and glomerulonephritis

(Christian & Sergent, 1976), these typically involve immune complex deposition (or reaction with planted antigens). Some of these models are considered further in Chapter 1 because of the insight they give into the pathogenesis of glomerulonephritis in general, but because of their dubious relevance will not be discussed further here. However, animal models have been helpful in the understanding of one of the more characteristic pathological features of this group of diseases, namely crescent formation.

Crescents can occur in a number of diseases with varying pathogenesis (see Table 8.2), and it therefore seems likely that there is a final common pathway leading to their formation. Although it was initially thought that the epithelial cell was the main cell contributing to the crescent, a number of lines of evidence now demonstrate that the macrophage is a key cell (for review see Atkins & Thomson, 1988). The main stimulus to macrophage migration is probably the presence of fibrin in Bowman's space. Any cause of damage to the glomerular basement membrane could allow exudation of fibrin, and this is the initial pathological event in experimental nephritis (Thomson et al., 1979). Because macrophages have procoagulant activity (Brentjens, 1987) there is the potential for a vicious circle to develop. Further confirmation of the important role of fibrin is provided by experimental defibrination with ancrod (Holdsworth et al., 1979). This abolishes crescent formation but does not affect glomerular inflammation (including accumulation of macrophages within the glomerulus). Although antibody-mediated experimental nephritis is the usual model of crescentic nephritis, it is also possible to produce crescents via a T cell-mediated response (Rennke, Klein & Mendrick, 1990; see also anti-GBM disease in chickens, Chapter 2).

Human studies

As with the animal models, the macrophage may be an important cell in crescent formation in human disease. Studies with monoclonal antibodies demonstrate that macrophages can account for about 35% of cells in cellular crescents, with polymorphs contributing 12% and epithelial cells 10%; the bulk of the remainder are probably fibroblasts (Hancock & Atkins, 1984). Further evidence for the extrinsic origin of crescent cells under some circumstances is provided by the development of crescentic nephritis in a graft from a female donor transplanted into a male recipient (Schiffer & Michael, 1978). Identification of male cells by Y body expression suggested that most of the cells in the crescent were of donor (extrinsic) origin. However, contrary evidence has also been obtained, demonstrating an absence of macrophage/monocyte staining in crescents (Yoshioka et al., 1987). One possible explanation for these discrepancies is that the major source of the cellular component depends on the integrity of Bowman's capsule: in one study when this was ruptured macrophages were indeed the predominant cell, but when the capsule was intact, epithelial cells made up the bulk of the crescent (Boucher *et al.*, 1987).

Although the mediation of glomerular damage in these diseases is understood to some extent by analogy with the animal models, little is known of the factors involved in precipitating disease. A preceding viral illness is often noted and this, together with a seasonal variation in incidence, suggests an infective trigger (Falk *et al.*, 1990*a*). Certainly, infective episodes are clearly documented as causing relapses of these diseases (Pinching *et al.*, 1983). In a small number of cases, certain drugs with known immunomodulatory properties (penicillamine, hydralazine) have precipitated a crescentic nephritis (Devogelaer *et al.*, 1987; Mason & Lockwood, 1986). The involvement of the immune system in pathogenesis has long been suspected on indirect grounds, such as the presence of elements of the cellular immune system within lesions and the response to immunosuppressive treatment. The discovery of an autoantibody system directly linked with these diseases has therefore led to a renewed interest in the immunopathology of these disorders.

Anti-neutrophil cytoplasm antibodies (ANCA)

ANCA were first described (although there are hints in the older literature; Yust, Schwartz & Dreyfuss, 1969) in cases of acute necrotising glomerulonephritis and thought to be related to an arbovirus infection (Davies *et al.*, 1982). Subsequently ANCA were found in a subgroup of patients with vasculitis and glomerulonephritis (Hall *et al.*, 1984), and then, in the publication that attracted the most attention, the striking association with Wegener's granulomatosis was reported (van der Woude *et al.*, 1985). The initial detection of ANCA used indirect immunofluorescence (IIF): serum from the patient is layered onto neutrophils fixed to a slide, and bound antibody subsequently detected with a fluorescinated anti-immunoglobulin reagent. At present, two main types are defined by IIF: a granular cytoplasmic staining pattern found on neutrophils and some monocytes (cytoplasmic ANCA, cANCA) and a perinuclear pattern (pANCA) (van der Woude, Daha & van Es, 1989). A number of groups have developed solid phase immunoassays (for review see van der Woude, Daha & van Es, 1989) using neutrophil extracts or purified antigens; these are currently being standardised.

Clinical correlates

The initial association with Wegener's granulomatosis has been confirmed by several groups (for review see van der Woude, Daha & van Es, 1989), and a retrospective analysis of 379 sera has demonstrated that cANCA have a positive predictive value of 89% for the diagnosis of Wegener's granulomatosis (van der Woude, Daha & van Es, 1989). Another study found a specificity of 99% and a sensitivity of 96% for the diagnosis of active Wegener's granulomatosis (Nölle *et al.*, 1989). This may be somewhat lower in subacute (D'Cruz *et al.*, 1989) or localised disease (Nölle *et al.*, 1989). ANCA are also found in microscopic polyarteritis: one study, using a radioimmunoassay with the appropriate controls for non-specific binding, found a sensitivity of 96% and a specificity of 97% for the diagnosis of systemic vasculitis (Wegener's granulomatosis and microscopic polyarteritis combined) (Savage *et al.*, 1987). In necrotising glomerulonephritis, ANCA are found in a similar proportion of cases whether there is an associated systemic vasculitis or not (Falk & Jennette, 1988; Cohen Tervaert *et al.*, 1990a). To summarise the types of ANCA found in these three conditions, results from a number of sources (Proceedings of the 2nd International Workshop on Antineutrophil Cytoplasmic Antibodies (ANCA), 1990; Jennette & Falk, 1990) suggest that over 90% of patients with Wegener's granulomatosis have cANCA, with only a small fraction having pANCA. Approximately half the patients with polyarteritis will have cANCA, and half pANCA. In idiopathic crescentic glomerulonephritis most patients have pANCA.

In addition to these main categories of ANCA-associated diseases, more limited data is available on a variety of other conditions. The autoantibodies have been found in Kawasaki disease (Savage *et al.*, 1989), Churg–Strauss syndrome (Wathen & Harrison, 1987; Cohen Tervaert, Elema & Kallenberg, 1990) and hepatitis B-associated polyarteritis nodosa (Guillevin *et al.*, 1990). Takayasu's disease does not seem to be associated with ANCA, but antibodies to other neutrophil components may be present (Lai *et al.*, 1990). IgA antibodies that react with neutrophils in a pattern distinct from both cANCA and pANCA have been described in Henoch–Schönlein purpura (van der Wall Bake *et al.*, 1987). The relationship of the granulocyte-specific anti-nuclear antibodies found in patients with rheumatoid arthritis (Wiik, Jensen & Friis, 1974) to pANCA is at present unclear. This is a rapidly developing field and no doubt further associations will be described.

As well as their use in diagnosis, ANCA are also useful in an individual patient as an index of disease activity. The original report of the occurrence of ANCA in Wegener's granulomatosis noted a correlation with disease activity (van der Woude *et al.*, 1985); this finding has subsequently been extended and confirmed (Jayne *et al.*, 1990a; Nölle *et al.*, 1989). Although some patients in remission have a stable raised ANCA titre, a clinical relapse is almost invariably preceded by a rise in ANCA titre (Cohen Tervaert *et al.*, 1989; Jayne *et al.*, 1990a). The converse is not true, in that a rise in titre does not always predict a relapse (Jayne *et al.*, 1990a; Cohen

Tervaert *et al.*, 1990*b*). However, the association of a rising ANCA titre with relapse is sufficiently close to allow pre-emptive reintroduction or intensification of immunosuppression (Cohen Tervaert *et al.*, 1990*b*). This study showed that such a strategy prevented clinical relapses and in addition led to lower cumulative doses of immunosuppressant drugs in the group randomised to receive pre-emptive treatment following a rise in ANCA titre as compared to the group left untreated until a relapse actually occurred.

Properties of ANCA

These can be considered in terms of the class and subclass of antibody, the antigen specificity, and the functional effects of antibody binding.

The initial descriptions of ANCA were of IgG antibodies, and the vast majority of cases are confined to this class. An interesting subset, characterised clinically by pulmonary haemorrhage (often catastrophic) and a variable degree of glomerulonephritis, is defined by ANCA of IgM class (Jayne *et al.*, 1989). A few of these patients have demonstrated a class switch from IgM to IgG ANCA in association with the development of a more typical vasculitic illness (Jayne *et al.*, 1989). The occurrence of IgA ANCA in Henoch–Schönlein purpura has already been mentioned.

Studies on the IgG subclass distribution of ANCA have produced variable results. One group, using quantitative techniques, found ANCA in all subclasses, but with a preponderance in IgG3 and a deficit in IgG2 in acute sera which was reversed in remission sera (Jayne, Weetman & Lockwood, 1991*b*). Other work demonstrates ANCA mostly restricted to IgG1 and IgG4 (Brouwer *et al.*, 1991).

The antigenic targets are clearly different for cANCA and pANCA. The cANCA target is located within the primary (alpha, azurophilic) granules of neutrophils, and there is now general agreement that it is a 29 kD protein, at least under reducing conditions (Goldschmeding *et al.*, 1989*b*; Lüdemann, Utecht & Gross, 1990; Niles *et al.*, 1989; Goldschmeding *et al.*, 1989*c*; Wieslander, Rasmussen & Bygren, 1989). Protein(s) of approximately 40 kD are also recognised by cANCA under some conditions (Lüdemann, Utecht & Gross, 1990; Jones & Lockwood, 1990), as is a 91 kD glycoprotein isolated from sputum (Daha *et al.*, 1990). Interestingly, monoclonal antibodies raised against this 91 kD protein also recognise a 29 kD antigen in neutrophil extracts. The precise relationship between these various species remains to be established. Further characterisation of the main 29 kD antigen has shown sequence homology with the serine protease family (Lüdemann, Utecht & Gross, 1990; Niles *et al.*, 1989). This is supported by an identical substrate specificity for both the 29 kD antigen and proteinase 3 (Lüdemann, Utecht & Gross, 1990), a serine proteinase found in neutrophils (Kao *et al.*, 1988). Following some initial confusion due to variations in

reported N-terminal sequences, it now seems highly probable that the
cANCA antigen is indeed proteinase 3 (Gupta *et al.*, 1990). Interestingly,
proteinase 3, the cDNA for which has now been cloned and sequenced
(Campanelli *et al.*, 1990), is identical, or highly homologous, to myeloblastin, a protein involved in the growth and differentiation of myeloid cells
(Bories *et al.*, 1989).

There is good evidence that myeloperoxidase is a major pANCA antigen
(Falk & Jennette, 1988). The perinuclear staining pattern is an artefact of
the fixation process, during which myeloperoxidase migrates from the
primary granules to the nuclear membrane (Falk *et al.*, 1990c). It seems
probable that pANCA antigens are more heterogeneous than is the case for
cANCA, as antibodies to elastase and lactoferrin may also produce a
perinuclear pattern (Goldschmeding *et al.*, 1989a; Thompson & Lee, 1989;
Lesavre *et al.*, 1990).

One quite different antigenic target for ANCA is the antigen-binding
region of other antibodies in the form of idiotypic–antiidiotypic interactions.
Such antiidiotypic antibodies with specificity for ANCA are present in
pooled normal human immunoglobulin and in the remission sera of certain
patients that were previously ANCA positive (Rossi *et al.*, 1991). The
possible significance of such antiidiotypic antibodies in immunoregulation
and therapy is considered further below. Lastly, there is some evidence that
ANCA-positive sera can bind to glomerular antigens (Abbott *et al.*, 1989),
although whether this is mediated by ANCA or by separate antibodies is
unknown. The *in vivo* relevance of this observation is uncertain, given the
usual lack of immune deposits in the glomerulus in the ANCA-associated
diseases.

A number of preliminary studies have shown that binding of ANCA to
neutrophils or myeloperoxidase *in vitro* may have functional effects, usually
stimulatory (Lee, Adu & Thompson, 1990; Falk *et al.*, 1990d). The *in vivo*
significance of this is uncertain, but it may be significant that ultrastructural
studies do show small amounts of antigen on the cell surface (Csernok *et al.*,
1990).

Whether ANCA are pathogenic or not is considered in the final section of
this chapter.

Other antigen–antibody systems

An association between hepatitis B and macroscopic polyarteritis nodosa
has been known for some time (Trepo & Thivolet, 1970; Gocke *et al.*, 1970).
Hepatitis antigens are present in the vessel walls (Gocke *et al.*, 1970) and in
circulating immune complexes in this condition (Gupta & Kohler, 1984).
This is only indirect evidence for a pathogenic role; in particular, non-
specific trapping of circulating antigen at sites of inflammation may contrib-

ute to the vessel wall deposition. Many of these patients have been drug abusers, and other factors, such as amphetamines (Citron *et al.*, 1970), may be involved in pathogenesis. In any event, the renal lesion found in these patients has usually been of the ischaemic type associated with macroscopic polyarteritis nodosa, rather than a glomerulonephritis. Furthermore, although ANCA have been described, changes in ANCA status follow the clinical state of the vasculitis, whilst the hepatitis serology remains unchanged (Guillevin *et al.*, 1990), suggesting that the latter is not directly involved in pathogenesis. Hepatitis B is, however, associated with other types of glomerular lesion, such as membranous nephropathy (see Chapter 3).

Anti-endothelial cell antibodies, identified first in Kawasaki disease (Leung *et al.*, 1986), have also been found in adult systemic vasculitis (Brasile *et al.*, 1989; Baguley & Hughes, 1988; Frampton *et al.*, 1990). These antibodies are found less frequently than ANCA (in approximately 30% of ANCA positive sera) but do correlate similarly with disease activity (Frampton *et al.*, 1990). The antigens recognised by these antibodies are unknown.

Cellular immunity

The role of the cellular immune system in the pathogenesis of this group of diseases is even less clear than that of the humoral system (discussed below). T cells are presumably involved in helping the production of ANCA and other autoantibodies, as these often possess the characteristics of T cell-dependent antibodies (IgG class, high affinity). Evidence for a more direct involvement of T cells is at present scanty and indirect. It has been inferred that they (or other cellular components of the immune system) are probably important because of the usual lack of immune deposits in the glomeruli in these diseases; this may, of course, simply reflect our ignorance of other possible mechanisms. However, T cells are present within the glomeruli in crescentic glomerulonephritis (Stachura, Si & Whiteside, 1984; Nolasco *et al.*, 1987; although not all agree: Hooke *et al.*, 1984), as are polymorphs and macrophages (Hooke *et al.*, 1984). It would clearly be of great interest to determine the antigen specificity of such T cells, but this presents formidable technical problems. The small amount of work in this area has therefore used the much more readily accessible peripheral blood lymphocyte (PBL). One group has reported, in brief outline, impressive proliferation of PBLs to both the cANCA antigen from azurophilic granules and the 91 kD antigen isolated from sputum (Daha *et al.*, 1990). This proliferation was seen in all four patients reported and in none of the five healthy controls. Other data, presented in abstract form, have also demonstrated T cell proliferation to an alpha granule extract in three out of seven patients with Wegener's granulomatosis and in none of ten controls (Petersen *et al.*, 1991). All three responders had active disease, and two were ANCA positive; all four non-responders were ANCA negative. The author's own experience in 30 patients, using as antigen an acid extract of neutrophils known to contain both the pANCA and cANCA antigens, has been uniformly negative (unpublished observations). Difference in antigen preparation is one obvious explanation for this discrepancy, but there are other possibilities. Further indirect evidence for the role of T cells comes from the response to anti-T cell therapy (see below).

Other vasculitic syndromes

Certain diseases considered elsewhere in this volume (e.g. lupus, cryoglobulinaemia) may be associated with a vasculitis, but are not discussed further here.

As mentioned above, ANCA have been found in some other vasculitic syndromes, such as Kawasaki disease and Churg–Strauss syndrome. Kawasaki disease does not typically affect the kidneys but Churg–Strauss syndrome may produce a variety of renal manifestations. Originally described in 1951 (Churg & Strauss, 1951) this condition is characterised by a systemic vasculitis with eosinophilia, usually occurring on a background of asthma. A review of the literature up to the early 1980s suggested that renal involvement was infrequent and mild (Lanham et al., 1984). However, the experience of one centre has shown that renal involvement was present in over 80% of cases and that the common lesion was a focal proliferative nephritis, often with necrosis and/or crescent formation (Clutterbuck, Evans & Pusey, 1990). Although cases with mild renal involvement (serum creatinine < 200 μmol l^{-1}) did well when treated with corticosteroids alone, the more severe cases often did not respond and required more aggressive treatment with cytotoxic drugs and plasma exchange. This experience could not all be accounted for by referral bias, and it seems clear that Churg–Strauss syndrome can often be associated with a severe glomerulonephritis.

Takayasu's disease, which may be associated with atypical anti-neutrophil antibodies (Lai et al., 1990), can also cause a crescentic nephritis (Hellman et al., 1987). This renal lesion has also been found occasionally in certain other conditions with a vasculitic component such as relapsing polychondritis (Chang-Miller et al., 1987) and Behçet's disease (Donnelly, Jothy & Barré, 1989; Tietjen & Moore, 1990).

Therapeutic aspects

There is no doubt that the prognosis in this group of diseases has improved considerably. Early experience was very unfavourable, with approximately three-quarters of patients with idiopathic crescentic nephritis either dying or going onto dialysis (for review see Couser, 1988), a mortality rate of approximately 80% at 1 year in Wegener's granulomatosis (Walton, 1958), and a mortality rate of almost 90% at 5 years in untreated polyarteritis, both macroscopic and microscopic (Frohnert & Sheps, 1967; Leib, Restivo & Paulus, 1979). By contrast, recent series show survival rates, off dialysis, in the region of 60%–70% (Hind et al., 1983; Fauci et al., 1983; Savage et al., 1985; Bolton & Sturgill, 1989). No doubt, many non-specific factors have contributed to this improved prognosis, such as improvements in dialysis, better control of sepsis and so on, but it seems probable that a major contribution has come from advances in the use of immunosuppression.

There are many difficulties in assessing studies in this area. In general, there is a dearth of controlled data, and there is no doubt that some patients can improve spontaneously (Maxwell et al., 1979; Coward et al., 1986). Numbers are usually small and the patient population heterogeneous, often including patients with anti-glomerular basement membrane disease which is known to behave differently (Hind et al., 1983; and see Chapter 2). Further heterogeneity is introduced by differences in known prognostic variables. At one stage, the degree of crescentic involvement on biopsy appeared to be a good guide to outcome (Whitworth et al., 1976), but this is no longer the case (Hind et al., 1983; Heilman et al., 1987), perhaps due to changes in management. A better prognostic indicator is provided by the degree of renal impairment at presentation, judged either by serum creatinine (Parfrey et al., 1985; Heilman et al., 1987) or need for dialysis (Bolton & Sturgill, 1989). With the above caveats in mind, it is possible to draw some general conclusions concerning the efficacy of various forms of immunosuppression.

Although no controlled data are available, oral corticosteroids are widely used (intravenous pulse steroid therapy is considered separately below). It is generally accepted that these are of value in polyarteritis (Frohnert & Sheps, 1967; Leib, Restivo & Paulus, 1979; Balow, 1985), but of only marginal benefit when used alone in Wegener's granulomatosis (Balow, 1985). It has been stated that there is no evidence that oral steroids used alone are of benefit in idiopathic crescentic nephritis (Atkins & Thomson, 1988), but this needs re-evaluation in view of the probable relationship with microscopic polyarteritis. However, these considerations are of largely theoretical interest, as present practice almost universally employs cytotoxic drugs in addition to corticosteroids, usually in the form of azathioprine or cyclophosphamide. Again, there are no controlled data, but experience from a number of centres suggests that the addition of cytotoxic therapy, and in particular cyclophosphamide, has led to a considerable improvement in outcome (Fauci et al., 1979, 1983; Hind et al., 1983; Bruns et al., 1989). Cyclophosphamide is usually given orally, but it is possible that intravenous pulses (as advocated in lupus nephritis; see Chapter 4) may be as (or more) efficacious in some situations (Fort & Abruzzo, 1988; Falk *et al.*, 1990*b*). Further uncontrolled studies, however, have suggested that, although pulse cyclophosphamide is highly effective at inducing remission, it is not as effective as daily oral cyclophosphamide at producing a sustained remission (Hoffman *et al.*, 1990 and discussed further in Cupps, 1990).

The main modalities of treatment being considered as additions to the basic therapy outlined above are plasma exchange and pulse methylprednisolone. There have been controlled attempts to evaluate additional plasma exchange. Preliminary results from one trial suggested that this was of benefit (Rifle *et al.*, 1981) and this has been confirmed by a more recent trial (Pusey *et al.*, 1991). This latter study showed that patients who were not dialysis dependent at entry did very well whether they received plasma exchange or not (28 out of 29 improved). In dialysis-dependent patients, ten out of eleven treated with additional plasma exchange improved, compared to three out of eight given steroids and cytotoxic drugs alone ($p < 0.04$). In contrast to these reports, another trial failed to show benefit (Glöckner *et al.*, 1988). However, this latter trial suffered from many of the problems mentioned at the beginning of this section, namely small numbers, heterogeneous diseases, and variable degrees of renal impairment in the study groups (e.g. the plasma exchange group had more dialysis-dependent patients). It is therefore difficult to assess the significance of the findings. The balance of the evidence at present, therefore, favours the additional use of plasma exchange in patients with severe renal impairment.

Pulse methylprednisolone has not been evaluated in the same way, but appears to give results comparable to those obtained with plasma exchange: compare 63% coming off dialysis with plasma exchange (Hind *et al.*, 1983) versus 70% with methylprednisolone (Bolton & Sturgill, 1989). A more direct comparison of the two modalities also suggested that they were of roughly equivalent benefit (Stevens, McConnell & Bone, 1983). Because pulse methylprednisolone, as compared to plasma exchange, is cheap, safe and probably as effective, it has been suggested by some authorities that this is the treatment of choice (Couser, 1988).

Turning now to less mainstream forms of therapy, the role of infection in triggering relapses (Pinching *et al.*, 1980) has already been mentioned. It is therefore of particular interest that antimicrobial therapy alone, usually with cotrimoxazole, has been found to be capable of inducing a remission in limited Wegener's granulomatosis (Deremee, 1989), although the anecdotal nature of the evidence has led to some criticism (Leavitt, Hoffman & Fauci, 1989).

Because of the evidence implicating the coagulation system in the causation of glomerular damage (see Chapter 1), a number of groups have used heparin and/or antiplatelet drugs, usually in combination with other forms of therapy (Atkins & Thomson, 1988). It is therefore difficult to evaluate the efficacy of anticoagulation or antiplatelet agents; however, they are not part of most current therapeutic regimes. There is, however, a possible connection with plasma exchange, as this is quite efficient at depleting fibrinogen; it has been suggested that such defibrination is an important mode of action of plasma exchange in this context (d'Apice & Kincaid-Smith, 1979, and ensuing discussion).

In an even smaller number of cases, the predominantly anti-T cell agent cyclosporin A has been used successfully, in some cases for disease which has failed to respond to cyclophosphamide (Schollmeyer & Grotz, 1990). One patient with a rather atypical form of systemic vasculitis resistant to more conventional therapy has been successfully treated with a combination of monoclonal antibodies directed at, amongst others, T cell antigens (Mathieson et al., 1990).

The occurrence of antiidiotypic antibodies with specificity for ANCA in pooled normal human immunoglobulin (IVIG; see above) has encouraged the therapeutic use of IVIG. Such treatment is certainly capable of producing a sustained fall in ANCA titres, and in some cases a clinical remission, although this may be short-lived (Jayne et al., 1991a). Whether the fall in ANCA titre causes the remission is unclear; IVIG has many other potential effects on the immune system.

All of the therapeutic options considered so far have been concerned with initial treatment, or 'induction' therapy. Relapses are frequent in this group of diseases (Fauci et al., 1983; Savage et al., 1985), in contrast to anti-glomerular basement membrane disease, in which relapses are rare (see Chapter 2), and 'maintenance' therapy is therefore a major consideration. The optimum form of such therapy is unclear, but it seems increasingly likely that serial estimations of ANCA titre will allow whatever form of maintenance treatment is chosen to be adjusted on an individual basis (Cohen Tervaert et al., 1990b). This should hopefully minimise the side effects commonly found in patients on long-term treatment with steroids and/or cyclophosphamide.

Concluding remarks

The classification of vasculitic syndromes and crescentic nephritis has at times been rather confusing (Falk, 1990). The measurement of anti-glomerular basement membrane antibodies and ANCA now allow most cases of crescentic nephritis to be divided into (reflected in Table 8.2) 1) anti-glomerular basement membrane disease; 2) ANCA-positive disease (Wegener's granulomatosis, microscopic polyarteritis, crescentic nephritis with few immune deposits; 3) a crescentic process superimposed on another pre-existing renal lesion (triggered, for example, by damage sufficient to cause breaches in the glomerular basement membrane and exudation of fibrin); 4) truly idiopathic crescentic glomerulonephritis (with or without immune deposits). No doubt this last category will include some cases of small vessel vasculitis, or renal vasculitis, which are ANCA negative, but further work is required on this point. Our own experience suggests that this last form of crescentic nephritis is very uncommon (one or two possible examples out of approximately 60 cases of glomerulonephritis associated with extracapillary proliferation seen over the last 3–4 years). Whether the rare cases of crescentic nephritis found in association with other vasculitic syndromes, such as relapsing polychondritis, are associated with ANCA is unknown.

The reasons for thinking that Wegener's granulomatosis, microscopic polyarteritis and crescentic nephritis with few immune deposits are closely related conditions were briefly mentioned at the beginning of this chapter. It is perhaps ironic that ANCA, having helped to lump these conditions together (Falk & Jennette, 1988; Jennette, Wilkman & Falk, 1989), is now helping to split them again on the basis of different antigenic targets.

Although ANCA have had a major impact on the diagnosis and classification of this group of diseases, it is still far from clear what role, if any, they play in pathogenesis. Such evidence as there is for the pathogenicity of ANCA is indirect. The antibodies are present at the site of tissue damage, as shown by their elution from post mortem kidney (Jayne et al., 1989); it is, however, difficult to generalise this finding given the usual paucity of immune deposits in the glomeruli in these diseases. The link between different immunoglobulin classes of ANCA and particular clinical syndromes is suggestive of a more fundamental role than their presence as a mere epiphenomenon, as are the functional effects that ANCA may have, at least in vitro. Clinical remissions induced by infusion of pooled immunoglobulin with ANCA-specific antiidiotypic activity may reflect inhibition of pathogenic autoantibody, although a number of other mechanisms are also possible. The often close relationship between ANCA titre and disease activity, and in particular the temporal association between rising titres and clinical relapse, is consistent with a role in pathogenesis. On the other hand, some patients in remission continue to have high titres on a long-term basis, so, even if ANCA are implicated, other factors must be involved. Direct attempts to test the pathogenicity of ANCA are hampered by the restricted phylogenetic distribution of some of the target antigens, which, at least in the case of proteinase 3, appears confined to primates (Lockwood, personal communication). One experiment that infused ANCA into baboons produced a transient neutropaenia but no evidence of vasculitis or glomerulonephritis (Lockwood, personal communication).

In addition to these empirical observations, hypotheses have been proposed as to possible mechanisms of ANCA pathogenesis. The anti-
endothelial cell antibodies found in Kawasaki disease are cytolytic, and it
has been proposed that cytokines from monocytes lead to induction of the
target antigens for such antibodies with resultant endothelial damage
(Leung *et al.*, 1989). As ANCA bind to monocytes and may stimulate them
to release cytokines, and as anti-endothelial cell antibodies are also found in
systemic vasculitis, a similar mechanism may be operating (Jayne & Lockwood, 1990*b*). Another hypothesis suggests that genetically predisposed
individuals make a cellular and humoral immune response to neutrophil
lysosomal enzymes released following infection (van der Woude, Daha &
van Es, 1989). The activated T cells may then contribute to granuloma
formation, whilst ANCA, by causing granulocyte lysis or activation, lead to
the release of more neutrophil enzymes with resulting tissue damage. It is
also possible that ANCA may form immune complexes with proteinases
which are then transported to the kidney where they may cause further
damage. These ideas are clearly speculative, but should serve as a further
stimulus to research in an area which will undoubtedly see much activity
over the next few years.

References

Abbott, F., Jones, S. J., Lockwood, C. M. & Rees, A. J. (1989). Autoantibodies to glomerular
  antigens in patients with Wegener's granulomatosis. *Nephrology Dialysis and Transplantation*, **4**, 1–8.
Andrews, M., Edmunds, M., Campbell, A., Walls, J. & Feehally, J. (1990). Systemic vasculitis
  in the 1980s – Is there an increasing incidence of Wegener's granulomatosis and microscopic
  polyarteritis? *Journal of the Royal College of Physicians of London*, **24**, 284–8.
Antonovych, T. T., Sabnis, S. G., Tuur, S. M., Sesterhenn, I. A. & Balow, J. E. (1989).
  Morphologic differences between polyarteritis and Wegener's granulomatosis using light,
  electron and immunohistochemical techniques. *Modern Pathology*, **2**, 349–59.
Atkins, R. C. & Thomson, N. M. (1988). Rapidly progressive glomerulonephritis. In *Diseases
  of the Kidney*, 4th edn, ed. R. W. Schrier & C. W. Gottschalk, pp. 1903–27. Boston/Toronto:
  Little, Brown and Company.
Baguley, E. & Hughes, G. R. V. (1988). Lytic IgG anti-endothelial cell antibodies in vasculitis.
  Lancet, **ii**, 907.
Balow, J. E. (1985). Renal vasculitis. *Kidney International*, **27**, 954–64.
Balow, J. E. & Fauci, A. S. (1988). Vasculitic diseases of the kidney: polyarteritis nodosa,
  Wegener's granulomatosis, allergic angiitis and granulomatosis, and other disorders. In
  Diseases of the Kidney, 4th edn, ed. R. W. Schrier & C. W. Gottschalk, pp. 2335–60. Boston/
  Toronto: Little, Brown and Company.
Bolton, W. K. & Sturgill, B. C. (1989). Methylprednisolone therapy for acute crescentic
  rapidly progressive glomerulonephritis. *American Journal of Nephrology*, **9**, 368–75.
Bories, D., Raynal, M-C., Solomon, D. H., Darzynkiewicz, Z. & Cayre, Y. E. (1989). Down-
  regulation of a serine protease, myeloblastin, causes growth arrest and differentiation of
  promyelocytic leukaemia cells. *Cell*, **59**, 959–68.

Boucher, A., Droz, D., Adafer, E. & Noel, L. H. (1987). Relationship between the integrity of Bowman's capsule and the composition of cellular crescents in human crescentic glomerulonephritis. *Laboratory Investigation*, **56**, 526–33.

Brasile, L., Kremer, J. M., Clarke, J. L. & Cerilli, J. (1989). Identification of an autoantibody to vascular endothelial cell-specific antigens in patients with systemic vasculitis. *American Journal of Medicine*, **87**, 74–80.

Brentjens, J. R. (1987). Glomerular procoagulant activity and glomerulonephritis. *Laboratory Investigation*, **57**, 107–11.

Brouwer, E., Cohen Tervaert, J. W., Horst, G. *et al.* (1991). Predominance of IgG1 and IgG4 subclasses of anti-neutrophil cytoplasmic autoantibodies (ANCA) in patients with Wegener's granulomatosis and clinically related disorders. *Clinical and Experimental Immunology*, **83**, 379–86.

Bruns, F. J., Adler, S., Fraley, D. S. & Segel, D. P. (1989). Long-term follow-up of aggressively treated idiopathic rapidly progressive glomerulonephritis. *American Journal of Medicine*, **86**, 400–6.

Campanelli, D., Melchior, M., Fu, Y. *et al.* (1990). Cloning of cDNA for proteinase 3: a serine protease, antibiotic and autoantigen from human neutrophils. *Journal of Experimental Medicine*, **172**, 1709–15.

Carrington, C. B. & Liebow, A. A. (1966). Limited forms of angiitis and granulomatosis of Wegener's type. *American Journal of Medicine*, **41**, 497–527.

Chang-Miller, A., Okamura, M., Torres, V. E. *et al.* (1987). Renal involvement in relapsing polychondritis. *Medicine*, **66**, 202–17.

Christian, C. L. & Sergent, J. S. (1976). Vasculitis syndromes: clinical and experimental models. *American Journal of Medicine*, **61**, 385–92.

Churg, J. & Strauss, L. (1951). Allergic granulomatosis, allergic angiitis and periarteritis nodosa. *American Journal of Pathology*, **27**, 277–301.

Citron, B. P., Halpern, M., McCarron, M. *et al.* (1970). Necrotizing angiitis associated with drug abuse. *New England Journal of Medicine*, **283**, 1003–11.

Clutterbuck, E. J., Evans, D. J. & Pusey, C. D. (1990). Renal involvement in Churg–Strauss syndrome. *Nephrology Dialysis and Transplantation*, **5**, 161–7.

Cohen Tervaert, J. W., Elema, J. D. & Kallenberg, C. G. M. (1990). Clinical and histopathological association of 29 kD-ANCA and MPO-ANCA. *APMIS*, **98** (suppl. 19), 35.

Cohen Tervaert, J. W., van der Woude, F. J., Fauci, A. S. *et al.* (1989). Association between active Wegener's granulomatosis and anticytoplasmic antibodies. *Archives of Internal Medicine*, **149**, 2461–5.

Cohen Tervaert, J. W., Goldschmeding, R., Elema, J. D. *et al.* (1990a). Autoantibodies against myeloid lysosomal enzymes in crescentic glomerulonephritis. *Kidney International*, **37**, 799–806.

Cohen Tervaert, J. W., Huitema, M. G., Hené, R. J. *et al.* (1990b). Prevention of relapses in Wegener's granulomatosis by treatment based on antineutrophil cytoplasmic antibody titre. *Lancet*, **ii**, 709–11.

Couser, W. G. (1988). Rapidly progressive glomerulonephritis: classification, pathogenetic mechanisms, and therapy. *American Journal of Kidney Disease*, **11**, 449–64.

Coward, R. A., Hamdy, N. A. T., Shortland, J. S. & Brown, C. B. (1986). Renal micropolyarteritis: a treatable condition. *Nephrology Dialysis and Transplantation*, **1**, 31–7.

Csernok, E., Ludemann, J., Gross, W. L. & Bainton, D. F. (1990). Ultrastructural localisation of proteinase 3, the target antigen of anti-cytoplasmic antibodies circulating in Wegener's granulomatosis. *American Journal of Pathology*, **137**, 1113–20.

Cupps, T. R. (1990). Cyclophosphamide: to pulse or not to pulse? *American Journal of Medicine*, **89**, 399–402.

d'Apice, A. J. F. & Kincaid-Smith, P. (1979). Plasma exchange in the treatment of glomerulo-nephritis. In *Progress in Glomerulonephritis*, ed. P. Kincaid-Smith, A. J. F. d'Apice & R. C. Atkins, pp. 371–84. New York: Wiley Medical.

D'Cruz, D. P., Baguley, E., Asherson, R. A. & Hughes, G. R. V. (1989). Ear, nose, and throat symptoms in subacute Wegener's granulomatosis. *British Medical Journal*, **299**, 419–22.

Daha, M. R., Leusen, J., Kramps, J. A., Schrama, E., van Es, L. A. & van der Woude, F. J. (1990). Isolation from purulent sputum of an antigen reactive with antibodies in serum of patients with Wegener's granulomatosis. *Netherlands Journal of Medicine*, **36**, 117–20.

Davies, D. J., Moran, J. E., Niall, J. F. & Ryan, G. B. (1982). Segmental necrotizing glomerulonephritis with antineutrophil antibody: possible arbovirus aetiology? *British Medical Journal*, **285**, 606–9.

Davson, J., Ball, J. & Platt, R. (1948). The kidney in periarteritis nodosa. *Quarterly Journal of Medicine*, **17**, 175–202.

Deremee, R. A., McDonald, T. J., Harrison, E. G. Jr. & Coles, D. T. (1976). Wegener's granulomatosis. Anatomic correlates, a proposed classification. *Mayo Clinic Proceedings*, **51**, 777–81.

Deremee, R. A. (1989). The treatment of Wegener's granulomatosis with trimethoprim/sulfamethoxazole: illusion or vision? *Arthritis and Rheumatism*, **31**, 1068–73.

Devogelaer, J. P., Pirson, Y., Vandenbroucke, J. M., Cosyns, J. P., Brichard, S. & Nagant de Deuxchaisnes, C. (1987). D-penicillamine induced crescentic glomerulonephritis: report and review of the literature. *Journal of Rheumatology*, **14**, 1036–41.

Donnelly, S., Jothy, S. & Barré, P. (1989). Crescentic glomerulonephritis in Behçet's syndrome – results of therapy and review of the literature. *Clinical Nephrology*, **31**, 213–18.

Elkon, K. B., Sutherland, D. C., Rees, A. J., Hughes, G. R. V. & Batchelor, J. R. (1983). HLA antigen frequencies in systemic vasculitis: increase in HLA-DR2 in Wegener's granulomatosis. *Arthritis and Rheumatism*, **26**, 102–4.

Falk, R. J. & Jennette, J. C. (1988). Anti-neutrophil cytoplasmic autoantibodies with specificity for myeloperoxidase in patients with systemic vasculitis and idiopathic necrotizing and crescentic glomerulonephritis. *New England Journal of Medicine*, **318**, 1651–7.

Falk, R. J., Hogan, S. L., Jennette, J. C. & NC Glomerular Disease Collaborative Network (1990a). A prospective cohort study of 70 patients with anti-neutrophil cytoplasmic antibody (ANCA)-associated glomerulonephritis (GN). *Kidney International*, **37**, 256.(Abstract).

Falk, R. J., Hogan, S., Carey, T. S. & Jennette, J. C. (1990b). Clinical course of anti-neutrophil cytoplasmic autoantibody-associated glomerulonephritis and systemic vasculitis. The Glomerular Disease Collaborative Network. *Annals of Internal Medicine*, **113**, 656–63.

Falk, R. J., Hogan, S. L., Wilkman, A. S. et al. (1990c). Myeloperoxidase specific anti-neutrophil cytoplasmic autoantibodies (MPO-ANCA). *Netherlands Journal of Medicine*, **36**, 121–5.

Falk, R. J., Terrell, R. S., Charles, L. A. & Jennette, J. C. (1990d). Anti-neutrophil cytoplasmic autoantibodies induce neutrophils to degranulate and produce oxygen radicals *in vitro*. *Proceedings of the National Academy of Sciences, USA*, **87**, 4115–19.

Falk, R. J. (1990). ANCA-associated renal disease. *Kidney International*, **38**, 998–1010.

Fauci, A. S., Katz, P., Haynes, B. F. & Wolff, S. M. (1979). Cyclophosphamide therapy of severe systemic necrotizing vasculitis. *New England Journal of Medicine*, **301**, 235–8.

Fauci, A. S., Haynes, B. F., Katz, P. & Wolff, S. M. (1983). Wegener's granulomatosis: prospective clinical and therapeutic experience with 85 patients for 21 years. *Annals of Internal Medicine*, **98**, 76–85.

Fort, J. G. & Abruzzo, J. L. (1988). Reversal of progressive necrotizing vasculitis with intravenous pulse cyclophosphamide and methylprednisolone. *Arthritis and Rheumatism*, **31**, 1194–8.

Frampton, G., Jayne, D. R. W., Lockwood, C. M. & Cameron, J. S. (1990). Autoantibodies to endothelial cells and neutrophil cytoplasmic antigens in systemic vasculitis. *Clinical and Experimental Immunology*, **82**, 227–32.

Frohnert, P. P. & Sheps, S. G. (1967). Long-term follow-up study of periarteritis nodosa. *American Journal of Medicine*, **43**, 8–14.

Glöckner, W. M., Sieberth, H. G., Wichmann, H. E. *et al.* (1988). Plasma exchange and immunosuppression in rapidly progressive glomerluonephritis: a controlled, multi-center study. *Clinical Nephrology*, **29**, 1–8.

Gocke, D. J., Hsu, K., Morgan, C., Bombardieri, S., Lockshin, M. & Christian, C. L. (1970). Association between polyarteritis and Australia antigen. *Lancet*, **ii**, 1149–53.

Goldschmeding, R., Cohen Tervaert, J. W., van der Schoot, C. E., van der Veen, C., Kallenberg, C. G. M. & von dem Borne, A. E. G. Kr. (1989*a*). ANCA, anti-myeloperoxidase and anti-elastase: three members of a novel class of autoantibodies against myeloid lysosomal enzymes. *APMIS*, **97** suppl. 6, 48–9.

Goldschmeding, R., van der Schoot, C. E., ten Bokkel Huinink, D. *et al.* (1989*b*). Wegener's granulomatosis autoantibodies identify a novel diisopropylflurophosphate-binding protein in the lysosomes of normal human neutrophils. *Journal of Clinical Investigation*, **84**, 1577–87.

Goldschmeding, R., ten Bokkel Huinink, D., Faber, N. *et al.* (1989*c*). Identification of the 'ANCA-antigen' as a novel myeloid lysosomal serine protease. *APMIS*, **97** suppl. 6, 46.

Guillevin, L., Visser, H., Oksman, F. & Pourrat, J. (1990). Antineutrophil cytoplasmic antibodies in polyarteritis nodosa related to hepatitis B virus. *Arthritis and Rheumatism*, **33**, 1871–2.

Gupta, R. C. & Kohler, P. F. (1984). Identification of HBsAg determinants in immune complexes from hepatitis B virus-associated vasculitis. *Journal of Immunology*, **132**, 1223–8.

Gupta, S. K., Niles, J. L., McCluskey, R. T. & Arnaout, M. A. (1990). Identity of Wegener's autoantigen (p29) with proteinase 3 and myeloblastin. *Blood*, **76**, 2162.

Hall, J. B., Wadham, B. McN., Wood, C. J., Ashton, V. & Adam, W. R. (1984). Vasculitis and glomerulonephritis: a subgroup with an antineutrophil cytoplasmic antibody. *Australian and New Zealand Journal of Medicine*, **14**, 277–8.

Hancock, W. W. & Atkins, R. C. (1984). Cellular composition of crescents in human rapidly progressive glomerulonephritis identified using monoclonal antibodies. *American Journal of Nephrology*, **3**, 177–81.

Heilman, R. L., Offord, K. P., Holley, K. E. & Velosa, J. A. (1987). Analysis of risk factors for patient and renal survival in crescentic glomerulonephritis. *American Journal of Kidney Disease*, **9**, 98–107.

Hellman, D. B., Hardy, K., Lindenfield, S. & Ring, E. (1987). Takayasu's arteritis associated with crescentic glomerulonephritis. *Arthritis and Rheumatism*, **30**, 451–4.

Hind, C. R. K., Paraskevakou, H., Lockwood, C. M., Evans, D. J., Peters, D. K. & Rees, A. J. (1983). Prognosis after immunosuppression of patients with crescentic nephritis requiring dialysis. *Lancet*, **i**, 263–5.

Hoffman, G. S., Leavitt, R. Y., Fleisher, T. A., Minor, J. R. & Fauci, A. S. (1990). Treatment of Wegener's granulomatosis with intermittent high-dose intravenous cyclophosphamide. *American Journal of Medicine*, **89**, 403–10.

Holdsworth, S. R., Thomson, N. M., Glasgow, E. F. & Atkins, R. C. (1979). The effect of defibrination on macrophage participation in rabbit nephrotoxic nephritis. *Clinical and Experimental Immunology*, **37**, 38–43.

Hooke, D. H., Hancock, W. W., Gee, D. C., Kraft, N. & Atkins, R. C. (1984). Monoclonal antibody analysis of glomerular hypercellularity in human glomerulonephritis. *Clinical Nephrology*, **22**, 163–8.

Hunder, G. G., Arend, W. P., Bloch, D. A. *et al.* (1990). The American College of Rheumatology 1990 criteria for the classification of vasculitis. Introduction. *Arthritis and Rheumatism*, **33**, 1065–7.

Jayne, D. R. W., Jones, S. J., Severn, A., Shaunak, S., Murphy, J. & Lockwood, C. M. (1989). Severe pulmonary hemorrhage and systemic vasculitis in association with circulating anti-neutrophil cytoplasm antibodies of IgM class only. *Clinical Nephrology*, **32**, 101–6.

Jayne, D. R. W., Heaton, A., Evans, D. B. & Lockwood, C. M. (1990a). Sequential anti-neutrophil cytoplasm antibody titres in the management of systemic vasculitis. *Nephrology Dialysis and Transplantation*, **4**, 309.(Abstract).

Jayne, D. R. W. & Lockwood, C. M. (1990b). Pathogenesis of acute Kawasaki disease (letter). *Lancet*, **335**, 410–11.

Jayne, D. R. W., Black, C. M., Davies, M., Fox, C. & Lockwood, C. M. (1991a). Treatment of systemic vasculitis with pooled intravenous immunoglobulin. *Lancet*, **337**, 1137–9.

Jayne, D. R. W., Weetman, A. P. & Lockwood, C. M. (1991b). IgG subclass distribution of autoantibodies to neutrophil cytoplasmic antigens in systemic vasculitis. *Clinical and Experimental Immunology*, **84**, 476–81.

Jennette, J. C. & Falk, R. J. (1990). Antineutrophil cytoplasmic autoantibodies and associated diseases: a review. *American Journal of Kidney Disease*, **15**, 517–29.

Jennette, J. C., Wilkman, A. S. & Falk, R. J. (1989). Anti-neutrophil cytoplasmic autoantibody-associated glomerulonephritis and vasculitis. *American Journal of Pathology*, **135**, 921–30.

Jones, S. J. & Lockwood, C. M. (1990). Characterisation of autoantigens in systemic vasculitis. *Kidney International*, **37**, 441.(Abstract).

Kao, R. C., Wehner, N. G., Skubitz, K. M., Gray, B. H. & Hoidal, J. R. (1988). Proteinase 3. A distinct human polymorphonuclear leukocyte proteinase that produces emphysema in hamsters. *Journal of Clinical Investigation*, **82**, 1963–73.

Katz, P., Alling, D. W., Haynes, B. F. & Fauci, A. S. (1979). Association of Wegener's granulomatosis with HLA-B8. *Clinical Immunology and Immunopathology*, **14**, 268–72.

Lai, K. N., Jayne, D. R. W., Brownlee, A. & Lockwood, C. M. (1990). The specificity of anti-neutrophil cytoplasm autoantibodies in systemic vasculitides. *Clinical and Experimental Immunology*, **82**, 233–7.

Lanham, J. G., Elkon, K. B., Pusey, C. D. & Hughes, G. R. (1984). Systemic vasculitis with asthma and eosinophilia: a clinical approach to the Churg–Strauss syndrome. *Medicine*, **63**, 65–81.

Leavitt, R. Y., Hoffman, G. S. & Fauci, A. S. (1989). Response: the role of trimethoprim/sulfamethoxazole in the treatment of Wegener's granulomatosis. *Arthritis and Rheumatism*, **31**, 1073–4.

Lee, S. S., Adu, D. & Thompson, R. A. (1990). Anti-myeloperoxidase antibodies in systemic vasculitis. *Clinical and Experimental Immunology*, **79**, 41–6.

Leib, E. S., Restivo, C. & Paulus, H. E. (1979). Immunosuppressive and corticosteroid therapy of polyarteritis nodosa. *American Journal of Medicine*, **67**, 941–5.

Lesavre, P., Chen, N., Nusbaum, P., Mecarelli, L. & Noël, L-H. (1990). Antineutrophil cytoplasm antibodies (ANCA) with antilactoferrin activity in vasculitis. *Kidney International*, **37**, 442.(Abstract).

Leung, D. Y. M., Collins, T., Lapierre, L. A., Geha, R. S. & Pober, J. S. (1986). Immunoglobulin M antibodies present in the acute phase of Kawasaki syndrome lyse cultured vascular endothelial cells stimulated with gamma interferon. *Journal of Clinical Investigation*, **77**, 1428–35.

Leung, D. Y. M., Cotran, R. S., Kurt-Jones, E., Burns, J. C., Newburger, J. W. & Pober, J. S. (1989). Endothelial cell activation and high interleukin-1 secretion in the pathogenesis of acute Kawasaki disease. *Lancet*, **i**, 1298–302.

Lüdemann, J., Utecht, B. & Gross, W. L. (1990). Anti-neutrophil cytoplasm antibodies in Wegener's granulomatosis recognise an elastinolytic enzyme. *Journal of Experimental Medicine*, **171**, 357–62.

Mason, P. D. & Lockwood, C. M. (1986). Rapidly progressive nephritis in patients taking hydralazine. *Journal of Clinical and Laboratory Immunology*, **20**, 151–3.

Mathieson, P. W., Cobbold, S. P., Hale, G. *et al.* (1990). Monoclonal antibody therapy in systemic vasculitis. *New England Journal of Medicine*, **323**, 250–4.

Maxwell, D. R., Ozawa, T., Nielsen, R. L. & Luft, F. C. (1979). Spontaneous recovery from rapidly progressive glomerulonephritis. *British Medical Journal*, **II**, 643.

Müller, G. A., Gebhardt, M., Kömpf, J., Baldwin, W. M., Ziegenhagen, D. & Bohle, A. (1984). Association between rapidly progressive glomerulonephritis and the properdin factor BfF and different HLA-D region products. *Kidney International*, **25**, 115–18.

Niles, J. L., McCluskey, R. T., Ahmed, M. F. & Arnaout, M. A. (1989). Wegener's granulomatosis autoantigen is a novel neutrophil serine proteinase. *Blood*, **74**, 1888–93.

Nolasco, F. E. B., Cameron, J. S., Hartley, B., Coelho, A., Hildreth, G. & Reuben, R. (1987). Intraglomerular T cells and monocytes in nephritis: study with monoclonal antibodies. *Kidney International*, **31**, 1160–6.

Nölle, B., Specks, U., Lüdemann, J., Rohrbach, M. S., Deremee, R. A. & Gross, W. L. (1989). Anticytoplasmic autoantibodies: their immunodiagnostic value in Wegener Granulomatosis. *Annals of Internal Medicine*, **111**, 28–40.

Parfrey, P. S., Hutchinson, T. A., Jothy, S. *et al.* (1985). The spectrum of diseases associated with necrotizing glomerulonephritis and its prognosis. *American Journal of Kidney Disease*, **6**, 387–96.

Petersen, J., Rasmussen, N., Szpirt, W., Hermann, E. & Mayet, W. (1991). T lymphocyte proliferation to neutrophil cytoplasmic antigen(s) in Wegener's granulomatosis (WG). *American Journal of Kidney Disease* (in press).

Pinching, A. J., Rees, A. J., Pussell, B. A., Lockwood, C. M., Mitchison, R. S. & Peters, D. K. (1980). Relapses in Wegener's granulomatosis: the role of infection. *British Medical Journal*, **281**, 836–8.

Pinching, A. J., Lockwood, C. M., Pussell, B. A. *et al.* (1983). Wegener's granulomatosis: observations on 18 patients with severe renal disease. *Quarterly Journal of Medicine*, **52**, 435–60.

Proceedings of the 2nd International Workshop on Antineutrophil Cytoplasmic Antibodies (ANCA) (1990). *Netherlands Journal of Medicine*, **36**, 87–175.

Pusey, C. D., Rees, A. J., Evans, D. J., Peters, D. K. & Lockwood, C. M. (1991). A randomised controlled trial of plasma exchange in rapidly progressive glomerulonephritis without anti-GBM antibodies. *Kidney International* (in press).

Rasmussen, N., Borregaard, N. & Wiik, A. (1987). Anti-neutrophil-cytoplasm antibodies in Wegener's granulomatosis are not directed against alkaline phosphatase. *Lancet*, **i**, 1488.

Rennke, H. G., Klein, P. S. & Mendrick, D. L. (1990). Cell-mediated immunity (CMI) in hapten-induced interstitial nephritis and glomerular crescent formation in the rat. *Kidney International*, **37**, 428.(Abstract).

Rifle, G., Chalopin, J. M., Zech, P. *et al.* (1981). Treatment of idiopathic acute crescentic glomerulonephritis by immunodepression and plasma-exchanges. A prospective randomised study. *Proceedings of the European Dialysis and Transplantation Association*, **18**, 493–502.

Rossi, F., Jayne, D. R. W., Lockwood, C. M. & Kazatchkine, M. D. (1991). Anti-idiotypes against anti-neutrophil cytoplasmic antigen autoantibodies in normal human polyspecific IgG for therapeutic use and in the remission sera of patients with systemic vasculitis. *Clinical and Experimental Immunology*, **83**, 298–303.

Savage, C. O. S., Winearls, C. J., Evans, D. J., Rees, A. J. & Lockwood, C. M. (1985). Microscopic polyarteritis: presentation, pathology and prognosis. *Quarterly Journal of Medicine*, **56**, 467–83.

Savage, C. O. S., Winearls, C. G., Jones, S., Marshall, P. D. & Lockwood, C. M. (1987). Prospective study of radioimmunoassay for antibodies against neutrophil cytoplasm in diagnosis of systemic vasculitis. *Lancet*, **i**, 1389–93.

Savage, C. O. S., Tizard, J., Jayne, D. R. W., Lockwood, C. M. & Dillon, M. J. (1989). Antineutrophil cytoplasm antibodies in Kawasaki disease. *Archives of Disease in Childhood*, **64**, 360–3.

Schiffer, M. S. & Michael, A. F. (1978). Renal cell turnover studied by Y chromosome (Y body) staining of the transplanted human kidney. *Journal of Laboratory and Clinical Medicine*, **92**, 841–8.

Schollmeyer, P. & Grotz, W. (1990). Ciclosporin in the treatment of Wegener's granulomatosis and related diseases. *APMIS*, **98** (Suppl. 19), 54–5.

Spencer, S. J., Burns, A., Gaskin, G., Pusey, C. D. & Rees, A. J. (1991). Influence of HLA class II genes on susceptibility to vasculitis. *Nephrology Dialysis and Transplantation* (in press).

Stachura, I., Si, L. & Whiteside, T. L. (1984). Mononuclear-cell subsets in human idiopathic crescentic glomerulonephritis (ICGN): analysis in tissue sections with monoclonal antibodies. *Journal of Clinical Immunology*, **4**, 202–8.

Stevens, M. E., McConnell, M. & Bone, J. M. (1983). Aggressive treatment with pulse methylprednisolone or plasma exchange is justified in rapidly progressive glomerulonephritis. *Proceedings of the European Dialysis and Transplantation Association*, **19**, 724–31.

Thompson, R. A. & Lee, S. S. (1989). Antineutrophil cytoplasmic antibodies. *Lancet*, **i**, 670–1.

Thomson, N. M., Holdsworth, S. R., Glasgow, E. F. & Atkins, R. C. (1979). The macrophage in the development of experimental crescentic glomerulonephritis. *American Journal of Pathology*, **94**, 223–40.

Tietjen, D. P. & Moore, W. J. (1990). Treatment of rapidly progressive glomerulonephritis due to Behçet's syndrome with intravenous cyclophosphamide. *Nephron*, **55**, 69–73.

Trepo, C. G. & Thivolet, J. (1970). Hepatitis associated antigen and periarteritis nodosa (PAN). *Vox Sanguinis*, **19**, 410–11.

van der Wall Bake, A. W. L., Lobatto, S., Jonges, L., Daha, M. R. & van Es, L. A. (1987). IgA antibodies directed against cytoplasmic antigens of polymorphonuclear leucocytes in patients with Henoch–Schonlein purpura. *Advances in Experimental and Medical Biology*, **216B**, 1593–8.

van der Woude, F. J., Daha, M. R. & van Es, L. A. (1989). The current status of neutrophil cytoplasmic antibodies. *Clinical and Experimental Immunology*, **78**, 143–8.

van der Woude, F. J., Rasmussen, N., Lobatto, S. *et al.* (1985). Autoantibodies against neutrophils and monocytes; tool for diagnosis and marker of disease activity in Wegener's granulomatosis. *Lancet*, **i**, 425–9.

Walton, E. W. (1958). Giant-cell granuloma of the respiratory tract (Wegener's granulomatosis). *British Medical Journal*, **II**, 265–70.

Wathen, C. W. & Harrison, D. J. (1987). Circulating anti-neutrophil antibodies in systemic vasculitis. *Lancet*, **i**, 1037.

Whitworth, J. A., Morel-Maroger, L., Mignon, F. & Richet, G. (1976). The significance of extracapillary proliferation. Clinicopathological review of 60 patients. *Nephron*, **16**, 1–19.

Wieslander, J., Rasmussen, N. & Bygren, P. (1989). An ELISA for ANCA and preliminary studies of the antigens involved. *APMIS*, **97** (suppl. 6), 42.

Wiik, A., Jensen, E. & Friis, J. (1974). Granulocyte-specific antinuclear factors in synovial fluids and sera from patients with rheumatoid arthritis. *Annals of Rheumatic Diseases*, **33**, 515–22.

Woodrow, G., Cook, J. A., Brownjohn, A. M. & Turney, J. H. (1990). Is renal vasculitis increasing in incidence? *Lancet*, **336**, 1583.

Woodworth, T. G., Abvelo, J. G., Austin, H. A. & Esparza, A. (1987). Severe glomerulonephritis with late emergence of classic Wegener's granulomatosis. *Medicine*, **66**, 181–91.

Yoshioka, K., Takemura, T., Akano, N., Miyamoto, H., Iseki, T. & Maki, S. (1987). Cellular and non-cellular compositions of crescents in human glomerulonephritis. *Kidney International*, **32**, 284–91.

Yust, I., Schwartz, J. & Dreyfuss, F. (1969). A cytotoxic serum factor in polyarteritis nodosa and related conditions. *American Journal of Medicine*, **48**, 472–6.

Zeek, P. M. (1952). Periarteritis nodosa: a critical review. *American Journal of Clinical Pathology*, **22**, 777–90.

–9–
Tubulointerstitial nephritis

A range of disorders of diverse pathogenesis may produce tubulointerstitial inflammation; this chapter deals only with those diseases in which there are reasonable grounds to assume that immunological mechanisms play a prominent role. In man, such diseases can be classified broadly into: 1) drug-induced; 2) associated with anti-tubular basement membrane (TBM) antibodies; 3) presumed immune complex disease-associated (e.g. lupus); and 4) a miscellaneous group with a presumed immunological basis. All of these categories usually manifest a common histological pattern of a predominantly mononuclear cell infiltrate composed primarily of T cells with some macrophages and plasma cells. In addition, immunofluorescence will often show granular deposits of immunoglobulins and complement in immune complex-associated disease, and linear staining for immunoglobulin along the TBM in the presence of anti-TBM antibodies. Depending on the chronicity of the lesion there may be varying degrees of fibrosis. Clinically, the presentation also depends on the acuteness of the lesion, ranging from acute renal failure on the one hand to varying degrees of tubular dysfunction (inability to concentrate or acidify the urine, glycosuria, aminoaciduria, etc) plus or minus chronic renal impairment on the other.

It is difficult to give precise incidence figures for these diseases. Interstitial nephritis as a whole may account for about 10% of cases of acute renal failure (Wilson et al., 1976; Naito & Sado, 1989), and a degree of interstitial involvement may be seen in up to 70% of cases of lupus (Brentjens et al., 1975); anti-TBM disease is certainly very rare. The incidence of drug-induced acute tubulointerstitial nephritis has been variously estimated as 0.8% (Richet et al., 1978; Grünfeld, Kleinknecht & Droz, 1988) and 8% (Linton et al., 1980) of cases of acute renal failure. It may occur in 1–2% of patients taking methicillin (Grünfeld, Kleinknecht & Droz, 1988), but this is seen much less frequently now with the declining use of methicillin.

Immunogenetics

Nothing appears to be known about the immunogenetics of drug-induced tubulointerstitial nephritis and anti-TBM disease in man. Because of the rarity of the latter condition it is unlikely that any substantial series will be studied, and the diverse range of drugs that can precipitate interstitial nephritis may be associated with a similarly diverse range of immunogenetic predispositions, making analysis very difficult. Perhaps the best approach would be to study a presumably relatively homogeneous group, such as the cases associated with beta-lactam antibiotics. However, such studies are not available, and with the decreasing use of methicillin, perhaps the principal agent in this category, it will be increasingly difficult to assemble a sizeable series.

The immunogenetics of lupus have been covered in Chapter 4; there is no information on whether interstitial involvement in this disease is associated with a particular immunogenetic background. Sjögren's syndrome (considered further below) is associated with DR3 and DRw52 (Arnett et al., 1988). As with lupus, certain autoantibodies are correlated with certain MHC alleles, and in the case of Sjögren's syndrome the presence of anti-Ro (usually accompanied by anti-La) appears to be mainly responsible for the DR3 association, with antibody-negative patients maintaining an association with DRw52 (Wilson et al., 1984). Interestingly, the highest amounts of autoantibody are found in patients who are DQw1/DQw2 heterozygotes (Harley et al., 1986). As with lupus there is no information on whether a particular immunogenetic background predisposes to the development of interstitial nephritis in Sjögren's syndrome.

Immunopathology

Animal studies

Animal models of tubulointerstitial nephritis (for review see Wilson, 1989) are usually considered under the main headings of anti-TBM, immune complex, and cell mediated disease, although there is considerable overlap between these categories in some cases. There are also some models which may not be immune mediated at all, such as the tubulointerstitial nephritis that follows the administration of the aminonucleoside of puromycin (Eddy & Michael, 1988).

Anti-TBM interstitial nephritis

The heading to this section purposely omits the qualification of a humoral or cellular anti-TBM response; although all the models considered here do exhibit an anti-TBM antibody response, in many cases the cellular immune system is intimately involved as well. However, one of the earliest models described is an example of a predominantly antibody mediated disease.

Immunisation of guinea pigs with rabbit TBM induces the production of anti-TBM antibodies and a severe interstitial nephritis (Steblay & Rudofsky, 1971). This disease can be passively transferred with antibodies (Steblay & Rudofsky, 1973) but not cells (van Zwieten et al., 1976), and there is evidence that the transferred antibodies are capable of initiating active autoimmunity (Hall et al., 1977). Heterologous antiidiotypic antibodies with specificity for anti-TBM antibodies can decrease the severity of interstitial nephritis (Brown, Carey & Colvin, 1979).

A rather similar disease is induced in Brown Norway rats and (Brown Norway × Lewis)F1 hybrids by immunisation with either homologous kidney extracts (Sugisaki et al., 1973) or heterologous (bovine) TBM (Lehman, Wilson & Dixon, 1974). As before, the anti-TBM antibody response seems to be a major factor in pathogenesis (Zanetti & Wilson, 1983), and the disease can be transferred with antibody (Sugisaki et al., 1973); only minor lesions are produced by transfer of cells (Lehman & Wilson, 1976). Antiidiotypic antibodies are again capable of down modulating disease expression (Zanetti, Mampaso & Wilson, 1983).

It is possible to inhibit the expression of experimental interstitial nephritis in the rat by the induction of suppressor cells using antigen in incomplete Freund's adjuvant (Kelly, Clayman & Neilson, 1986). This approach does not affect the production of anti-TBM antibodies. Further evidence for a role for cellular immunity is provided by immunisation with T cells specific for TBM antigens; this produces antibodies, presumably antiidiotypic, that can suppress the nephritis produced by immunisation with rabbit TBM (Neilson & Phillips, 1982).

The disease in rats is strain dependent. Lewis rats, for instance, do not possess the relevant nephritogenic tubular antigen, and are resistant to disease induction (Krieger, Thoenes & Günther, 1981). Transplantation of a (Brown Norway × Lewis)F1 kidney into a Lewis host results in the production of anti-TBM antibodies and nephritis, because the Lewis rat is not tolerant of the nephritogenic antigen contributed to the donor kidney by the Brown Norway parent (Lehman et al., 1974). This may provide a close analogy to the formation of anti-TBM antibodies following some human allografts (Wilson et al., 1974). Lack of involvement of the cellular immune system may be critical in other strains which possess the antigen and make anti-TBM antibodies, and yet fail to develop disease (Neilson et al., 1983).

Mice will also make an anti-TBM response to immunisation with heterologous TBM. All strains will make anti-TBM antibodies, but there are marked differences with respect to the development of interstitial nephritis, with SJL and BALB/c mice being the most susceptible (Rudofsky, Dilworth & Tung, 1980; Neilson & Phillips, 1982). Although both antibody and T cells may be involved in the pathogenesis (transfer of either will produce disease, albeit of differing pattern; Zakheim et al., 1984) it seems likely that the T cell response is the most critical (Ueda *et al.*, 1988; Evans *et al.*, 1988), at least in strains other than SJL (Clayman, Michaud & Neilson, 1987). Murine interstitial nephritis is of particular interest because of the considerable data available on immunomodulatory therapies. Thus treatment with an anti-idiotype against the major idiotype present on anti-TBM antibodies prevents renal injury (Clayman *et al.*, 1988). The treatment is also effective if administered two weeks into the disease. The T cell responses are attenuated, but the anti-TBM antibody titre is only very slightly lowered. This emphasises the role of T cells in this disease, but also implies some form of (presumably idiotypic) connection between the cellular and humoral compartments. It is also possible to induce antigen-specific suppressor cells by immunisation with syngeneic lymphocytes coupled to tubular antigens (Neilson *et al.*, 1985). Again, such treatment can even be effective once disease is established, in this case at up to six weeks into the disease (Mann & Neilson, 1986).

Immune complex-mediated interstitial nephritis

Models with a presumed immune complex immunopathogenesis can be induced by immunisation with exogenous or endogenous antigens, or occur in the setting of spontaneous autoimmunity. The classical model of serum sickness produced in rabbits by repeated injections of bovine serum albumin may exhibit an interstitial nephritis characterised by granular immune deposits along the TBM and in the interstitium (Brentjens *et al.*, 1974). Such lesions were only found in high responder animals given high doses of antigen. In an attempt to model drug-induced interstitial nephritis, mice have been immunised with a cephalosporin antibiotic and then a cephalosporin-protein conjugate injected into the renal cortex (Joh *et al.*, 1989). This does indeed produce interstitial nephritis, which can be shown by transfer experiments to be antibody dependent. Immunisation of rats with a known autoantigen, Tamm–Horsfall protein, results in a tubulointerstitial nephritis which is most prominent around the thick limb of the ascending loop of Henle, a major site of Tamm–Horsfall protein production (Hoyer, 1980). A similar lesion is produced by the administration of heterologous antisera to Tamm–Horsfall protein (Friedman, Hoyer & Seiler, 1982). Finally, spontaneous immune deposits and interstitial infiltrates develop late in the course of some murine models of systemic lupus erythematosus (McCluskey, 1983).

Cell-mediated interstitial nephritis

Although cellular mechanisms are clearly involved in a number of the models discussed above, there are also examples of pure cell-mediated disease. The earliest of these involved the injection of exogenous antigens into the kidney of pre-sensitised recipients (van Zwieten *et al.*, 1977; Vargas Arenas & Turner, 1982). More recently, Lewis rats have been shown to develop a tubulointerstitial nephritis when immunised with homologous TBM (Sugisaki *et al.*, 1980). As mentioned above, Lewis rats lack the principal nephritogenic tubular antigen recognised by anti-TBM antibodies, and, indeed, sera from the immunised animals do not bind to the TBM and are incapable of passively transferring the disease; such transfer can, however, be successfully accomplished with lymphocytes (Bannister, Ulich & Wilson, 1987). A spontaneous cell-mediated nephritis develops in kdkd strain mice (Kelly & Neilson, 1987*b*). Analysis of this system has revealed the presence of contra-suppressor cells, which act, as their name implies, by reducing the action of suppressor cells, which in turn facilitates the develop-ment of autoimmunity. Analogies, both histological and in inheritance pattern, between this animal model and the human medullary cystic disease/ juvenile nephronopthisis complex have produced the suggestion that similar regulatory abnormalities may underlie the human disease (Kelly & Neilson, 1987*a*).

Human studies

Drug-induced acute interstitial nephritis

Numerous drugs have been implicated (Cotran, Rubin & Tolkoff-Rubin, 1986; Grünfeld, Kleinknecht & Droz, 1988). Perhaps the most characteristic picture is seen in the case of β-lactam antibiotics, and in particular methicil-lin. A hypersensitivity response is suggested by the latent period (2–60 days), the co-existence in some cases of fever, rash and eosinophilia, and a raised total serum IgE concentration (Ooi *et al.*, 1978; Linton *et al.*, 1980).

A wide variety of tests have been employed in an attempt to provide more specific evidence for drug hypersensitivity (Grünfeld, Kleinknecht & Droz, 1988) with generally inconclusive results. Circulating antibodies to the drug are very occasionally found, notably in the case of rifampicin (Kleinknecht, Homberg & Decroix, 1972). Similarly there are occasional reports of positive skin tests (Baldwin *et al.*, 1968; Hyman, Ballow & Knieser, 1978) and a cell-mediated response (Watson *et al.*, 1983) to the offending agent. In many cases, there is no firm direct evidence for drug-specific hypersensiti-vity, although one series did find evidence (using lymphocyte stimulation) for such hypersensitivity in all ten cases studied (Joh *et al.*, 1990).

In non-specific terms, it seems unlikely that the humoral response is important in pathogenesis. Immunofluorescence generally does not reveal any immune deposits, and although anti-TBM antibodies have been found in a few cases, for reasons discussed in the next section these are unlikely to

be pathogenetic. The histological findings would certainly support a prominent role for cell-mediated immunity, with a predominance of T cells, which
may be CD4⁺ or CD8⁺ (Grünfeld, Kleinknecht & Droz, 1988), and the
occasional presence of granulomas and giant cells (Magil, 1983). Increased
expression of MHC class II molecules on tubular cells may contribute to the
localisation or activation of interstitial T cells (Cheng *et al.*, 1989).

In addition to the typical form of drug-induced interstitial nephritis a
relatively distinct syndrome is occasionally seen following the use of non-
steroidal anti-inflammatory drugs (NSAIDS) (Porile, Bakris & Garella,
1990). This is separate from the acute decline in renal function presumed to
be due to the inhibition of prostaglandin synthesis, and consists of an
interstitial nephritis together with heavy proteinuria. The glomeruli are
usually normal to light microscopy and immunofluorescence, suggesting
minimal change nephropathy. As it is common to this class of drugs, this
syndrome presumably reflects a causal role for the common prostaglandin
synthesis inhibitory effects, but the details remain speculative. Prostaglandins certainly affect T lymphocyte and macrophage function, and there is
indirect evidence for the involvement of T cells in the pathogenesis of
minimal change nephropathy (see Chapter 7).

Anti-TBM antibodies and tubulointerstitial nephritis

Anti-TBM antibodies have been found in a number of situations. As
mentioned above, some cases of drug-induced tubulointerstitial nephritis
are associated with such antibodies; examples include methicillin (Border *et
al.*, 1974) and phenytoin (Hyman, Ballow & Knieser, 1978). These clearly
represent a very small proportion of all cases of drug-induced interstitial
nephritis. Furthermore, there is no correlation between the titre of anti-
TBM antibody and interstitial inflammation, and attempts at passive transfer of disease to rats have been unsuccessful (Ooi *et al.*, 1978). Although this
last point must be interpreted with caution (cellular as well as humoral anti-
TBM activity is often required in experimental models for full disease
expression) the evidence is therefore against a significant role for these
antibodies in the pathogenesis of drug-induced interstitial nephritis. It is
perhaps more likely that they represent a secondary immune response to
neoantigens released by the interstitial inflammation.

Anti-TBM antibodies have been found in association with primary
glomerular diseases, including poststreptococcal glomerulonephritis
(Morel-Maroger *et al.*, 1974), membranous nephropathy (Levy *et al.*, 1978),
and anti-glomerular basement membrane (GBM) disease (Lehman, Wilson
& Dixon, 1975; Andres *et al.*, 1978), as well as in a number of other renal
conditions (Mahieu, Dardenne & Bach, 1972). It is possible that the anti-
TBM activity in the context of anti-GBM disease simply reflects the tubular

distribution of the Goodpasture antigen: anti-GBM sera appear to recognise the same epitope(s) in TBM as seen in GBM, albeit with lower avidity (Yoshioka *et al.*, 1986). A contribution of such anti-TBM activity to pathogenesis in some of the above situations is supported by the presence of tubular lesions in some of the membranous nephropathy-associated cases (Levy *et al.*, 1978) and the correlation between the presence of antibodies and the presence of severe tubulointerstitial lesions in crescentic nephritis (Andres *et al.*, 1978). However, as with drug-induced interstitial nephritis, it is impossible to exclude the possibility that the presence of anti-TBM antibodies is secondary to severe interstitial damage, and this is presumably the explanation for the occurrence of such antibodies in conditions such as cortical necrosis (Mahieu, Dardenne & Bach, 1972).

The presence of anti-TBM activity in patients with renal allografts is of uncertain significance. Although some such cases may represent an immune response to a tubular alloantigen (Wilson *et al.*, 1974; Neilson, 1989) or autoantigen (Klassen *et al.*, 1973), the occurrence of linear TBM immuno-fluorescence in 20% of allografts (Cotran, Rubin & Tolkoff-Rubin, 1986) suggests that in many cases this is a relatively non-specific phenomenon.

Finally, very occasional cases of interstitial nephritis have been described in which anti-TBM antibodies are the only apparent abnormality (Bergstein & Litman, 1975; Clayman *et al.*, 1986; Fliger *et al.*, 1987; Neilson, 1989; Brentjens *et al.*, 1989). Further evidence for a pathogenetic role is provided by characterisation of the target antigen: as with some of the animal models of anti-TBM disease discussed above, this appears to be the 3M–1 glyco-protein (Yoshioka *et al.*, 1986; Clayman *et al.*, 1986; Fliger *et al.*, 1987). Furthermore, there is idiotypic sharing between human and animal anti-TBM antibodies (Clayman *et al.*, 1988), providing further evidence for the close relationship between the experimental models and the human disease. This relationship is discussed further in the final section of the chapter. Although interstitial nephritis with renal failure is the usual manifestation, there are occasional reports of renal tubular acidosis occurring in the presence of anti-tubular antibodies (Pasternack & Linder, 1970; Chanarin *et al.*, 1974); the relationship between these antibodies and the anti-TBM antibodies discussed above is unclear.

Systemic lupus erythematosus and other immune complex diseases

Interstitial involvement is common in lupus nephritis, and was originally attributed to interstitial deposition of immune complexes (Brentjens *et al.*, 1975). Such deposits may be found in association with capillaries, within the interstitium, or along or within the TBM. They are often associated with inflammation and tubular damage (Schwartz, Fennell & Lewis, 1982), suggesting a pathogenetic role. However, other reports have found no correlation between the presence of tubulointerstitial deposits and an inflammatory interstitial infiltrate (Magil & Tyler, 1984), suggesting that the cellular immune system may also be important. Whatever the aetiology, further evidence for the clinical importance of this extra-glomerular inflammation in lupus nephritis is provided by the occurrence of renal failure in which glomerular involvement is mild or absent (Gur, Kopolovic & Gross, 1987), and the correlation between the degree of renal impairment and extent of interstitial damage (O'Dell *et al.*, 1985). The interstitial changes could also contribute to the tubular dysfunction that may be found in lupus (Yeung *et al.*, 1984; Kozeny *et al.*, 1987).

Mixed essential cryoglobulinaemia (see Chapter 10) is associated with large amounts of circulating immune complexes, and it is perhaps not surprising that a presumed immune complex-mediated interstitial nephritis has been described in this condition (McCluskey, 1983), in addition to the more typical glomerular lesion (see Chapter 10). However, as in lupus, there are also reports of cases in which interstitial inflammation occurs in the apparent absence of immune deposits (Steinmuller *et al.*, 1979).

Other conditions with a possible immune complex contribution to pathogenesis in which interstitial deposits have been noted include IgA nephropathy (Frascà *et al.*, 1982), mesangiocapillary glomerulonephritis, the glomerulonephritis associated with infectious endocarditis, and membranous nephropathy (Cotran, Rubin & Tolkoff-Rubin, 1986).

Miscellaneous tubulointerstitial nephritides

The principal entity in this category is Sjögren's syndrome. This disease is characterised by a chronic inflammatory infiltrate (lymphocytes and plasma cells) of exocrine glands, most notably of the salivary and lacrimal glands causing a dry mouth and eyes (sicca syndrome). The syndrome may occur in isolation (primary Sjögren's) or in association with a connective tissue disorder, which is most commonly rheumatoid arthritis but may also be systemic lupus erythematosus, poly- or dermatomyositis, or systemic sclerosis. The commonest renal manifestation is a chronic tubulointerstitial nephritis, with a very similar infiltrate to that seen in the exocrine glands (Rosenberg *et al.*, 1988; Matsumura *et al.*, 1988); this may occur in a high proportion of cases (e.g. six out of nine in one biopsy series; Tu *et al.*, 1968). This infiltrate may be composed of Ig-containing B and plasma cells (Gerhardt, Loebl & Rao, 1978), and in some cases is associated with granular deposits of immunoglobulin and C3 along the TBM (Winer *et al.*, 1977); in others, the immunofluorescent findings are negative (Feest *et al.*, 1978). Some evidence for the pathogenicity of immunoglobulin is provided by the transient induction of distal renal tubular dysfunction in a neonate by transplacental passage of IgG (with reactivity for a renal tubular antigen) from a mother with Sjögren's syndrome (Jordan *et al.*, 1985). Perhaps because of the chronic nature of this disease, the clinical manifestations are often those of tubular impairment (renal tubular acidosis, problems with concentrating the urine, and rarely the Fanconi syndrome), with significant renal impairment being rather unusual. For completeness, it is worth noting that glomerular involvement has also been described in Sjögren's syndrome. This may be a focal segmental glomerular sclerosis, which is probably secondary to severe tubulointerstitial disease, or a glomerular lesion typical of an associated connective tissue disease, e.g. lupus (Steinberg & Talal, 1971) or mixed cryoglobulinaemia (Case records of the Massachusetts General Hospital, 1975), but an apparently primary glomerulopathy (with a mesangiocapillary or membranous pattern) has also been reported (Moutsopoulos *et al.*, 1978). The aetiology of Sjögren's syndrome is unknown, although there has been recent interest in the possibility that a virus (Epstein Barr virus or a retrovirus) may be involved (for review see Flescher & Talal, 1991).

The association of tubulointerstitial nephritis with uveitis (TINU syndrome) is a rare but intriguing entity (Dobrin, Vernier & Fish, 1975; Burghard *et al.*, 1984); possibly linked with this, in that patients combining all features have been reported, is the association between interstitial nephritis and bone marrow granulomas (Nakamoto, Kida & Mizumura, 1979). In many of these cases, eosinophils have been prominent in the interstitial infiltrate. This combination of features, and the response to corticosteroid therapy (Steinman & Silva, 1984; Cacoub *et al.*, 1989), clearly implies a significant immunopathogenesis, but no details are known.

Finally, acute tubulointerstitial nephritis may occur with no obvious precipitating factors (Spital, Panner & Sterns, 1987); in one series this accounted for 10 out of 30 cases of biopsy-proven interstitial nephritis (Laberke & Bohle, 1980).

Therapeutic aspects

There are no randomised controlled trials available to guide therapy in this condition, no doubt reflecting its heterogeneity and the relative rarity of well-defined subtypes. However, the immunopathology and the animal models provide a good rationale for the use of immunosuppression. One study compared eight patients who received steroids with six that did not; the creatinine fell to a new baseline in an average of 9.3 days in the treated group, whereas this took 54 days in the untreated group (Galpin *et al.*, 1978). There is anecdotal evidence to support the efficacy of steroids in other cases (Linton *et al.*, 1980). However, there are also some reports of patients in which steroids had no apparent influence on the course of the disease (Ditlove *et al.*, 1977; Richmond *et al.*, 1979).

A general scheme of treatment has been outlined (Neilson, 1989). This involves the use of corticosteroids, unless renal function improves after removal of any precipitating factors such as drugs, or unless extensive interstitial fibrosis is present on the biopsy. If anti-TBM antibodies are present, or if there is no response to 7–10 days of corticosteroid therapy, then consideration is given to the addition of cyclophosphamide, together with plasma exchange in the case of anti-TBM antibodies. The efficacy of cyclosporin in experimental models (Shih, Hines & Neilson, 1988) suggests this as another possible agent, particularly if cyclophosphamide is poorly tolerated or ineffective.

Concluding remarks

As with many other human renal diseases, the evidence for an immunological basis to the pathogenesis of tubulointerstitial nephritis is indirect, albeit persuasive. The lymphocytic infiltrate, the presence of anti-TBM antibodies, the analogies with the animal models and the response to immunosuppressive treatment all contribute to the case for an immunopathogenesis. This case is perhaps best established in the case of anti-TBM antibody nephritis. Although it is possible that such antibodies are formed as a secondary phenomena in the response to neoantigens exposed by pre-existing interstitial inflammation, the fact that similar antibodies in animals directed against the same epitope are pathogenetic argues strongly for a similar role in man. However, anti-TBM antibodies are rare in man, and the analysis of antigen recognition is based on a very small number of cases. Some caution is therefore warranted in attempting to generalise to all such cases. In particular, the anti-TBM reactivity found in some cases of drug-induced interstitial nephritis and in a high proportion of renal allografts is probably not of pathogenetic significance. A prediction from this is that these latter antibodies will recognise a different epitope(s), or even a different antigen(s), from that recognised by primary anti-TBM antibodies; this prediction does not appear to have been tested.

A role for interstitial immune complexes in the aetiology of interstitial inflammation in lupus is also plausible. Little is known of the mechanisms involved in such interstitial deposition; does it represent 'overflow' following saturation of glomerular sites? Is there primary *in situ* immune complex formation? Or are cellular mechanisms in fact more important, with the immune deposits a non-specific phenomenon reflecting leakage from damaged vessels?

Unfortunately, the commonest type of human interstitial nephritis, that due to drugs, is also the type about which least is known. Although in many cases a hypersensitivity response to the drug appears likely, attempts to produce direct evidence for this have not produced consistent results. The general lack of immune deposits and the character of the infiltrate lends support to the idea that this is a predominantly cell-mediated lesion. There are no particularly relevant animal models, but the existence of purely cell-mediated experimental interstitial nephritis is at least some evidence that such a pathogenesis is possible.

The therapeutic strategies that are successful in experimental tubulointerstitial nephritis are potentially of considerable importance. The attraction lies in the specificity: it appears possible to selectively turn off just the autoreactive response via suppressive mechanisms without resorting to hazardous non-specific immunosuppression. The concept of suppressor cells has come in for considerable criticism recently (Möller, 1988). Elaborate suppressor cell networks, linked by poorly characterised (at least in molecular terms) suppressor factors, are a feature of a number of suppressor cell systems (Asherson, Colizzi & Zembala, 1986), but their relationship to physiological *in vivo* suppression is unclear. It is no longer satisfactory to refer uncritically to 'I-J restriction' of suppressor cell systems, as it is clear that I-J does not exist as originally proposed, namely as a separate major histocompatibility complex locus (Murphy, 1985). However, these criticisms are to a certain extent beside the point, as whatever the mechanism experimental manoeuvres such as the injection of derivatised syngeneic lymphocytes are undoubtedly effective at down-regulating an immune response in a number of experimental systems, e.g. Sherr *et al.*, 1980. Because autologous cells can be used, such an approach may be feasible in man.

References

Andres, G. A., Brentjens, J., Kohli, R. *et al.* (1978). Histology of human tubulo-interstitial nephritis associated with antibodies to renal basement membranes. *Kidney International*, 13, 480–91.

Arnett, F. C., Goldstein, R., Duvic, M. & Reveille, J. D. (1988). Major histocompatibility complex genes in systemic lupus erythematosus, Sjögren's syndrome, and polymyositis. *American Journal of Medicine*, 85 suppl. 6A, 38–41.

Asherson, G. L., Colizzi, V. & Zembala, M. (1986). An overview of T-suppressor cell circuits. *Annual Review of Immunology*, 4, 37–68.

Baldwin, D. S., Levine, B. B., McCluskey, R. T. & Gallo, G. R. (1968). Renal failure and interstitial nephritis due to penicillin and methicillin. *New England Journal of Medicine*, 279, 1245–52.

Bannister, K. M., Ulich, T. R. & Wilson, C. B. (1987). Induction, characterization, and cell transfer of autoimmune tubulointerstitial nephritis. *Kidney International*, 32, 642–51.

Bergstein, J. & Litman, N. (1975). Interstitial nephritis with anti-tubular-basement-membrane antibody. *New England Journal of Medicine*, **292**, 875–8.

Border, W. A., Lehman, D. H., Egan, J. D., Sass, H. J., Glode, J. E. & Wilson, C. B. (1974). Antitubular basement-membrane antibodies in methicillin-associated interstitial nephritis. *New England Journal of Medicine*, **291**, 381–4.

Brentjens, J. R., O'Connell, D. W., Pawlowski, I. B. & Andres, G. A. (1974). Extraglomerular lesions associated with deposition of circulating antigen–antibody complexes in kidneys of rabbits with chronic serum sickness. *Clinical Immunology and Immunopathology*, **3**, 112–26.

Brentjens, J. R., Sepulveda, M., Baliah, T. *et al.* (1975). Interstitial immune complex nephritis in patients with systemic lupus erythematosus. *Kidney International*, **7**, 342–50.

Brentjens, J. R., Matsuo, S., Fukatsu, A. *et al.* (1989). Immunologic studies in two patients with antitubular basement membrane nephritis. *American Journal of Medicine*, **86**, 603–8.

Brown, C. A., Carey, K. & Colvin, R. B. (1979). Inhibition of autoimmune tubulointerstitial nephritis in guinea pigs by heterologous antisera containing anti-idiotype antibodies. *Journal of Immunology*, **123**, 2102–7.

Burghard, R., Brandis, M., Hoyer, P. F., Ehrich, J. H. H., Galaske, R. G. & Brodehl, J. (1984). Acute interstitial nephritis in childhood. *European Journal of Paediatrics*, **142**, 103–10.

Cacoub, P., Deray, G., Le Hoang, P. *et al.* (1989). Idiopathic acute interstitial nephritis associated with anterior uveitis in adults. *Clinical Nephrology*, **31**, 307–10.

Case records of the Massachusetts General Hospital (1975). *New England Journal of Medicine*, **292**, 1285–90.

Chanarin, I., Loewi, G., Tavill, A. S., Swain, C. P. & Tidmarsh, E. (1974). Defect of renal tubular acidification with antibody to loop of Henle. *Lancet*, **ii**, 317–18.

Cheng, H-F., Nolasco, F., Cameron, J. S., Hildreth, G., Neild, G. & Hartley, B. (1989). HLA-DR display by renal tubular epithelium and phenotype of infiltrate in interstitial nephritis. *Nephrology Dialysis and Transplantation*, **4**, 205–15.

Clayman, M. D., Michaud, L., Brentjens, J., Andres, G. A., Kefalides, N. A. & Neilson, E. G. (1986). Isolation of the target antigen of human anti-tubular basement membrane antibody-associated interstitial nephritis. *Journal of Clinical Investigation*, **77**, 1143–7.

Clayman, M. D., Michaud, L. & Neilson, E. G. (1987). Murine interstitial nephritis. VI. Characterization of the B cell response in anti-tubular basement membrane disease. *Journal of Immunology*, **139**, 2242–9.

Clayman, M. D., Sun, M. J., Michaud, L., Brill-Dashoff, J., Riblet, R. & Neilson, E. G. (1988). Clonotypic heterogeneity in experimental interstitial nephritis. Restricted specificity of the anti-tubular basement membrane B cell repertoire is associated with a disease-modifying crossreactive idiotype. *Journal of Experimental Medicine*, **167**, 1296–312.

Cotran, R. S., Rubin, R. H. & Tolkoff-Rubin, N. E. (1986). Tubulointerstitial diseases. In *The Kidney*, 3rd edn, ed. B. M. Brenner & F. C. Rector, pp. 1143–73. Philadelphia: W. B. Saunders Company.

Ditlove, J., Weidmann, P., Bernstein, M. & Massry, S. G. (1977). Methicillin nephritis. *Medicine*, **56**, 483–91.

Dobrin, R. S., Vernier, R. L. & Fish, A. J. (1975). Acute eosinophilic interstitial nephritis and renal failure with bone marrow-lymph node granulomas and anterior uveitis. A new syndrome. *American Journal of Medicine*, **59**, 325–33.

Eddy, A. A. & Michael, A. F. (1988). Acute tubulointerstitial nephritis associated with aminonucleoside nephrosis. *Kidney International*, **33**, 14–23.

Evans, B. D., Dilwith, R. L., Balaban, S. L. & Rudofsky, U. H. (1988). Lack of passive transfer of renal tubulointerstitial disease by serum or monoclonal antibody specific for renal tubular antigens in the mouse. *International Archives of Allergy and Applied Immunology*, **86**, 238–42.

Feest, T. G., Lockwood, C. M., Morley, A. R. & Uff, J. S. (1978). Renal histology and immunopathology in distal renal tubular acidosis. *Clinical Nephrology*, 10, 187–90.

Flescher, E. & Talal, N. (1991). Do viruses contribute to the development of Sjögren's syndrome? *American Journal of Medicine*, 90, 283–5.

Fliger, F. D., Wieslander, J., Brentjens, J. R., Andres, G. & Butkowski, R. J. (1987). Identification of a target antigen in human anti-tubular basement membrane nephritis. *Kidney International*, 31, 800–7.

Frascà, G., Vangelista, A., Biagini, G. & Bonomini, V. (1982). Immunological tubulo-interstitial deposits in IgA nephropathy. *Kidney International*, 22, 184–91.

Friedman, J., Hoyer, J. R. & Seiler, M. W. (1982). Formation and clearance of tubulointerstitial immune complexes in kidneys of rats immunized with heterologous antisera to Tamm–Horsfall protein. *Kidney International*, 21, 575–82.

Galpin, J. E., Shinaberger, J. H., Stanley, T. M. *et al.* (1978). Acute interstitial nephritis due to methicillin. *American Journal of Medicine*, 65, 756–65.

Gerhardt, R. E., Loebl, D. H. & Rao, R. N. (1978). Interstitial immunofluorescence in nephritis of Sjögren's syndrome. *Clinical Nephrology*, 10, 201–7.

Grünfeld, J-P., Kleinknecht, D. & Droz, D. (1988). Acute interstitial nephritis. In *Diseases of the Kidney*, 4th edn, ed. R. W. Schrier & C. W. Gottschalk, pp. 1461–87. Boston/Toronto: Little, Brown and Company.

Gur, H., Kopolovic, Y. & Gross, D. J. (1987). Chronic predominant interstitial nephritis in a patient with systemic lupus erythematosus: a follow up of three years and review of the literature. *Annals of the Rheumatic Diseases*, 46, 617–23.

Hall, C. L., Colvin, R. B., Carey, K. & McCluskey, R. T. (1977). Passive transfer of autoimmune disease with isologous IgG_1 and IgG_2 antibodies to the tubular basement membrane in strain XIII guinea pigs. Loss of self-tolerance induced by autoantibodies. *Journal of Experimental Medicine*, 146, 1246–60.

Harley, J. B., Reichlin, M., Arnett, F. C., Alexander, E. L., Bias, W. B. & Provost, T. T. (1986). Gene interaction at HLA-DQ enhances autoantibody production in primary Sjögren's syndrome. *Science*, 232, 1145–7.

Hoyer, J. R. (1980). Tubulointerstitial immune complex nephritis in rats immunized with Tamm–Horsfall protein. *Kidney International*, 17, 284–92.

Hyman, L. R., Ballow, M. & Knieser, M. R. (1978). Diphenylhydantoin interstitial nephritis. Roles of cellular and humoral immunologic injury. *Journal of Pediatrics*, 92, 915–20.

Joh, K., Shibasaki, T., Azuma, T. *et al.* (1989). Experimental drug-induced allergic nephritis mediated by antihapten antibody. *International Archives of Allergy and Applied Immunology*, 88, 337–44.

Joh, K., Aizawa, S., Yamaguchi, Y. *et al.* (1990). Drug-induced hypersensitivity nephritis: lymphocyte stimulation testing and renal biopsy in 10 cases. *American Journal of Nephrology*, 10, 222–30.

Jordan, S. C., Sakai, R., Tabak, M. A., Ettenger, R. B., Cohen, H. & Fine, R. N. (1985). Induction of neonatal renal tubular dysfunction by transplacentally acquired IgG from a mother with Sjögren syndrome. *Journal of Pediatrics*, 107, 566–9.

Kelly, C. J., Clayman, M. D. & Neilson, E. G. (1986). Immunoregulation in experimental interstitial nephritis: immunization with renal tubular antigen in incomplete Freund's adjuvant induces major histocompatibility complex-restricted, $OX8^+$ suppressor T cells which are antigen-specific and inhibit the expression of disease. *Journal of Immunology*, 136, 903–7.

Kelly, C. J. & Neilson, E. G. (1987a). Medullary cystic disease: an inherited form of autoimmune interstitial nephritis? *American Journal of Kidney Disease*, 10, 389–95.

Kelly, C. J. & Neilson, E. G. (1987b). Contrasuppression in autoimmunity. Abnormal contrasuppression facilitates expression of nephritogenic effector T cells and interstitial nephritis in kdkd mice. *Journal of Experimental Medicine*, 165, 107–23.

Klassen, J., Kano, K., Milgrom, F. *et al.* (1973). Tubular lesions produced by autoantibodies to tubular basement membrane in human renal allografts. *International Archives of Allergy and Applied Immunology*, 45, 674–89.

Kleinknecht, D., Homberg, J. C. & Decroix, G. (1972). Acute renal failure after rifampicin. *Lancet*, i, 1238–9.

Kozeny, G. A., Barr, W., Bansal, V. K. *et al.* (1987). Occurrence of renal tubular dysfunction in lupus nephritis. *Archives of Internal Medicine*, 147, 891–5.

Krieger, A., Thoenes, G. H. & Günther, E. (1981). Genetic control of autoimmune tubulointerstitial nephritis in rats. *Clinical Immunology and Immunopathology*, 21, 301–8.

Laberke, H-G. & Bohle, A. (1980). Acute interstitial nephritis: correlations between clinical and morphological findings. *Clinical Nephrology*, 14, 263–73.

Lehman, D. H., Wilson, C. B. & Dixon, F. J. (1974). Interstitial nephritis in rats immunized with heterologous tubular basement membrane. *Kidney International*, 5, 187–95.

Lehman, D. H., Lee, S., Wilson, C. B. & Dixon, F. J. (1974). Induction of antitubular basement membrane antibody in rats by renal transplantation. *Transplantation*, 17, 429–31.

Lehman, D. H. & Wilson, C. B. (1976). Role of sensitized cells in antitubular basement membrane interstitial nephritis. *International Archives of Allergy and Applied Immunology*, 51, 168–74.

Lehman, D. H., Wilson, C. B. & Dixon, F. J. (1975). Extraglomerular immunoglobulin deposits in human nephritis. *American Journal of Medicine*, 58, 765–86.

Levy, M., Gagnadoux, M-F., Beziau, A. & Habib, R. (1978). Membranous glomerulonephritis associated with anti-tubular and anti-alveolar basement membrane antibodies. *Clinical Nephrology*, 10, 158–65.

Linton, A. L., Clark, W. F., Driedger, A. A., Turnbull, D. I. & Lindsay, R. M. (1980). Acute interstitial nephritis due to drugs. Review of the literature with a report of nine cases. *Annals of Internal Medicine*, 93, 735–41.

Magil, A. B. (1983). Drug-induced acute interstitial nephritis with granulomas. *Human Pathology*, 14, 36–41.

Magil, A. B. & Tyler, M. (1984). Tubulo-interstitial disease in lupus nephritis. A morphometric study. *Histopathology*, 8, 81–7.

Mahieu, P., Dardenne, M. & Bach, J. F. (1972). Detection of humoral and cell-mediated immunity to kidney basement membranes in human renal diseases. *American Journal of Medicine*, 53, 185–92.

Mann, R. & Neilson, E. G. (1986). Murine interstitial nephritis. V. The auto-induction of antigen-specific Lyt-2+ suppressor T cells diminishes the expression of interstitial nephritis in mice with antitubular basement membrane disease. *Journal of Immunology*, 136, 908–12.

Matsumura, R., Kondo, Y., Sugiyama, T. *et al.* (1988). Immunohistochemical identification of infiltrating mononuclear cells in tubulointerstitial nephritis associated with Sjögren's syndrome. *Clinical Nephrology*, 30, 335–40.

McCluskey, R. T. (1983). Immunologically mediated tubulointerstitial nephritis. In *Tubulointerstitial Nephropathies*, ed. R. S. Cotran, B. M. Brenner & J. H. Stein, pp. 121–49. New York: Churchill Livingstone.

Morel-Maroger, L., Kourilsky, O., Mignon, F. *et. al.* (1974). Antitubular basement membrane antibodies in rapidly progressive poststreptococcal glomerulonephritis: report of a case. *Clinical Immunology and Immunopathology*, 2, 185–94.

Moutsopoulos, H. M., Balow, J. E., Lawley, T. J., Stahl, N. I., Antonovych, T. T. & Chused, T. M. (1978). Immune complex glomerulonephritis in sicca syndrome. *American Journal of Medicine*, 64, 955–60.

Murphy, D. B. (1985). Commentary on the genetic basis for control of I-J determinants. *Journal of Immunology*, 135, 1543–7.

Möller, G. (1988). Do suppressor T cells exist? *Scandinavian Journal of Immunology*, **27**, 247–50.

Naito, I. & Sado, Y. (1989). Early changes of rat experimental autoimmune glomerulonephritis induced with the nephritogenic antigen from bovine renal basement membranes. *Journal of Clinical and Laboratory Immunology*, **28**, 187–93.

Nakamoto, Y., Kida, H. & Mizumura, Y. (1979). Acute eosinophilic interstitial nephritis with bone marrow granulomas. Report of a case. *Clinical Immunology and Immunopathology*, **14**, 379–83.

Neilson, E. G. & Phillips, S. M. (1982). Suppression of interstitial nephritis by auto-anti-idiotypic immunity. *Journal of Experimental Medicine*, **155**, 179–89.

Neilson, E. G., Gasser, D. L., McCafferty, E., Zakheim, B. & Phillips, S. M. (1983). Polymorphism of genes involved in anti-tubular basement membrane disease in rats. *Immunogenetics*, **17**, 55–65.

Neilson, E. G., McCafferty, E., Mann, R., Michaud, L. & Clayman, M. (1985). Tubular antigen-derivatized cells induce a disease-protective, antigen-specific, and idiotype-specific suppressor T cell network restricted by I-J and Igh-V in mice with experimental interstitial nephritis. *Journal of Experimental Medicine*, **162**, 215–30.

Neilson, E. G. (1989). Pathogenesis and therapy of interstitial nephritis. *Kidney International*, **35**, 1257–70.

Neilson, E. G. & Phillips, S. M. (1982). Murine interstitial nephritis. I. Analysis of disease susceptibility and its relationship to pleiomorphic gene products defining both immune-response genes and a restrictive requirement for cytotoxic T cells at H-2K. *Journal of Experimental Medicine*, **155**, 1075–85.

O'Dell, J. R., Hays, R. C., Guggenheim, S. J. & Steigerwald, J. C. (1985). Tubulointerstitial renal disease in systemic lupus erythematosus. *Archives of Internal Medicine*, **145**, 1996–9.

Ooi, B. S., Ooi, Y. M., Mohini, R. & Pollak, V. E. (1978). Humoral mechanisms in drug-induced acute interstitial nephritis. *Clinical Immunology and Immunopathology*, **10**, 330–4.

Pasternack, A. & Linder, E. (1970). Renal tubular acidosis: an immunopathological study on four patients. *Clinical and Experimental Immunology*, **7**, 115–23.

Porile, J. L., Bakris, G. L. & Garella, S. (1990). Acute interstitial nephritis with glomerulopathy due to nonsteroidal anti-inflammatory agents: a review of its clinical spectrum and effects of steroid therapy. *Journal of Clinical Pharmacology*, **30**, 468–75.

Richet, G., Sraer, J. D., Kourilsky, O. *et al.* (1978). La ponction biopsie rénale dans les insuffisances rénales aiguës. *Annales de Medecine Interne*, **129**, 445–7.

Richmond, J. M., Whitworth, J. A., Fairley, K. F. & Kincaid-Smith, P. (1979). Co-trimoxazole nephrotoxicity (letter). *Lancet*, **i**, 493.

Rosenberg, M. E., Schendel, P. B., McCurdy, F. A. & Platt, J. L. (1988). Characterization of immune cells in kidneys from patients with Sjogren's syndrome. *American Journal of Kidney Disease*, **11**, 20–2.

Rudofsky, U. H., Dilworth, R. L. & Tung, K. S. K. (1980). Susceptibility differences of inbred mice to induction of autoimmune renal tubulointerstitial lesions. *Laboratory Investigation*, **43**, 463–70.

Schwartz, M. M., Fennell, J. S. & Lewis, E. J. (1982). Pathologic changes in the renal tubule in systemic lupus erythematosus. *Human Pathology*, **13**, 534–47.

Sherr, D. H., Heghinian, K. M., Benacerraf, B. & Dorf, M. E. (1980). Immune suppression in vivo with antigen-modified syngeneic cells. IV. Requirement for Ia$^+$ adherent cells for induction. *Journal of Immunology*, **124**, 1389–95.

Shih, W., Hines, W. H. & Neilson, E. G. (1988). Effects of cyclosporin A on the development of immune-mediated interstitial nephritis. *Kidney International*, **33**, 1113–18.

Spital, A., Panner, B. J. & Sterns, R. H. (1987). Acute idiopathic tubulointerstitial nephritis: report of two cases and review of the literature. *American Journal of Kidney Disease*, **9**, 71–8.

Steblay, R. W. & Rudofsky, U. (1971). Renal tubular disease and autoantibodies against tubular basement membrane induced in guinea pigs. *Journal of Immunology*, **107**, 589–94.

Steblay, R. W. & Rudofsky, U. (1973). Transfer of experimental autoimmune renal cortical tubular and interstitial disease in guinea pigs by serum. *Science*, **180**, 966–8.

Steinberg, A. D. & Talal, N. (1971). The coexistence of Sjögren's syndrome and systemic lupus erythematosus. *Annals of Internal Medicine*, **74**, 55–61.

Steinman, T. I. & Silva, P. (1984). Acute interstitial nephritis and iritis. Renal-ocular syndrome. *American Journal of Medicine*, **77**, 189–91.

Steinmuller, D. R., Bolton, W. K., Stilmant, M. M. & Couser, W. G. (1979). Chronic interstitial nephritis and mixed cryoglobulinemia associated with drug abuse. *Archives of Pathology & Laboratory Medicine*, **103**, 63–6.

Sugisaki, T., Klassen, J., Milgrom, F., Andres, G. A. & McCluskey, R. T. (1973). Immunopathologic study of an autoimmune tubular and interstitial renal disease in Brown Norway rats. *Laboratory Investigation*, **28**, 658–71.

Sugisaki, T., Yoshida, T., McCluskey, R. T., Andres, G. A. & Klassen, J. (1980). Autoimmune cell-mediated tubulointerstitial nephritis induced in Lewis rats by renal antigen. *Clinical Immunology and Immunopathology*, **15**, 33–43.

Tu, W. H., Shearn, M. A., Lee, J. C. & Hopper, J. (1968). Interstitial nephritis in Sjögren's syndrome. *Annals of Internal Medicine*, **69**, 1163–70.

Ueda, S., Wakashin, M., Wakashin, Y. *et al.* (1988). Autoimmune interstitial nephritis induced in inbred mice. Analysis of mouse tubular basement membrane antigen and genetic control of immune response to it. *American Journal of Pathology*, **132**, 304–18.

van Zwieten, M. J., Bhan, A. K., McCluskey, R. T. & Collins, A. B. (1976). Studies on the pathogenesis of experimental anti-tubular basement membrane nephritis in the guinea pig. *American Journal of Pathology*, **83**, 531–46.

van Zwieten, M. J., Leber, P. D., Bhan, A. K. & McCluskey, R. T. (1977). Experimental cell-mediated interstitial nephritis induced with exogenous antigens. *Journal of Immunology*, **118**, 589–93.

Vargas Arenas, R. E. & Turner, D. R. (1982). Pathology of interstitial nephritis induced in guinea pigs by exoantigens. *Nephron*, **32**, 170–9.

Watson, A. J. S., Dalbow, M. H., Stachura, I. *et al.* (1983). Immunologic studies in cimetidine-induced nephropathy and polymyositis. *New England Journal of Medicine*, **308**, 142–5.

Wilson, C. B., Lehman, D. H., McCoy, R. C., Gunnells, J. C. & Stickel, D. L. (1974). Antitubular basement membrane antibodies after renal transplantation. *Transplantation*, **18**, 447–52.

Wilson, C. B. (1989). Study of the immunopathogenesis of tubulointerstitial nephritis using model systems. *Kidney International*, **35**, 938–53.

Wilson, D. M., Turner, D. R., Cameron, J. S., Ogg, C. S., Brown, C. B. & Chantler, C. (1976). Value of renal biopsy in acute intrinsic renal failure. *British Medical Journal*, **II**, 459–61.

Wilson, R. W., Provost, T. T., Bias, W. B. *et al.* (1984). Sjögren's syndrome. Influence of multiple HLA-D region alloantigens on clinical and serologic expression. *Arthritis and Rheumatism*, **27**, 1245–53.

Winer, R. L., Cohen, A. H., Sawhney, A. S. & Gorman, J. T. (1977). Sjögren's syndrome with immune-complex tubulointerstitial renal disease. *Clinical Immunology and Immunopathology*, **8**, 494–503.

Yeung, C. K., Wong, K. L., Ng, R. P. & Ng, W. L. (1984). Tubular dysfunction in systemic lupus erythematosus. *Nephron*, **36**, 84–8.

Yoshioka, K., Morimoto, Y., Iseki, T. & Maki, S. (1986). Characterization of tubular basement membrane antigens in human kidney. *Journal of Immunology*, **136**, 1654–60.

Zakheim, B., McCafferty, E., Phillips, S. M., Clayman, M. & Neilson, E. G. (1984). Murine interstitial nephritis. II. The adoptive transfer of disease with immune T lymphocytes produces a phenotypically complex interstitial lesion. *Journal of Immunology*, **133**, 234–9.

Zanetti, M., Mampaso, F. & Wilson, C. B. (1983). Anti-idiotype as a probe in the analysis of autoimmune tubulointerstitial nephritis in the Brown Norway rat. *Journal of Immunology*, **131**, 1268–73.

Zanetti, M. & Wilson, C. B. (1983). Characterization of anti-tubular basement membrane antibodies in rats. *Journal of Immunology*, **130**, 2173–9.

-10-
Other renal diseases of immunological interest

Infections and immunologically mediated renal disease

A wide range of infections have been associated with renal pathology which is probably immunologically mediated (Wilson & Dixon, 1986; Glassock *et al.*, 1986). This section will not attempt to be comprehensive, but will concentrate on those conditions of particular importance or immunological interest.

Poststreptococcal glomerulonephritis

Although the link between acute nephritis and infections has been recognised for two centuries, and the particular association with streptococcal disease for a number of decades (Rodríquez-Iturbe, 1988), there are still unanswered questions concerning the pathogenesis of this condition.

The onset of acute nephritis (as manifested by haematuria and fluid retention) typically occurs two to three weeks following infection (usually pharyngeal, but may be cutaneous) with a nephritogenic strain of Group A streptococcus. Such strains are defined on the basis of their M protein, with type 12, amongst others, being particularly nephritogenic (Stetson *et al.*, 1955). The prognosis is good, with less than 1% mortality in the acute attack, and a similar proportion progressing eventually to chronic renal failure (Rodríquez-Iturbe, 1988), although there is some controversy concerning the size of this latter subgroup, particularly in adults (Cameron, 1988). Histology in the acute phase shows an endocapillary proliferative glomerulonephritis, with an increase in mesangial and endothelial cells (Ludwigsen

194

& Sorensen, 1978), as well as infiltration with polymorphonuclear leuko-cytes. The most characteristic lesion on electron microscopy is the subepith-elial 'hump', an electron-dense deposit projecting outward from the base-ment membrane. A number of immunofluorescence patterns (principally for C3, IgG and/or IgM) have been defined (Sorger et al., 1983), with varying degrees of deposition in the mesangium and capillary walls.

Immunogenetics

The possibility of a genetic contribution to susceptibility is supported by an increased attack rate amongst siblings as compared to the general popu-lation (Rodríquez-Iturbe, Rubio & García, 1981). The proportion of affec-ted siblings is compatible with an autosomal recessive trait (Rodríquez-Iturbe et al., 1982), but no genetic markers that might support this hypoth-esis have been identified. Studies of MHC associations have shown an increased incidence of DR4 (Layrisse et al., 1983), a link with another D antigen known as DEn (Sasazuki et al., 1979), or no significant differences between patients and controls (Read et al., 1980; Naito, Kohara & Arak-awa, 1987).

Immunopathology: animal studies

Acute 'one-shot' serum sickness in rabbits bears some similarity to post-streptococcal glomerulonephritis in man; serum sickness is considered further in Chapter 1. A number of studies have used streptococcal antigens to induce renal disease in animals, but it is far from clear what relationship (if any) the resulting models bear to human poststreptococcal glomerulonep-ritis. Thus prolonged exposure to streptococci within diffusion chambers results in a predominantly tubular lesion, probably due to the toxic effects of streptolysin S (Tan & Kaplan, 1962). Repeated immunisation with M protein alone can produce proteinuria and renal impairment (Kantor, 1965), but this is not associated with a glomerulonephritis. However, repeated streptoccocal infection of rabbits does produce a lesion rather similar to poststreptococcal glomerulonephritis in man (Becker & Murphy, 1968). Immunisation of monkeys with streptoccocal antigens may also result in a short-lived glomerulonephritis (Markowitz et al., 1971). Perhaps the model with the closest relationship to human poststreptococcal glomerulo-nephritis is produced by nephritogenic strains of streptococci in sub-cutaneous cages in rabbits (Holm, 1988). The resulting glomerulonephritis is very similar to the human disease. Furthermore, the relevant antigen is only found in nephritogenic strains, and administration of this antigen in isolation is capable of inducing the renal lesion. It may well be that this antigen is the same as one of the proteins proposed as a candidate for the nephritogenic antigen in man (Villareal *et al.*, 1979 and see below).

Immunopathology: human studies

Topics of interest here are the nature of the nephritogenic antigen(s), the means by which immunopathology is produced, and the resulting abnormalities of serology and cellular immunity.

Three criteria have been proposed that should be met by potential nephritogenic antigens (Rodríquez-Iturbe, 1984): the antigen should be found only in nephritogenic strains; the antigen should be identifiable within the glomerulus; and antibodies should be present to the antigen in convalescent sera. The M protein was an obvious candidate, particularly given the experimental models mentioned above. However, the development during convalescence of an antibody that probably identifies the nephritogenic antigen is independent of the M type of the precipitating infection (Treser *et al.*, 1971). In addition, the observation that one episode of poststreptococcal glomerulonephritis provides lasting immunity against a second episode argues for the existence of a common immunising nephritogenic antigen other than the variable M protein. There are a number of other antigens that are more likely candidates, in that they meet (to a variable extent) the three criteria referred to above. These include an extract from disrupted streptococci termed endostreptosin (Lange *et al.*, 1976; Lange, Seligson & Cronin, 1983; Cronin *et al.*, 1989); a protein from streptococcal culture supernatants that has very similar physicochemical characteristics to endostreptosin, although the relationship between the two is undefined (Villareal *et al.*, 1979); a series of cationic proteins also produced from culture supernatants (Vogt *et al.*, 1983); and a protein identified by its heparin-inhibitable binding to basement membrane (Bergey & Stinson, 1988).

The production of immunopathology could, in principle, be due to antigenic crossreactivity between streptococcal components and self-glomerular antigens, deposition of circulating immune complexes, or *in situ* formation of such complexes. Autoantibodies are certainly present in the sera of patients with poststreptococcal glomerulonephritis, and of particular interest are antibodies to basement membrane collagen and laminin, as these could clearly react with renal autoantigens (Kefalides *et al.*, 1986). Whether such antibodies arise due to crossreactivity with streptococcal components is less clear; they could simply represent a response to antigens released from damaged basement membrane. It is possible to produce antibodies, both polyclonal (Kraus & Beachey, 1988) and monoclonal (Zelman & Lange, 1989), that react with both streptococcal and renal antigens, but at least in the case of the polyclonal antisera such reactivity does not appear to be directed against laminin, type IV collagen or heparan-sulfate proteoglycan (Kraus & Beachey, 1988). One final variation on this theme is provided by a possible role for certain M proteins as superantigens (Tomai et al., 1990). Such antigens are able to activate large numbers of T cells of varying specificity, probably by crosslinking MHC molecules to T cell receptors belonging to particular families (such families usually being defined by usage of particular Vβ genes). The suggestion is that such stimulation of subsets of T cells with a degree of potential autoreactivity may allow activation beyond the threshold required for a damaging autoimmune response.

It is difficult to exclude a contribution from the deposition of circulating immune complexes; however, the fact that immunopathology is confined to the kidney, that circulating immune complexes do not correlate with nephritis (see below), that glomerular localisation of some of the candidate nephritogenic antigens mentioned above has been demonstrated (Lange, Seligson & Cronin, 1983; Cronin & Lange, 1990), and that haematuria may be detected at the time of infection before immune complexes could have been formed (Stetson et al., 1955) all suggests that streptococcal components can bind to glomerular structures and act as planted antigen for in situ complex formation. As discussed in Chapter one, this does not exclude some contribution from deposition, or accretion, of circulating complexes.

The serological abnormalities accompanying poststreptococcal glomeru-lonephritis include polyclonal increases in IgG and IgM (Rodríquez-Iturbe et al., 1980) as well as increases in specific antibodies to a number of streptococcal components (e.g. streptolysin O, DNAse B, hyaluronidase), increased amounts of immune complexes (Rodríquez-Iturbe et al., 1980) and cryoglobulins (McIntosh et al., 1970), the presence of rheumatoid factors (McIntosh et al., 1979), and hypocomplementaemia. Some of these abnormalities are probably non-specific. In particular, increased amounts of immune complexes are found following streptococcal infections that do not result in nephritis (van de Rijn et al., 1978). Similarly, the presence of cryoglobulins is probably a reflection of the polyclonal B cell activation and immune complex formation. With respect to the formation of rheumatoid factors, there has been some interest in the possibility that streptococcal neuraminidase may alter the carbohydrate composition of IgG, rendering it immunogenic (McIntosh et al., 1979; Mosquera et al., 1985). It has also been suggested that interactions between IgG and Fc receptors on streptococcal structures may result in an immunogenic complex, and there is some experimental evidence that shows that such complexes can be formed (Schalén et al., 1985). However, polyclonal B cell activation from any cause would be expected to be associated with the presence of rheumatoid factors, and the relevance of these more exotic explanations for their formation is uncertain. Hypocomplementaemia is a particular feature of poststreptococ-cal glomerulonephritis: serum C3 concentrations are reduced in almost 90%

of cases (Rodríquez-Iturbe *et al.*, 1980). Activation appears to be mainly via the alternative pathway (McLean & Michael, 1973), although in some cases there is also evidence for classical pathway activation (Wyatt *et al.*, 1988).

T cells are certainly present in the glomeruli in poststreptococcal glomerulonephritis (Parra *et al.*, 1984), but the significance of this observation is unknown. The *in vitro* T cell responsiveness to glomerular basement antigens found in some cases is almost certainly non-specific, as it is also seen in a range of other glomerulonephritides (Fillit & Zabriskie, 1982). The depressed cellular immune response to streptococcal antigens found in poststreptococcal glomerulonephritis (Reid *et al.*, 1984), in some cases years after the acute event (Bhat, Gombos & Baldwin, 1977), is similarly of uncertain significance.

Infective endocarditis

The incidence of significant glomerulonephritis in infective endocarditis has almost certainly been reduced by effective treatment, but in certain subgroups, such as the endocarditis associated with intravenous drug abuse, it may still occur in more than 15% of cases (Pelletier & Petersdorf, 1977). The clinical manifestations are usually urinary abnormalities, but occasionally an acute nephritic syndrome, a rapidly progressive glomerulonephritis, or, even more rarely, the nephrotic syndrome may develop. The lesions classically described include a focal glomerulonephritis, a diffuse proliferative glomerulonephritis (Bell, 1932), and a possibly distinct proliferative lesion seen in association with acute staphylococcal endocarditis (Tu, Shearn & Lee, 1969).

The focal glomerulonephritis usually consists of areas of necrosis, but immunofluorescence demonstrates diffuse deposits of IgG, IgM and complement components in a predominantly mesangial location (Boulton-Jones *et al.*, 1974). Electron microscopy also shows mesangial deposits. The diffuse proliferative lesion may include duplication of basement membrane and thickening of capillary walls, resembling in some cases mesangiocapillary glomerulonephritis. Immunofluorescence and electron microscopy again show mesangial deposits, together with deposits in subendothelial and subepithelial locations (Gutman *et al.*, 1972). A very few of the cases described have had negative findings on immunofluorescence (Morel-Maroger *et al.*, 1972; Boulton-Jones *et al.*, 1974); the explanation is unclear, but it is possible that the renal lesion was caused by the development of an ANCA positive vasculitis (Wagner, Andrassy & Ritz, 1991; and see Chapter 8), rather than being directly related to the endocarditis. The lesion found in association with acute endocarditis is very similar to that of poststreptococcal glomerulonephritis, including the presence on electron microscopy of subepithelial humps (Tu, Shearn & Lee, 1969). A review of the literature demonstrates a striking association between subepithelial and intramembranous deposits with acute staphylococcal endocarditis on the one hand, and between subendothelial and mesangial deposits with subacute endocarditis on the other (Neugarten & Baldwin, 1984).

The serological abnormalities in infective endocarditis are very similar to those found in poststreptococcal glomerulonephritis, with polyclonal increases in immunoglobulins (Gutman et al., 1972) and increases in antibodies specific for the infecting organism (Laxdal et al., 1968), increased amounts of immune complexes (Bayer & Theofilopoulos, 1989), the presence of rheumatoid factors (Williams & Kunkel, 1962) and cryoglobulins (Hurwitz, Quismorio & Friou, 1975), and hypocomplementaemia. The latter finding usually appears to be due to classical pathway activation, with depression of C4 in addition to C3, but on occasion there is only evidence of alternative pathway activation (O'Connor, Weisman & Fierer, 1978), which may be due to non-immune interactions with bacterial products such as staphylococcal protein A.

The analogies between the abnormalities found in infective endocarditis and poststreptococcal glomerulonephritis suggest similarities in pathogenesis, and this is indeed likely to be the case. Although not as well defined as for streptococci, bacterial antigens (Perez, Rothfield & Williams, 1976) and corresponding antibody (Levy & Hong, 1973) can be found in the glomeruli of patients with infective endocarditis, and the circumstantial evidence that the disease is mediated by immune complexes is strong. Again, the same question as to whether these complexes deposit from the circulation or are formed in situ is relevant here. The lack of a correlation between the amount of circulating complexes and the severity of glomerulonephritis (Cabane et al., 1979) is some evidence for the latter mechanism, but, as previously discussed, the two processes are not mutually exclusive. Differences between the glomerulonephritis of infective endocarditis and poststreptococcal glomerulonephritis are plausibly explained by the more prolonged exposure to antigen in the former condition.

Other bacterial infections

The glomerulonephritis seen in association with infected ventriculo-atrial shunts (Arzee et al., 1983) has a number of factors in common with the glomerulonephritis of infective endocarditis and no doubt has a similar immunopathogenesis. Both share the features secondary to chronic stimulation of the immune system, with polyclonal increases in immunoglobulins, immune complex formation, the presence of rheumatoid factors and cryoglobulins, and hypocomplementaemia. Bacterial antigens, usually from coagulase-negative staphylococci, have been found in the glomeruli (Kaufman & McIntosh, 1971). The typical histological pattern is that of a type I mesangiocapillary glomerulonephritis, although occasionally only mesangial proliferation is seen. Immune deposits are seen by immunofluorescence and electron microscopy, predominantly in the capillary walls. The major point of difference between the renal lesions of infective endocarditis and infected ventriculo-atrial shunts is clinical: the nephrotic syndrome is much more frequent in the latter condition, and in some series is present in the majority of patients (Stickler et al., 1968).

Many other bacterial infections have been implicated in the immunopathogenesis of presumed immune complex-mediated glomerulonephritis (Wilson & Dixon, 1986); two examples will be briefly mentioned. The glomerulonephritis found in association with visceral sepsis (Beaufils et al., 1977) is clearly closely related to that found in cases of infective endocarditis and infected ventriculo-atrial shunts, although a presentation with acute renal failure is perhaps more common. Syphilis, both congenital (Sanchez-Bayle et al., 1983) and acquired (Gamble & Reardon, 1975), may be associated with a membranous or mesangiocapillary nephropathy (Weiner & Northcutt, 1989) and the nephrotic syndrome. The elution of anti-treponemal antibodies (Gamble & Reardon, 1975) and the demonstration of treponemal antigens within the glomerulus (Sanchez-Bayle et al., 1983) lends support to the concept of an immune complex pathogenesis, but the possibility of non-specific trapping must be borne in mind (see Chapter 3).

Other infections

Although a number of protozoal infections are associated with a glomerulopathy (Wilson & Dixon, 1986) the most important is malaria, and, in particular, malaria caused by plasmodium malariae (quartan malaria) (Houba, 1979). The presentation is with the nephrotic syndrome, and in endemic areas the incidence of the nephrotic syndrome is considerably raised (Kibukamusoke, Hutt & Wilks, 1967). Histologically, the appearances are not typical of a conventional category but show a combination of features (capillary wall thickening, segmental glomerular sclerosis) which are said to be characteristic (Hendrickse et al., 1972). Parasite antigens have been detected by immunofluorescence in affected glomeruli (Hendrickse et al., 1972), and specific antibody found in renal eluates (Allison et al., 1969). However, treatment of the underlying infection, in general, does not lead to significant improvement in the renal lesion, although prolonged prophylactic therapy together with steroids may be beneficial (Kibukamusoke, 1968). Thus, although parasite antigen–antibody complexes are clearly implicated, other ill-defined immunopathological processes may also be involved. A rather similar situation exists with respect to the nephropathy (a mesangioproliferative or mesangiocapillary glomerulonephritis) seen in association with schistosomiasis (Sobh *et al.*, 1988), which is unaffected by anti-parasite or immunosuppressive treatment (Martinelli *et al.*, 1989).

Hepatitis B is perhaps the virus most frequently linked to renal immunopathology; specific instances are discussed further in the chapters on membranous nephropathy, IgA nephropathy, and systemic vasculitis. More recently, human immunodeficiency virus (HIV) has been associated with a range of glomerular lesions, most frequently a focal glomerulosclerosis (Rao *et al.*, 1984; Pardo *et al.*, 1984); the pathogenesis is unknown, although direct renal infection by the virus is a possibility (Seney, Burns & Silva, 1990).

Cryoglobulins and other abnormal B cell products

The conditions considered under this heading are often the reflection of an underlying monoclonal B cell proliferation, and may indeed be frankly neoplastic. This latter group is only mentioned very briefly for completeness, but there is much of interest in the immunopathology associated with cryoglobulins, which may or may not be associated with neoplasia.

Cryoglobulinaemia

Immunoglobulins that precipitate in the cold can be classified into three types (Brouet *et al.*, 1974). Electrophoresis of a type I cryoglobulin reveals a single monoclonal band; this type is usually the product of obvious neoplastic disease such as myeloma or Waldenström's macroglobulinaemia. Types II and III are both associated with the presence of rheumatoid factors which bind to and precipitate a polyclonal IgG population; in type II the rheumatoid factor is monoclonal, whereas in type III it is polyclonal. In both cases the rheumatoid factor is usually (but not always: Wager, Mustakallio & Räsänen, 1968) IgM. As with type I, type II cryoglobulinaemia may be associated with an underlying neoplasm, or with Sjögren's syndrome which may itself sometimes evolve into lymphoma. Type III cryoglobulins are usually found in diseases that involve chronic stimulation of the immune system, such as chronic infections and autoimmune conditions. With respect to chronic infections, hepatitis B is often featured, although this relationship is controversial (Levo, 1981; D'Amico *et al.*, 1989). In both types II and III there may be no obvious underlying disease, and the condition is then termed mixed essential cryoglobulinaemia. Although renal involvement may occur in all types of cryoglobulinaemia, this is most frequent in type II mixed cryoglobulinaemia (D'Amico *et al.*, 1989), which will be the main subject of the rest of this section.

Type II cryoglobulinaemia is a systemic disease, often associated with a vasculitis. Arthralgias, a purpuric skin rash, and hepatomegaly are the commonest extra-renal features (Tarantino *et al.*, 1981; Montagnino, 1988); renal manifestations may range from haematuria and proteinuria to the nephrotic syndrome or an acute nephritic picture. Histologically, there is a proliferative glomerulonephritis, very often with thickening and double contouring of the basement membrane giving a mesangiocapillary pattern. Characteristic features are a heavy infiltration with monocytes (Castiglione *et al.*, 1988; D'Amico *et al.*, 1989) and the presence of large subendothelial and/or intraluminal deposits. Immunofluorescence reveals deposits of C3 and immunoglobulins (the latter usually corresponding to the composition of the circulating cryoglobulin) predominantly localised to the capillary walls in a subendothelial position; when present, the intraluminal deposits also stain for immunoglobulin. On electron microscopy, the subendothelial and intraluminal deposits may have a crystalline or fibrillar appearance (Feiner & Gallo, 1977).

Immunopathology

Topics of interest here are a consideration of the factors that lead to the formation of cryoglobulins, the reasons for their particular properties, and the means by which they produce pathology.

It seems reasonably clear that the production of a type I cryoglobulin reflects the secretory activity of a neoplastic B cell clone, and that the production of a type III cryoglobulin is due to chronic polyclonal stimulation, in which the production of rheumatoid factors may be a normal part of this type of response. What is less clear is the status of type II cryoglobulins. In some cases it seems likely that this also reflects an underlying neoplastic state, as overt lymphoma may develop with time (Brouet *et al.*, 1974), although this is by no means always the case (Gorevic *et al.*, 1980). On the other hand, type II cryoglobulins may also be seen in conditions characterised by polyclonal activation, such as rheumatoid arthritis or Sjögren's syndrome. The observation that many of the monoclonal components of type II cryoglobulins from different individuals share crossreactive idiotypes (Abraham *et al.*, 1983; Ono *et al.*, 1987) may be relevant here. Genes encoding rheumatoid factors appear to be common among humans (Carson *et al.*, 1987), and in many cases share common germline sequences (Chen *et al.*, 1986). The conservation of such genes implies that they are performing an important function, although the nature of this remains speculative. Whatever their function, paraneoplastic transformation of cells expressing products of such genes (perhaps due in some cases to the Epstein Barr virus: Fiorini *et al.*, 1988), or possibly prolonged antigenic stimulation, could result in the expansion of a single clone, with the resultant formation of a type II cryoglobulin.

The physicochemical factors responsible for the phenomenon of cryoprecipitation are unclear (Wang, 1988). Both components of a mixed cryoglobulin have been found to be needed for cryoprecipitability (Klein et al., 1968), so that properties of individual immunoglobulins (class, subclass, charge, carbohydrate content), although they may be necessary, are not sufficient. A number of additional factors such as Fc–Fc interactions, antigen/antibody ratio and fibronectin content may also be implicated (Wang, 1988).

The immunopathology of cryoglobulinaemia is that of an immune complex disease. There may, however, be an interesting dissociation between the pathology produced by complexes formed by virtue of rheumatoid factor activity, and that produced by complexes presumably formed as a result of the cryoprecipitable properties of the immunoglobulin; studies in a murine system demonstrate that both rheumatoid factor activity and cryoglobulin activity are required for the development of cutaneous vasculitis, whereas cryoglobulin activity alone suffices for the development of glomerulonephritis (Reininger et al., 1990). As is often the case, the relative contribution from deposition of preformed circulating complexes on the one hand, versus that from complexes formed in situ on the other, is uncertain. Circulating immune complexes are (unsurprisingly) present, although the correlation with amount of cryoglobulin is imperfect (Winfield, 1983), and the characteristic complement abnormalities (very low C1, C4 and C2, slightly low C3: Tarantino et al., 1978; Gorevic et al., 1980) are suggestive of generalised activation via the classical pathway. However, the massive deposits not uncommonly found within the glomeruli must be the result of in situ accretion. Of interest is the fact that, although C3 is routinely found in association with glomerular deposits, earlier complement components are only found in about half the cases (Tarantino et al., 1981). It is possible that two separate processes are occurring. The classical pathway is involved in the inhibition of immune precipitation (Schifferli, Steiger & Schapira, 1985), and this function may be responsible for the systemic complement abnormalities. In particular, the complexes in type II mixed essential cryoglobulinaemia are able to fix sufficient C4 to form a fluid phase C3 convertase, but are relatively inefficient at fixing C3 (Ng, Peters & Walport, 1988). As a result, clearance via the normal CR1 receptor mechanism on red blood cells is impeded, leading to persistence of phlogistic complexes. Precipitated, aggregated immunoglobulin, however, can activate the alternative pathway, which would normally lead to solubilization (Fujita, Takata & Tamura, 1981); this could explain the relative deficiency of deposited early complement components.

Therapeutic aspects in cryoglobulinaemia

Problems with assessing the effect of treatment arise from the appreciable rate of spontaneous recovery of patients with deteriorating renal function (approximately 45%; De Vecchi *et al.*, 1983) and the lack of controlled studies. However, it appears that the use of oral steroids, plus or minus cytotoxic agents, is associated with a recovery rate of about 50% (De Vecchi *et al.*, 1983), suggesting that these agents are of no additional benefit. Most interest in attempting to modify the course of renal impairment in this disease has focused on the use of intravenous pulse methylprednisolone or plasmapheresis. The former therapy certainly leads to an improvement in extrarenal features, and, in one study, was also followed by an improvement in renal function in nine out of ten cases (De Vecchi *et al.*, 1983). Plasmapheresis is attractive because of its ability to remove circulating cryoglobulin, and a number of reports attest to its effectiveness, usually when combined with steroids and/or cytotoxic drugs (for review see D'Amico *et al.*, 1989). There is a report of a prolonged remission produced by intravenous immunoglobulin in a patient with limited response to immunosuppression and plasmapheresis (Boom *et al.*, 1988).

Paraproteins

A variety of more or less malignant monoclonal B cell disorders may be associated with the production of paraproteins with the potential for renal deposition. These include Waldenström's macroglobulinaemia (Morel-Maroger *et al.*, 1970), light chain nephropathy, AL type amyloidosis (Ganeval *et al.*, 1984), and myeloma, which may be associated with either of the two proceeding entities as well as with the intratubular deposits of paraprotein producing 'myeloma kidney' (Pirani *et al.*, 1987). In general, the damage caused by these deposits is not caused by immunopathological mechanisms.

References

Abraham, G. N., Podell, D. N., Welch, E. H. & Johnston, S. L. (1983). Idiotypic relatedness of human monoclonal IgG cryoglobulins. *Immunology*, **48**, 315–20.

Allison, A. C., Houba, V., Hendrickse, R. G., De Petris, S., Edington, G. M. & Adeniyi, A. (1969). Immune complexes in the nephrotic syndrome of African children. *Lancet*, i, 1232–8.

Arzee, R. S., Rashid, H., Morley, R., Ward, M. K. & Kerr, D. N. S. (1983). Shunt nephritis: report of two cases and review of the literature. *Clinical Nephrology*, **19**, 48–53.

Bayer, A. S. & Theofilopoulos, A. N. (1989). Immune complexes in infective endocarditis. *Springer Seminars in Immunopathology*, **11**, 457–69.

Beaufils, M., Morel-Maroger, L., Sraer, J-D., Kanfer, A., Kourilsky, O. & Richet, G. (1977). Acute renal failure of glomerular origin during visceral abscesses. *New England Journal of Medicine*, **295**, 185–9.

Becker, E. G. & Murphy, G. E. (1968). The experimental induction of glomerulonephritis like that in man by infection with Group A streptococci. *Journal of Experimental Medicine*, **127**, 1–24.

Bell, E. T. (1932). Glomerular lesions associated with endocarditis. *American Journal of Pathology*, **8**, 639–64.

Bergey, E. J. & Stinson, M. W. (1988). Heparin-inhibitable basement membrane-binding protein of *Streptococcus pyogenes*. *Infection and Immunity*, **56**, 1715–21.

Bhat, J. G., Gombos, E. A. & Baldwin, D. S. (1977). Depressed cellular immune response to streptococcal antigens in poststreptococcal glomerulonephritis. *Clinical Immunology and Immunopathology*, **7**, 230–9.

Boom, B. W., Brand, A., Bavinck, J-N. B., Eernisse, J. G., Daha, M. R. & Vermeer, B. J. (1988). Severe leukocytoclastic vasculitis of the skin in a patient with essential mixed cryoglobulinemia treated with high-dose gamma-globulin intravenously. *Archives of Dermatology*, **124**, 1550–3.

Boulton-Jones, J. M., Sissons, J. G. P., Evans, D. J. & Peters, D. K. (1974). Renal lesions of subacute infective endocarditis. *British Medical Journal*, **2**, 11–14.

Brouet, J-C., Clauvel, J-P., Danon, F., Klein, M. & Seligmann, M. (1974). Biologic and clinical significance of cryoglobulins. A report of 86 cases. *American Journal of Medicine*, **57**, 775–88.

Cabane, J., Godeau, P., Herreman, G., Acar, J., Digeon, M. & Bach, J-F. (1979). Fate of circulating immune complexes in infective endocarditis. *American Journal of Medicine*, **66**, 277–82.

Cameron, J. S. (1988). The long-term outcome of glomerular disease. In *Diseases of the Kidney*, 4th edn, ed. R. W. Schrier & C. W. Gottschalk, pp. 2127–89. Boston/Toronto: Little, Brown and Company.

Carson, D. A., Chen, P. P., Kipps, T. J. et. al. (1987). Idiotypic and genetic studies of human rheumatoid factors. *Arthritis and Rheumatism*, **30**, 1321–5.

Castiglione, A., Bucci, A., Fellin, G., D'Amico, G. & Atkins, R. C. (1988). The relationship of infiltrating renal leucocytes to disease activity in lupus and cryoglobulinaemic glomerulonephritis. *Nephron*, **50**, 14–23.

Chen, P. P., Albrandt, K., Orida, N. K. et al. (1986). Genetic basis for the cross-reactive idiotypes on the light chains of human IgM anti-IgG autoantibodies. *Proceedings of the National Academy of Sciences, USA*, **83**, 8318–22.

Cronin, W., Deol, H., Azadegan, A. & Lange, K. (1989). Endostreptosin: isolation of the probable immunogen of acute poststreptococcal glomerulonephritis (PSGN). *Clinical and Experimental Immunology*, **76**, 198–203.

Cronin, W. J. & Lange, K. (1990). Immunologic evidence for the *in situ* deposition of a cytoplasmic streptococcal antigen (endostreptosin) on the glomerular basement membrane in rats. *Clinical Nephrology*, **34**, 143–6.

D'Amico, G., Colasanti, G., Ferrario, F. & Sinico, R. A. (1989). Renal involvement in essential mixed cryoglobulinemia. *Kidney International*, **35**, 1004–14.

De Vecchi, A., Montagnino, G., Pozzi, C., Tarantino, A., Locatelli, F. & Ponticelli, C. (1983). Intravenous methylprednisolone pulse therapy in essential mixed cryoglobulinemia nephropathy. *Clinical Nephrology*, **19**, 221–7.

Feiner, H. & Gallo, G. (1977). Ultrastructure in glomerulonephritis associated with cryoglobulinemia. A report of six cases and review of the literature. *American Journal of Pathology*, **88**, 145–62.

Fillit, H. M. & Zabriskie, J. B. (1982). Cellular immunity in glomerulonephritis. *American Journal of Pathology*, **109**, 227–43.

Fiorini, G. F., Sinico, R. A., Winearls, C., Custode, P., De Giuli-Morghen, C. & D'Amico, G. (1988). Persistent Epstein-Barr virus infection in patients with type II essential mixed cryoglobulinemia. *Clinical Immunology and Immunopathology*, **47**, 262–9.

Fujita, T., Takata, Y. & Tamura, N. (1981). Solubilization of immune precipitates by six isolated alternative pathway proteins. *Journal of Experimental Medicine*, **154**, 1743–51.

Gamble, C. N. & Reardon, J. B. (1975). Immunopathogensis of syphilitic glomerulonephritis. Elution of antitreponemal antibody from glomerular immune-complex deposits. *New England Journal of Medicine*, **292**, 449–54.

Ganeval, D., Noël, L-H., Preud'homme, J-L., Droz, D. & Grünfeld, J-P. (1984). Light-chain deposition disease: its relation with AL-type amyloidosis. *Kidney International*, **26**, 1–9.

Glassock, R. J., Cohen, A. H., Adler, S. G. & Ward, H. J. (1986). Secondary glomerular disease. In *The Kidney*, 3rd edn, ed. B. M. Brenner & F. C. Rector, pp. 1014–84. Philadelphia: W.B. Saunders Company.

Gorevic, P. D., Kassab, H. J., Levo, Y. *et al.* (1980). Mixed cryoglobulinemia: clinical aspects and long-term follow-up of 40 patients. *American Journal of Medicine*, **69**, 287–308.

Gutman, R. A., Striker, G. E., Gilliland, B. C. & Cutler, R. E. (1972). The immune complex glomerulonephritis of bacterial endocarditis. *Medicine*, **51**, 1–25.

Hendrickse, R. G., Glasgow, E. F., Adeniyi, A., White, R. H. R., Edington, G. M. & Houba, V. (1972). Quartan malarial nephrotic syndrome. Collaborative clinicopathological study in Nigerian children. *Lancet*, i, 1143–9.

Holm, S. E. (1988). The pathogenesis of acute poststreptococcal glomerulonephritis in new lights. *APMIS*, **96**, 189–93.

Houba, V. (1979). Immunologic aspects of renal lesions associated with malaria. *Kidney International*, **16**, 3–8.

Hurwitz, D., Quismorio, F. P. & Friou, G. J. (1975). Cryoglobulinaemia in patients with infectious endocarditis. *Clinical and Experimental Immunology*, **19**, 131–41.

Kantor, F. S. (1965). Fibrinogen precipitation by streptococcal M protein. II. Renal lesions induced by intravenous injection of M protein into mice and rats. *Journal of Experimental Medicine*, **121**, 861–72.

Kaufman, D. B. & McIntosh, R. (1971). The pathogenesis of the renal lesion in a patient with streptococcal disease, infected ventriculoatrial shunt, cryoglobulinemia and nephritis. *American Journal of Medicine*, **50**, 262–8.

Kefalides, N. A., Pegg, M. T., Ohno, N., Poon-King, T., Zabriskie, N. & Fillit, H. (1986). Antibodies to basement membrane collagen and laminin are present in sera from patients with poststreptococcal glomerulonephritis. *Journal of Experimental Medicine*, **163**, 585–602.

Kibukamusoke, J. (1968). Malaria prophylaxis and immunosuppressant therapy in management of nephrotic syndrome associated with quartan malaria. *Archives of Disease in Childhood*, **43**, 598–600.

Kibukamusoke, J. W., Hutt, M. S. R. & Wilks, N. E. (1967). The nephrotic syndrome in Uganda and its association with quartan malaria. *Quarterly Journal of Medicine*, **36**, 393–408.

Klein, F., van Rood, J. J., van Furth, R. & Radema, H. (1968). IgM–IgG cryoglobulinaemia with IgM paraprotein component. *Clinical and Experimental Immunology*, **3**, 703–16.

Kraus, W. & Beachey, E. M. (1988). Renal autoimmune epitope of group A streptococci specified by M protein tetrapeptide Ile–Arg–Leu–Arg. *Proceedings of the National Academy of Sciences, USA*, **85**, 4516–20.

Lange, K., Ahmed, U., Kleinberger, H. & Treser, G. (1976). A hitherto unknown streptococcal antigen and its probable relation to acute poststreptococcal glomerulonephritis. *Clinical Nephrology*, **5**, 207–15.

Lange, K., Seligson, G. & Cronin, W. (1983). Evidence for the *in situ* origin of poststreptococcal glomerulonephritis: glomerular localization of endostreptosin and the clinical significance of the subsequent antibody response. *Clinical Nephrology*, **19**, 3–10.

Laxdal, T., Messner, R. P., Williams, R. C. & Quie, P. G. (1968). Opsonic, agglutinating, and complement-fixing antibodies in patients with subacute bacterial endocarditis. *Journal of Laboratory and Clinical Medicine*, **71**, 638–53.

Layrisse, Z., Rodríquez-Iturbe, B., García, R., Rodríquez, Z. & Tiwari, J. (1983). Family studies of the HLA system in acute poststreptococcal glomerulonephritis. *Human Immunology*, **7**, 177–85.

Levo, Y. (1981). Hepatitis B virus and essential mixed cryoglobulinemia. *Annals of Internal Medicine*, **94**, 282.

Levy, R. L. & Hong, R. (1973). The immune nature of subacute bacterial endocarditis (SBE) nephritis. *American Journal of Medicine*, **54**, 645–52.

Ludwigsen, E. & Sorensen, F. H. (1978). Poststreptococcal glomerulonephritis. A quantitative glomerular investigation. *APMIS*, **86A**, 319–24.

Markowitz, A. S., Horn, D., Aseron, C., Novak, R. & Battifora, H. A. (1971). Streptococcal related glomerulonephritis. III. Glomerulonephritis in Rhesus monkeys immunologically induced both actively and passively with a soluble fraction from nephritogenic streptococcal protoplasmic membranes. *Journal of Immunology*, **107**, 504–11.

Martinelli, R., Noblat, A. C. B., Brito, E. & Rocha, H. (1989). *Schistosoma mansoni*-induced mesangiocapillary glomerulonephritis: influence of therapy. *Kidney International*, **35**, 1227–33.

McIntosh, R. M., Kaufman, D. B., Kulvinskas, C. & Grossman, B. J. (1970). Cryoglobulins. I. Studies on the nature, incidence, and clinical significance of serum cryoproteins in glomerulonephritis. *Journal of Laboratory and Clinical Medicine*, **75**, 566–77.

McIntosh, R. M., Rabideau, D., Allen, J. E. *et al.* (1979). Acute poststreptococcal glomerulonephritis in Maracaibo. II. Studies on the incidence, nature, and significance of circulating anti-immunoglobulins. *Annals of the Rheumatic Diseases*, **38**, 257–61.

McLean, R. H. & Michael, A. F. (1973). Properdin and C3 proactivator: alternate pathway components in human glomerulonephritis. *Journal of Clinical Investigation*, **52**, 634–44.

Montagnino, G. (1988). Reappraisal of the clinical expression of mixed cryoglobulinemia. *Springer Seminars in Immunopathology*, **10**, 1–19.

Morel-Maroger, L., Basch, A., Danon, F., Verroust, P. & Richet, G. (1970). Pathology of the kidney in Waldenström's macroglobulinemia. Study of sixteen cases. *New England Journal of Medicine*, **283**, 123–9.

Morel-Maroger, L., Sraer, J-D., Herreman, G. & Godeau, P. (1972). Kidney in subacute endocarditis. Pathological and immunofluorescence findings. *Archives of Pathology*, **94**, 205–13.

Mosquera, J. A., Katiyar, V. N., Coello, J. & Rodríquez-Iturbe, B. (1985). Neuraminidase production by streptococci from patients with glomerulonephritis. *Journal of Infectious Disease*, **151**, 259–63.

Naito, S., Kohara, M. & Arakawa, K. (1987). Association of Class II antigens of HLA with primary glomerulopathies. *Nephron*, **45**, 111–4.

Neugarten, J. & Baldwin, D. S. (1984). Glomerulonephritis in bacterial endocarditis. *American Journal of Medicine*, **77**, 297–304.

Ng, Y. C., Peters, D. K. & Walport, M. J. (1988). Monoclonal rheumatoid factor-IgG immune complexes. Poor fixation of opsonic C4 and C3 despite efficient complement activation. *Arthritis and Rheumatism*, **31**, 99–107.

O'Connor, D. T., Weisman, M. H. & Fierer, J. (1978). Activation of the alternate complement pathway in *Staph. aureus* infective endocarditis and its relationship to thrombocytopenia, coagulation abnormalities, and acute glomerulonephritis. *Clinical and Experimental Immunology*, **34**, 179–87.

Ono, M., Winearls, C. G., Amos, N. *et al.* (1987). Monoclonal antibodies to restricted and cross-reactive idiotopes on monoclonal rheumatoid factors and their recognition of idiotope positive cells. *European Journal of Immunology*, **17**, 343–9.

Pardo, V., Aldana, M., Colton, R. M. et al. (1984). Glomerular lesions in the acquired immunodeficiency syndrome. Annals of Internal Medicine, 101, 429–34.

Parra, G., Platt, J. L., Falk, R. J., Rodríquez-Iturbe, B. & Michael, A. F. (1984). Cell populations and membrane attack complex in glomeruli of patients with poststreptococcal glomerulonephritis: identification using monoclonal antibodies by indirect immunofluorescence. Clinical Immunology and Immunopathology, 33, 324–32.

Pelletier, L. L. & Petersdorf, R. G. (1977). Infective endocarditis: a review of 125 cases from the University of Washington Hospitals, 1963–72. Medicine, 56, 287–313.

Perez, G. O., Rothfield, N. & Williams, R. C. (1976). Immune-complex nephritis in bacterial endocarditis. Archives of Internal Medicine, 136, 334–6.

Pirani, C. L., Silva, F., D'Agati, V., Chander, P. & Striker, L. M. M. (1987). Renal lesions in plasma cell dyscrasias: ultrastructural observations. American Journal of Kidney Disease, 10, 208–21.

Rao, T. K. S., Filippone, E. J., Nicastri, A. D. et al. (1984). Associated focal and segmental glomerulosclerosis in the acquired immunodeficiency syndrome. New England Journal of Medicine, 310, 669–73.

Read, S. E., Poon-King, T., Reid, H. F. M. & Zabriskie, J. B. (1980). HLA and group A streptococcal sequelae. In Streptoccoal Diseases and the Immune Response, ed. S. E. Read & J. B. Zabriskie, pp. 347–53. New York: Academic Press.

Reid, H. F. M., Read, S. E., Zabriskie, J. B., Ramkissoon, R. & Poon-King, T. (1984). Suppression of cellular reactivity to Group A streptococcal antigens in patients with acute poststreptococcal glomerulonephritis. Journal of Infectious Disease, 149, 841–50.

Reininger, L., Berney, T., Shibata, T., Spertini, F., Merino, R. & Izui, S. (1990). Cryoglobulinemia induced by a murine IgG3 rheumatoid factor: skin vasculitis and glomerulonephritis arise from distinct pathogenic mechanisms. Proceedings of the National Academy of Sciences, USA, 87, 10038–42.

Rodríquez-Iturbe, B., Carr, R. I., García, R., Rabideau, D., Rubio, L. & McIntosh, R. M. (1980). Circulating immune complexes and serum immunoglobulins in acute poststreptococcal glomerulonephritis. Clinical Nephrology, 13, 1–4.

Rodríquez-Iturbe, B., Rubio, L. & García, R. (1981). Attack rate of poststreptococcal nephritis in families. A prospective study. Lancet, i, 401–3.

Rodríquez-Iturbe, B., Moreno-Fuenmayor, H., Rubio, L., García, R. & Layrisse, Z. (1982). Mendelian recessive ratios in acute poststreptococcal glomerulonephritis. Experientia, 38, 918–19.

Rodríquez-Iturbe, B. (1984). Epidemic poststreptococcal glomerulonephritis. Kidney International, 25, 129–36.

Rodríquez-Iturbe, B. (1988). Acute poststreptococcal glomerulonephritis. In Diseases of the Kidney, 4th edn, ed. R. W. Schrier & C. W. Gottschalk, pp. 1929–47. Boston/Toronto: Little, Brown and Company.

Sanchez-Bayle, M., Ecija, J. L., Estepa, R., Cambronero, M. J. & Martinez, M. A. (1983). Incidence of glomerulonephritis in congenital syphilis. Clinical Nephrology, 20, 27–31.

Sasazuki, T., Hayase, R., Iwamoto, I. & Tsuchida, H. (1979). HLA and acute poststreptococcal glomerulonephritis. New England Journal of Medicine, 301, 1184–5.

Schalén, C., Truedsson, L., Christensen, K. K. & Christensen, P. (1985). Blocking of antibody complement-dependent effector functions by streptococcal IgG Fc-receptor and staphylococcal protein A. APMIS, 93B, 395–400.

Schifferli, J. A., Steiger, G. & Schapira, M. (1985). The role of C1, C1-inactivator and C4 in modulating immune precipitation. Clinical and Experimental Immunology, 60, 605–12.

Seney, F. D., Burns, D. K. & Silva, F. G. (1990). Acquired immunodeficiency syndrome and the kidney. American Journal of Kidney Disease, 16, 1–13.

Sobh, M. A., Moustafa, F. E., Sally, S. M., Deelder, A. M. & Ghoniem, M. A. (1988). Characterisation of kidney lesions in early schistosomal-specific nephropathy. *Nephrology Dialysis and Transplantation*, 3, 392–8.

Sorger, K., Gessler, U., Hübner, F. K. et al. (1983). Subtypes of acute postinfectious glomerulonephritis. Synopsis of clinical and pathological features. *Clinical Nephrology*, 17, 114–28.

Stetson, C. A., Rammelkamp, C. H., Krause, R. M., Kohen, R. J. & Perry, W. D. (1955). Epidemic acute nephritis: studies on etiology, natural history and prevention. *Medicine*, 34, 431–50.

Stickler, G. B., Shin, M. H., Burke, E. C., Holley, K. E., Miller, R. H. & Segar, W. E. (1968). Diffuse glomerulonephritis associated with infected ventriculoatrial shunt. *New England Journal of Medicine*, 279, 1077–82.

Tan, E. M. & Kaplan, M. H. (1962). Renal tubular lesions in mice produced by streptococci in intraperitoneal diffusion chambers. Role of streptolysin S. *Journal of Infectious Disease*, 110, 55–62.

Tarantino, A., Anelli, A., Costantino, A., De Vecchi, A., Monti, G. & Massaro, L. (1978). Serum complement pattern in essential mixed cryoglobulinaemia. *Clinical and Experimental Immunology*, 32, 77–85.

Tarantino, A., De Vechi, A., Montagnino, G. et al. (1981). Renal disease in essential mixed cryoglobulinaemia. Long-term follow-up in 44 patients. *Quarterly Journal of Medicine*, 50, 1–30.

Tomai, M., Kotb, M., Majumdar, G. & Beachey, E. H. (1990). Superantigenicity of streptococcal M protein. *Journal of Experimental Medicine*, 172, 359–62.

Treser, G., Semar, M., Sagel, I. et al. (1971). Independence of the nephritogenicity of group A streptococci from their M types. *Clinical and Experimental Immunology*, 9, 57–62.

Tu, W. H., Shearn, M. A. & Lee, J. C. (1969). Acute diffuse glomerulonephritis in acute staphylococcal endocarditis. *Annals of Internal Medicine*, 71, 335–41.

van de Rijn, I., Fillit, H., Brandeis, W. E. et al. (1978). Serial studies on circulating immune complexes in poststreptococcal sequelae. *Clinical and Experimental Immunology*, 34, 318–25.

Villareal, H., Fischetti, V. A., van de Rijn, I. & Zabriskie, J. B. (1979). The occurrence of a protein in the extracellular products of streptococci isolated from patients with acute glomerulonephritis. *Journal of Experimental Medicine*, 149, 459–72.

Vogt, A., Batsford, S., Rodríquez-Iturbe, B. & García, R. (1983). Cationic antigens in poststreptococcal glomerulonephritis. *Clinical Nephrology*, 20, 271–9.

Wager, O., Mustakallio, K. K. & Räsänen, J. A. (1968). Mixed IgA–IgG cryoglobulinemia. Immunological studies and case reports of three patients. *American Journal of Medicine*, 44, 179–87.

Wagner, J., Andrassy, K. & Ritz, E. (1991). Is vasculitis in subacute bacterial endocarditis associated with ANCA? *Lancet*, 337, 799–800.

Wang, A-C. (1988). Molecular basis for cryoprecipitation. *Springer Seminars in Immunopathology*, 10, 21–34.

Weiner, I. D. & Northcutt, A. D. (1989). Leprosy and glomerulonephritis: case report and review of the literature. *American Journal of Kidney Disease*, 13, 424–9.

Williams, R. E. & Kunkel, H. G. (1962). Rheumatoid factor, complement, and conglutinin aberrations in patients with subacute bacterial endocarditis. *Journal of Clinical Investigation*, 41, 666–75.

Wilson, C. B. & Dixon, F. J. (1986). The renal response to immunological injury. In *The Kidney*, 3rd edn, ed. B. M. Brenner & F. C. Rector, pp. 800–89. Philadelphia: W.B.Saunders Company.

Winfield, J. B. (1983). Cryoglobulinemia. *Human Pathology*, 14, 350–4.

Wyatt, R. J., Forristal, J., West, C. D., Sugimoto, S. & Curd, J. G. (1988). Complement profiles in acute poststreptococcal glomerulonephritis. *Pediatric Nephrology*, 2, 219–23.
Zelman, M. E. & Lange, C. F. (1989). Isolation and partial characterization of antigens from basement membranes and streptococcal cell membrane (SCM) employing anti-SCM monoclonal antibody. *Molecular Immunology*, 26, 915–23.

–11–
Therapeutic aspects

Aspects of therapy pertinent to individual diseases have been dealt with in the appropriate chapters. This final chapter attempts to unify and summarise these aspects, and to discuss some of the general principles that might underlie future (or at present experimental) therapeutic strategies for immune-mediated renal disease, using where necessary examples from other autoimmune models or diseases. Mirroring the structure of the introductory chapter, such strategies can be classified broadly into those that attempt to re-establish a state of tolerance, which may be somewhat artificial when achieved by immunosuppression, and those that interfere with the various non-specific mediators of tissue damage. Again, attempts to engage endogenous immunoregulatory mechanisms are considered under the first of these categories.

Re-establishment of the 'tolerant' state

Non-specific immunosuppression

In most cases in which a remission of autoimmunity is induced by immuno-suppression, the resulting 'tolerant' state is artificial and dependent on continuing immunosuppression. A good examples of this is immunotherapy for new onset insulin dependent diabetes mellitus: it is perfectly possible to induce a remission, but the disease eventually relapses, and does so rapidly if treatment is stopped (Feutren et al., 1988). However, in certain diseases it may be possible to establish a true state of tolerance. Thus if treatment in anti-glomerular basement membrane (GBM) disease is stopped once anti-GBM antibodies have disappeared, recurrence is very unusual (Rees & Lockwood, 1988). It has been hypothesised that any manoeuvre that weakens the interaction between T cell and antigen presenting cell is potentially tolerogenic (Waldmann, 1989). This could be achieved by a variety of approaches, although perhaps most easily with anti-T cell strate-gies (see next section). In this sense, non-specific immunosuppression, if we only knew how to use it, might be capable of inducing a state of true tolerance in a much wider range of autoimmune diseases.

Therapy directed against T cells

The key role played by T cells in the maintenance and breakdown of tolerance makes them a particularly attractive target. Furthermore, although there are exceptions, such as the autonomous production of rheumatoid factor in mixed essential cryoglobulinaemia, autoantibody production is usually T cell dependent, and such therapy may therefore also be effective in autoantibody-mediated disease.

Considering possible approaches in order of increasing specificity, the first is a non-selective attack on all T cells. Cyclosporin A is an agent that falls into this category, and has been used with some success in autoimmunity (Sandoz Medical Documentation, 1989). Apart from its lack of selectivity, the main problem is that the drug is nephrotoxic, a particular disadvantage for its use in renal disease. The appearance of FK506, which may have an action similar to cyclosporin A (see below) but is considerably more potent and less nephrotoxic, has therefore aroused interest. Experience is limited, but early use in transplantation has been encouraging (Starzl et al., 1989) and there seems no reason why it should not be similarly effective in autoimmunity (McCauley et al., 1990; see Chapter 7). Less is known about the mode of action of FK506 as compared to cyclosporin A, but both bind to intracellular receptors that possess peptidyl–prolyl isomerase activity (Harding et al., 1989). The connection between this and their immunosuppressive effect is obscure, but it suggests that FK506 will similarly inhibit a wide range of T cell functions.

The next step in selective immunosuppression is to focus on particular subsets of T cells. Activated T cells express the IL2 receptor. Antibodies against this receptor, or engineered conjugates of IL2 with toxins, are effective immunosuppressants (Strom & Kelley, 1989). Other subsets of T cells are defined by the CD4 and CD8 molecules. CD4$^+$ cells are usually helper/inducer cells and are particularly important in the initiation and boosting of an immune response. Antibodies to the CD4 molecule can reverse advanced lupus nephritis in a mouse model (Wofsey & Seaman, 1987). In man there is one case report in which a similar antibody was used, in conjunction with a more general anti-T cell antibody, to induce a prolonged remission in a case of systemic vasculitis resistant to more conventional therapy (Mathieson et al., 1990). As the role of the CD4 molecule is to interact with MHC class II molecules on antigen presenting cells, the use of anti-class II antibodies is a closely related approach. This has the added advantage that, in some experimental systems at least, an autoimmune response is associated with only one of two alleles present in a heterozygote. It is possible to block only this disease-associated allele, introducing further selectivity (McDevitt, Perry & Steinman, 1987). Such anti-class II antibodies may function purely passively by inhibiting the interaction between T cells and antigen presenting cells, but in some situations there is evidence for a more active mechanism via the induction of suppression (McDevitt, Perry & Steinman, 1987). There is therefore an overlap here with more direct approaches to the generation of suppression (see section on endogenous immunoregulation).

There is further heterogeneity within the subsets considered so far. For instance the CD4$^+$ subset can be further divided on the basis of the molecular weight of the CD45 molecule (Dexter et al., 1987; Akbar et al., 1988). This is the subject of debate, but the high molecular weight form of CD45 appears to be a marker for either a suppressor/inducer cell and/or an unactivated cell. In any event, a possible future therapeutic target in autoimmunity would be the reciprocal CD4$^+$ subset, expressing the low molecular weight form.

Although further progress in defining yet more restricted subsets of T cells is likely, the ultimate specificity is to target only the autoreactive T cell clones. This ideal appears to have been achieved in an animal model, experimental allergic encephalomyelitis (EAE). In mice and rats this disease is known to be mediated, and transferable, by T cells. These pathogenic T cells all use a very restricted set of variable (V) region genes in their T cell receptors, and recognise a particular myelin basic protein peptide in association with a particular MHC class II molecule (Janeway, 1989). It is possible to prevent disease by immunising an animal using peptides derived from the disease-associated V regions (Vandenbark, Hashim & Offner, 1989), administering antibodies that recognise those particular T cell receptors (Acha-Orbea et al., 1988), or administering peptides that bind to the relevant MHC class II molecule and compete with the pathogenic peptide (Sakai et al., 1989). Although it is uncertain that these approaches are working in quite this straightforward way (Janeway, 1989), there is no doubting their efficacy. It is unclear as to whether this approach is only applicable to diseases in which the T cells employ a restricted set of receptor genes, and, if so, which human diseases fall into this category. It is, however, a very attractive form of therapy because of its exquisite selectivity. Progress in this area in human renal disease will presumably require the isolation and characterisation of autoreactive T cells and/or the relevant T cell autoantigens.

Therapy directed against B cells and their products

This approach is clearly logical for conditions in which autoantibodies are of proven pathogenicity. Anti-glomerular basement membrane (GBM) disease falls into this category and plasma exchange is undoubtedly effective at removing anti-GBM antibodies (see Chapter 2). Indeed, the main determinant of prognosis in this condition is the extent of target organ damage that has occurred by the time of presentation (Savage *et al.*, 1986). Thus to improve the outcome, earlier diagnosis is a major requirement. Of other renal diseases, cryoglobulinaemia, lupus nephritis and possibly ANCA positive proliferative nephritis may also have a significant autoantibody-mediated component to their pathogenesis, and the use of plasma exchange in these conditions has been discussed in the appropriate chapters. In all of these diseases, the specificity of such treatment could in principle be improved by adopting an antigen-specific approach: given that the identity of the relevant autoantigen is known (which it probably now is for all these diseases), it would be possible to construct autoantigen columns that could be used to remove autoantibody from the circulation. The main obstacles to such an approach are technical, not least the difficulty of producing large enough quantities of autoantigen (with the exception of DNA). Once the molecular structure of the various autoantigens is confirmed, recombinant proteins should become available to circumvent this problem. However, given the relative safety and efficacy of plasma exchange, it is debatable as to whether, in practice, the theoretical benefits of the more specific approach would outweigh the increased costs that this would incur.

Another potential method for specifically targeting autoantibodies is to use antiidiotypic antibodies, either by direct administration or used in a similar way to autoantigen for extra-corporeal immunoadsorption. Although the role of antiidiotypic antibodies in human autoimmune disease is controversial (see below), it would, in principle, be possible to produce such antibodies by appropriate immunisation strategies in animals even if they do not occur naturally in man. The most convincing demonstration of the importance of antiidiotypic antibodies is in acquired anti-factor VIII disease (Sultan, Rossi & Kazatchkine, 1987). In renal disease, one might expect them to be important in anti-GBM disease because of the known idiotype restriction, but an exhaustive search for antiidiotypes in this condition yielded negative results (Savage, 1986). There is evidence for their existence in systemic vasculitis (Rossi *et al.*, 1991). Pooled normal human immunoglobulin is an effective treatment in anti-factor VIII disease (Sultan *et al.*, 1984) and in immune thrombocytopaenic purpura (Imbach *et al.*, 1981) and it is postulated that this is because it contains antiidiotypes, although other possible explanations are Fc receptor blockade of the reticulo-endothelial system or the presence of anti-MHC class II antibodies. Pooled normal immunoglobulin has some benefits in systemic vasculitis (Jayne *et al.*, 1991), but, at present, it is unclear what place this will have in therapy. The use of antiidiotypic treatment in experimental interstitial nephritis has been covered in Chapter 9, and is dealt with further in the next section.

Immunoregulatory therapy

As discussed in the first chapter, the role of a breakdown in immunoregulatory mechanisms in the aetiology of autoimmunity is controversial. However, whether or not immunoregulation is involved in the natural remission of autoimmunity, it may still be possible to engage it for therapeutic purposes. An experimental example is the control of anti-tubular basement membrane (TBM) nephritis in mice (see Chapter 9). In this system it is possible to activate antigen-specific suppressor cells by injecting the animals with syngeneic lymphocytes that have been conjugated with the TBM antigen used to initiate the disease (Neilson et al., 1985). These suppressor cells are able to attenuate the renal injury even when induced at up to six weeks after the onset of the autoimmune process. A close connection with idiotypic-antiidiotypic regulation is suggested by the idiotype specificity of the resulting suppressor cells, and by the similar therapeutic effect of antiidiotypic antibodies (Clayman et al., 1988). Such an approach is, in principle, feasible in man but will depend on the availability of sufficient amounts of the relevant autoantigen.

As discussed already, antiidiotypic effects may explain the efficacy of pooled normal immunoglobulin (IVIG) in the treatment of anti-factor VIII disease. This example is particularly interesting because the effect lasts for much longer than can be explained by persistence of the IVIG, suggesting that some form of endogenous immunoregulation has been engaged (Sultan et al., 1984; Sultan, Rossi & Kazatchkine, 1987). There is preliminary evidence of a similar prolonged suppressive effect by IVIG on anti-neutrophil cytoplasmic antibodies in systemic vasculitis (Jayne et al., 1991).

Clearance therapy

A common immunopathological theme in a number of renal diseases is deposition of immune complexes with resultant fixation of complement, antibody-dependent cellular cytotoxicity and tissue damage. This process is well illustrated by the nephritides associated with systemic lupus erythematosus (SLE), mixed essential cryoglobulinaemia and subacute infective endocarditis. The role of the normal complement system in the disposal of immune complexes, and contribution that hereditary deficiencies of complement components make to the aetiology of SLE, has been discussed in Chapter 4.

These considerations suggest that replacement of complement components would be a rational treatment for certain disorders. There are obvious problems with this approach, not least the expense involved. However, it may be possible to demonstrate a cost/benefit advantage in certain patients with hereditary complement deficiencies who experience a high frequency of immune complex-related disease. There is clearly a close relationship between this activation of endogenous mechanisms for the clearance of immune complexes and their exogenous clearance by plasma exchange (see section on B cells).

Interference with non-specific mediator systems

A variety of approaches aimed at some of the non-specific mediator systems mentioned in the first chapter have been used with some success in both animal models and man. Decomplementation can ameliorate experimental nephritis, but this approach is unlikely to prove feasible in man. Interference with the coagulation system, principally by defibrination with ancrod but also (less successfully) by anticoagulation with heparin, can prevent crescentic change and ameliorate renal damage in both nephrotoxic nephritis (Thomson, Simpson & Peters, 1975) and immune complex nephritis (Thomson et al., 1975). As might be expected, streptokinase, which as well as lysing fibrin also causes systemic defibrination, has a similar effect to ancrod (Tipping & Holdsworth, 1986). In addition, there has been interest in the use of ancrod in lupus nephritis, both in experimental models and in man (see Chapter 4). The use of ancrod in man is limited by its antigenicity, which would be a problem in a relapsing disease such as lupus. It may be possible to circumvent this by using natural inhibitors of the coagulation system produced by recombinant DNA technology. Tissue plasminogen activator is an obvious candidate, but initial experience with this agent in the treatment of nephrotoxic nephritis has been somewhat mixed (Zoja et al., 1990; Mathieson et al., 1991).

Manipulation of arachidonic acid metabolism, both by direct antagonism and by alteration of dietary lipids, is a promising approach which has been particularly successful in animal models of lupus nephritis. Early experience suggests that such an approach may be useful in a number of chronic glomerulonephritides in man. Work on reactive oxygen species is interesting but not sufficiently well advanced to assess the role of treatment aimed at these mediators.

There is rather limited scope for a direct attack on the non-specific cells involved in mediating tissue damage (polymorphonuclear leukocytes, monocytes, platelets). Such cells subserve vital functions, and, although depletion in experimental models may be very effective, this is unlikely to be applicable to man. However, such cells may effect damage via a number of the mediator systems considered elsewhere in this section, and interference with these represents an indirect attack on these cells. It is also worth mentioning here the use of anti-MHC class II antibodies (dealt with in the section on anti-T cell therapy) to directly interfere with the antigen presenting capabilities of monocytes.

Attempts have been made to influence various of the cytokines and growth factors that are produced by the above cell types and that might be involved in the mediation of damage. Cytokines such as interleukin-1 and tumour necrosis factor (TNF) are integral components of inflammatory reactions and their production by mononuclear cells may be amenable to dietary manipulation (Endres et al., 1989). This may be part of the explanation (in addition to the effects on arachidonic acid metabolism) for the beneficial effect on experimental lupus nephritis of diets supplemented with polyunsaturated fatty acids (Prickett, Robinson & Steinberg, 1981). Specific polyclonal and monoclonal antibodies to individual cytokines are now available and preliminary evidence in experimental nephritis suggests that anti-TNF antibodies ameliorate renal injury (Tomosugi et al., 1989). Such antibodies offer further therapeutic selectivity, but it is worth noting that in at least one situation, TNF is protective, possibly by release of prostaglandins (Jacob & McDevitt, 1988). There is some evidence that peptide growth factors such as platelet-derived growth factor (PDGF) and the insulin-like growth factors are important in renal disease (Frampton et al., 1988; Segal & Fine, 1989), but few selective antagonists of these agents are available. There is one report of the use of a PDGF antagonist in nephrotoxic nephritis in rabbits, without significant benefit (Shinkai & Cameron, 1987), but this is an area where further research is likely to be fruitful.

References

Acha-Orbea, H., Mitchell, D. J., Timmerman, L. et al. (1988). Limited heterogeneity of T cell receptors from lymphocytes mediating autoimmune encephalomyelitis allows specific immune intervention. Cell, 54, 263–73.

Akbar, A. N., Terry, L., Timms, A., Beverley, P. C. L. & Janossy, G. (1988). Loss of CD45R and gain of UCHL1 reactivity is a feature of primed T cells. Journal of Immunology, 140, 2171–8.

Clayman, M. D., Sun, M. J., Michaud, L., Brill-Dashoff, J., Riblet, R. & Neilson, E. G. (1988). Clonotypic heterogeneity in experimental interstitial nephritis. Restricted specificity of the anti-tubular basement membrane B cell repertoire is associated with a disease-modifying crossreactive idiotype. Journal of Experimental Medicine, 167, 1296–312.

Dexter, M., Marvel, J., Merkenschlager, M. et al., (1987). Progress in T cell biology. Immunology Letters, 16, 171–8.

Endres, S., Ghorbani, R., Kelley, V. E. et al. (1989). The effect of dietary supplementation with n-3 polyunsaturated fatty acids on the synthesis of interleukin-1 and tumor necrosis factor by mononuclear cells. New England Journal of Medicine, 320, 265–71.

Feutren, G., Boitard, C., Assan, R. & Bach, J-F. (1988). Therapeutic immunosuppression in type I (insulin-dependent) diabetes. *Journal of Autoimmunity*, 1, 603–14.

Frampton, G., Hildreth, G., Hartley, B., Cameron, J. S., Heldin, C-H. & Wasteson, A. (1988). Could platelet-derived growth factor have a role in the pathogenesis of lupus nephritis? *Lancet*, ii, 343.

Harding, M. W., Galat, A., Uehling, D. E. & Schreiber, S. L. (1989). A receptor for the immunosuppressant FK506 is a *cis–trans* peptidyl–prolyl isomerase. *Nature*, London, 341, 758–60.

Imbach, P., Barandun, S., D'Apuzo, V. *et al.* (1981). High-dose intravenous gammaglobulin for idiopathic thrombocytopenic purpura in childhood. *Lancet*, i, 1228–31.

Jacob, C. O. & McDevitt, H. O. (1988). Tumour necrosis factor-alpha in murine autoimmune 'lupus' nephritis. *Nature*, London, 331, 356–8.

Janeway, C. A. , Jr. (1989). Immunotherapy by peptides?. *Nature*, London, 341, 482–3.

Jayne, D. R. W., Black, C. M., Davies, M., Fox, C. & Lockwood, C. M. (1991). Treatment of systemic vasculitis with pooled intravenous immunoglobulin. *Lancet*, 337, 1137–9.

Mathieson, P. W., Cobbold, S. P., Hale, G. *et al.* (1990). Monoclonal antibody therapy in systemic vasculitis. *New England Journal of Medicine*, 323, 250–4.

Mathieson, P. W., Thiru, S., Peters, D. K. & Oliveira, D. B. G. (1991). Effects of ancrod and rTPA on fibrin accumulation, glomerular inflammation and renal function in nephrotoxic nephritis. *International Journal of Experimental Pathology* (in press).

McCauley, J., Tzakis, A. G., Fung, J. J., Todo, S. & Starzl, T. E. (1990). FK506 in steroid-resistant focal sclerosing glomerulonephritis of childhood. *Lancet*, 335, 674.

McDevitt, H. O., Perry, R. & Steinman, L. A. (1987). Monoclonal anti-Ia antibody therapy in animal models of autoimmune disease. In *Autoimmunity and Autoimmune Disease (Ciba Foundation Symposium 129)*, ed. D. Evered & J. Whelan, pp. 184–93. Chichester, UK: John Wiley & Sons.

Neilson, E. G., McCafferty, E., Mann, R., Michaud, L. & Clayman, M. (1985). Tubular antigen-derivatized cells induce a disease-protective, antigen-specific, and idiotype-specific suppressor T cell network restricted by I-J and Igh-V in mice with experimental interstitial nephritis. *Journal of Experimental Medicine*, 162, 215–30.

Prickett, J. D., Robinson, D. R. & Steinberg, A. D. (1981). Dietary enrichment with the polyunsaturated fatty acid eicosapentaenoic acid prevents proteinuria and prolongs survival in NZBxNZW F_1 mice. *Journal of Clinical Investigation*, 68, 556–9.

Rees, A. J. & Lockwood, C. M. (1988). Antiglomerular basement membrane antibody-mediated nephritis. In *Diseases of the Kidney*, 4th edn, ed. R. W. Schrier & C. W. Gottschalk, pp. 2091–126. Boston/Toronto: Little, Brown and Company.

Rossi, F., Jayne, D. R. W., Lockwood, C. M. & Kazatchkine, M. D. (1991). Anti-idiotypes against anti-neutrophil cytoplasmic antigen autoantibodies in normal human polyspecific IgG for therapeutic use and in the remission sera of patients with systemic vasculitis. *Clinical and Experimental Immunology*, 83, 298–303.

Sakai, K., Mitchell, D. J., Hodgkinson, S. J., Zamvil, S. S., Rothbard, J. B. & Steinman, L. (1989). Prevention of experimental allergic encephalomyelitis with peptides blocking T cell-MHC interaction. *Proceedings of the National Academy of Sciences, USA*, 86, 9470–4.

Sandoz Medical Documentation (1989). *Sandimmune(e) (ciclosporin) in Autoimmune Diseases*. Basle: Med. Documentation Sandoz.

Savage, C. O. S. (1986). Regulation of autoantibody production in man. The role of idiotype-antiidiotype network interactions in anti-glomerular basement membrane antibody mediated disease. University of London: PhD Thesis.

Savage, C. O. S., Pusey, C. D., Bowman, C., Rees, A. J. & Lockwood, C. M. (1986). Antiglomerular basement membrane antibody mediated disease in the British Isles 1980–4. *British Medical Journal*, 292, 301–4.

Segal, R. & Fine, L. G. (1989). Polypeptide growth factors and the kidney. *Kidney International*, **36** suppl. 27, s2–10.

Shinkai, Y. & Cameron, J. S. (1987). Trial of platelet-derived growth factor antagonist, trapidil, in accelerated nephrotoxic nephritis in the rabbit. *British Journal of Experimental Pathology*, **68**, 847–52.

Starzl, T. E., Todo, S., Fung, J., Demetris, A. J., Venkataramman, R. & Jain, A. (1989). FK506 for liver, kidney, and pancreas transplantation. *Lancet*, **ii**, 1000–4.

Strom, T. B. & Kelley, V. E. (1989). Towards more selective therapies to block undesired immune responses. *Kidney International*, **35**, 1026–33.

Sultan, Y., Kazatchkine, M. D., Maisonneuve, P. & Nydegger, U. E. (1984). Anti-idiotypic suppression of autoantibodies to factor VIII (anti-haemophilic factor) by high dose intravenous gammaglobulin. *Lancet*, **ii**, 765–8.

Sultan, Y., Rossi, F. & Kazatchkine, M. D. (1987). Recovery from anti-VIII:c (anti-haemophilic factor) autoimmune disease is dependent on generation of anti-idiotypes against anti-VIII:c autoantibodies. *Proceedings of the National Academy of Sciences, USA*, **84**, 828–31.

Thomson, N. M., Simpson, I. J., Evans, D. J. & Peters, D. K. (1975). Defibrination with ancrod in experimental chronic immune complex nephritis. *Clinical and Experimental Immunology*, **20**, 527–35.

Thomson, N. M., Simpson, I. J. & Peters, D. K. (1975). A quantitative evaluation of anticoagulants in experimental nephrotoxic nephritis. *Clinical and Experimental Immunology*, **19**, 301–8.

Tipping, P. G. & Holdsworth, S. R. (1986). Fibrinolytic therapy with streptokinase for established experimental glomerulonephritis. *Nephron*, **43**, 258–64.

Tomosugi, N. I., Cashman, S. J., Hay, H. *et al.* (1989). Modulation of antibody-mediated glomerular injury *in vivo* by bacterial lipopolysaccharide, tumour necrosis factor, and IL-1. *Journal of Immunology*, **142**, 3083–90.

Vandenbark, A. A., Hashim, G. & Offner, H. (1989). Immunization with a synthetic T-cell receptor V-region peptide protects against experimental autoimmune encephalomyelitis. *Nature*, London, **341**, 541–4.

Waldmann, H (1989). Manipulation of T-cell responses with monoclonal antibodies. *Annual Review of Immunology*, **7**, 407–44.

Wofsey, D. & Seaman, W. E. (1987). Reversal of advanced murine lupus in NZB/NZW F1 mice by treatment with monoclonal antibody to L3T4. *Journal of Immunology*, **138**, 3247–53.

Zoja, C., Corna, D., Macconi, D., Zilio, P., Bertani, T. & Remuzzi, G. (1990). Tissue plasminogen activator therapy of rabbit nephrotoxic nephritis. *Laboratory Investigation*, **62**, 34–40.

Index

adipsin 119
  partial lipodystrophy, role in 124
Aleutian disease of mink 92
Alport's syndrome
  anti-GBM antibodies following
    transplantation 29
  collagen defect in 31
  Goodpasture epitope and 29
amyloid and renal involvement 204
ANCA, see anti-neutrophil cytoplasm
  antibodies
Ancrod 13, 216
  crescent formation, effect on 158
  lupus, human, treatment with 75
  lupus, murine, treatment with 70
animal models
  adriamycin induced proteinuria 136
  aminonucleoside of puromycin induced
    proteinuria 136
  chickens, T cell-mediated nephritis 27
  crescent formation, mechanisms of 158
  glomerulosclerosis 136
  Heymann nephritis 45; antigen 45;
    cellular immunity 46; immune
    complexes 47; immunogenetics 45;
    immunoregulation 47; membrane
    attack complex 46; pathogenesis
    46
  horses, anti-GBM antibody in 27
  IgA nephropathy: alcohol abuse 93;
    Aleutian disease of mink 92; ddY
    mice 93; dextran immunisation 92;
    liver dysfunction 93; lymphocytic
    choriomeningitis virus 92; oral
    immunisation 92; preformed
    complexes, administration of 91
  interstitial nephritis, see animal models,
    tubulointerstitial nephritis
  lupus: autoantibodies 67; cellular
    immunity 69; coagulation system
    70; dog 67; gamma interferon 70;

idiotypes on anti-DNA antibodies
  68; inflammatory mediators 70;
  mouse 67; suppression 69;
  treatment 70; tumour necrosis
  factor, role in 70
membranous nephropathy: cationic
  immunoglobulin induced 47; serum
  sickness and 47; mouse 47;
  mercuric chloride induced 47; see
  also animal models, Heymann
  nephritis
mercuric chloride in Brown Norway
  rat 27
mesangiocapillary glomerulonephritis:
  dogs 117; Finnish Landrace lambs
  117; haemolytic anaemia in mice 117
nephrotoxic nephritis (Masugi
  nephritis) 25; antigens 26; cellular
  immune system, involvement in 26;
  complement and 26; Guinea pig
  12, 25; leukotrienes, antagonism of
  13; polymorphonuclear neutrophils,
  role in 26; pulmonary
  haemorrhage 26; reactive oxygen
  species, role in 26
poststreptococcal glomerulonephritis
  195
prostaglandins and 13
serum sickness 9
Steblay nephritis 27
tubulointerstitial nephritis: anti-tubular
  basement membrane antibody
  mediated 178, 179; cell mediated
  181; immune complex mediated 180
anti-DNA antibodies
  affinity and histological correlates 71
  charge, role in pathogenicity 69
  cross-reactivity of 68, 69
  idiotypes of 71; see also 16/6 idiotype
  lupus, human, and 70, 71
  lupus, murine, and 67

220

suppression 5
IgA-specific, defect in IgA
nephropathy 97
lupus, human, defects in 72
lupus, murine, defects in 69
mercuric chloride/Brown Norway
model, role in 28
minimal change nephropathy,
abnormalities in 138
tubulointerstitial nephritis, modulation
of 179, 180, 187
syphilis and glomerular involvement 200
systemic lupus erythematosus
cellular immunity, role in 72
drug-induced 73
familial immunological abnormalities
66
suppression, defects of 72
treatment: total lymphoid irradiation
75
see also lupus nephritis

T cell
autoantigen specific 11
autoreactive, in mercuric chloride/
Brown Norway model 28, 35
chickens, nephritis, role in 27
glomerulonephritis, presence in 11
murine tubulointerstitial nephritis and
179
poststreptococcal glomerulonephritis
and 198
tolerance 4
tolerance induction as therapy 211
treatment directed against 212
vasculitis, involvement in 163
T cell receptor genes
lupus, associations with 66
membranous nephropathy, associations
with 45
Takayasu's arteritis 164
antibodies to neutrophil components
in 160
Tamm–Horsfall protein, immunisation
with 180
tissue plasminogen activator 216
TNF, *see* tumour necrosis factor
tolerance 1
antiidiotypic mechanisms 6
B cell 3
peripheral 5
sequestration of autoantigens 2
suppression as a mechanism of 5

T cell: negative selection 4; positive
selection 4; tolerance induction as
therapy 211
thymic 4
treatment of immunologically mediated
disease 211
antiidiotypic antibodies 214
B cell, directed against 213
coagulation system, interference with
216
cytokines, antagonism of 217
dietary lipids 216
immunoadsorption 143, 214
immunosuppression, non-specific 211
intravenous immunoglobulin 214
plasma exchange 214
suppression, activation of 215
T cell, directed against 212
tubulointerstitial nephritis 177
animal models 178
anti-TBM antibodies and 182
classification of 177
drug-induced 181, 187
idiopathic 185
lupus, presence in 183
Sjögren's syndrome and 184
T cell involvement in 182
treatment 185
uveitis and (TINU syndrome) 185
tumour necrosis factor 217
antibodies to as therapy 217
lupus nephritis, role in 65
murine lupus, role in 70

uveitis
lens-induced 2
tubulointerstitial nephritis and (TINU
syndrome) 185

vasculitis 154
anti-endothelial antibodies and 163
classification of 154
idiopathic crescentic nephritis,
connection with 155
T cell involvement in 163
treatment 164; corticosteroids 165;
cyclosporin 167; cytotoxic agents
165; intravenous immunoglobulin
167; methylprednisolone, pulse 166;
plasma exchange 166
see also anti-neutrophil cytoplasm
antibodies